How Technology, Social Media, and Current Events Profoundly Affect Adolescents

T0293457

How Technology, Social Media, and Current Events Profoundly Affect Adolescents

MARK A. GOLDSTEIN

AND

MYRNA CHANDLER GOLDSTEIN

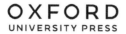

OXFORD
UNIVERSITY PRESS

OXFORD
UNIVERSITY PRESS

Oxford University Press is a department of the University of Oxford. It furthers
the University's objective of excellence in research, scholarship, and education
by publishing worldwide. Oxford is a registered trade mark of Oxford University
Press in the UK and certain other countries.

Published in the United States of America by Oxford University Press
198 Madison Avenue, New York, NY 10016, United States of America.

CIP data is on file at the Library of Congress

ISBN 978-0-19-764073-9

DOI: 10.1093/med/9780197640739.001.0001

This material is not intended to be, and should not be considered, a substitute for medical or other professional
advice. Treatment for the conditions described in this material is highly dependent on the individual
circumstances. And, while this material is designed to offer accurate information with respect to the subject
matter covered and to be current as of the time it was written, research and knowledge about medical and health
issues is constantly evolving and dose schedules for medications are being revised continually, with new side
effects recognized and accounted for regularly. Readers must therefore always check the product information
and clinical procedures with the most up-to-date published product information and data sheets provided by
the manufacturers and the most recent codes of conduct and safety regulation. The publisher and the authors
make no representations or warranties to readers, express or implied, as to the accuracy or completeness of this
material. Without limiting the foregoing, the publisher and the authors make no representations or warranties as
to the accuracy or efficacy of the drug dosages mentioned in the material. The authors and the publisher do not
accept, and expressly disclaim, any responsibility for any liability, loss, or risk that may be claimed or incurred as a
consequence of the use and/or application of any of the contents of this material.

Printed by Marquis Book Printing, Canada

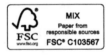

This book is dedicated to the clinicians, nurses, and staff at the Division of Adolescent and Young Adult Medicine, Massachusetts General Hospital, who provide exceptional, compassionate, and comprehensive care to adolescents.

Contents

LIFE EVENTS

PART IV. CURRENT EVENTS

Acknowledgments

With very great appreciation, I acknowledge my spouse and coauthor Myrna Chandler Goldstein. Her superb writing and editing skills and her overwhelming patience with me during this process have made this manuscript much more cohesive, flowing, and readable. Without her considerable assistance from the book's inception, this undertaking would not have moved forward.

At Oxford University Press, editor Emma Hodgton reviewed the entire manuscript with great skill and provided extraordinary input. I am also grateful to Andrea Knobloch of Oxford, who provided the initial interest and enthusiasm and encouraged us to begin this work.

The vast amount of research for this book could not have been undertaken without the generous support of the Harvard University library system and especially the Countway Library of Medicine. The staff answered countless queries and were able to quickly retrieve research papers that were not in the Harvard collections.

In addition, I want to thank the many thousands of adolescent patients for whom I have provided medical care over five decades. My relationships with them established the groundwork for this book, and I learned so much from our interactions.

And finally, I am eternally grateful to the late Robert Masland, MD, chief emeritus of the Division of Adolescent/Young Adult Medicine at Boston Children's Hospital. He introduced me to the care of adolescents and mentored me throughout my career. Dr. Masland continually encouraged me to seek and to understand the biological, psychological, and social aspects of each adolescent who presented for care.

Introduction

From 1973 to 1974, as part of my military service commitment, I practiced family medicine in Gallup, New Mexico. Gallup was a multiethnic city that was dotted with trading posts, pawnshops, an abundance of bars, and the Sante Fe railroad. Located in the high desert plateau of western New Mexico proximal to Route 66, this city of 20,000 bordered the Navajo reservation, which served as home to about 165,000 residents.

Although alcohol was not sold on the Navajo reservation, it was readily available in Gallup. At the time, it was not unusual for an adolescent of any ethnicity to die from hypothermia. Adolescents who drank excessive amounts of alcohol were at risk of losing consciousness, often in a desolate part of the city. With the wildly fluctuating nighttime temperatures, inebriated youth could easily drift into a hypothermic state.

Myrna and I were fortunate to rent a house that was heated and electrified and had hot and cold running water. But, while every White and Hispanic person whom we knew also had homes with these basic necessities, many Navajo homes did not. About one-quarter mile south of our rental stood Hogback Mountain. When I walked our dog in that area, I noticed a Navajo hogan, a round one-room structure on a plain just before the mountain's cliff. The hogan lacked electricity and running water. Wood was used to heat and cook. The surrounding land was arid and could not be cultivated or support livestock.

Within weeks of our arrival, it became clear to Myrna and me that the Navajo families were frequently desperately poor. Often, they subsisted on the jewelry they sold for nominal prices to the trading posts or on low-paying jobs. Frequently, they were subjected to predatory lending.

Like their parents, many Navajo adolescents faced poverty, racism, and discrimination and endured difficult living conditions; substance abuse, especially alcohol, was not a rare event. Some adolescents had a history of adverse childhood experiences, including physical and sexual abuse; many were removed from their homes and forced to attend Indian residential schools. At these schools, they were not allowed to speak their native language and were forced to wear military-style uniforms and obey harsh rules. Little family contact was permitted. It has been reported that students may have died from infections, especially tuberculosis. White individuals who never even tried to hide their prejudicial, anti-Indian rhetoric administered government rules, policies, and laws.

Though we are now living in the 21st century, adolescents worldwide continue to face serious issues, including bullying and sexual and gender identity concerns. And it is well known that there are problems associated with technological advances from the internet to cell phones to social media platforms. Divorce rates have increased, politics is sometimes frighteningly polarized, and school violence is rampant. While writing this introduction, I learned that a first grader apparently shot his teacher in Virginia. COVID-19 only added to these problems, impacting adolescents and their social and educational lives, as well as levels of daily stress. Because illegal drugs may be contaminated with fentanyl, adolescent overdose deaths have increased. And climate change is taking a toll on adolescent physical and mental health.

During the past two decades, more American youth have become obese, anxious, depressed, and violent. Larger numbers of males have developed eating disorders, emergency departments are overrun with suicidal teens, and more youth are addicted to the internet. Transgender adolescents, who seek medical and mental health services, often encounter obstacles to their care, and there are widely differing policies and politics on gender identity. While many of the technological advances have been positive, some have not. For example, young adolescents who keep checking social media sites experience changes in the brain's sensitivity to social rewards and punishments. And the wars in Ukraine and Israel-Gaza have not only shattered the lives of youth in those countries but also indirectly upended the lives of many youth throughout the world. During the last decade of my practice of adolescent and young adult medicine at Massachusetts General Hospital in Boston, at least half of my patients had at least one mental health issue.

This book is organized into 18 chapters; each chapter reviews important biological, psychological, and social issues that are interconnected and influence the lives of adolescents throughout the world. The primary goal of this book is to help clinicians, adolescents, parents, and others involved with youth navigate these often-difficult challenges. Family members, peers, neighborhoods, schools, communities, society at large, and governments at all levels can work to create stronger, healthier adolescents and young adults. And of course, each chapter has sections on treatments and preventive measures. For example, in the chapter on depression, it is noted that something as simple as increasing an adolescent's physical activities may help alleviate depressive symptoms.

There are recurrent themes throughout the text. I cannot sufficiently stress the critical importance that role modeling from parents, teachers, counselors, coaches, medical providers, clergy, politicians, and others plays in helping teens emerge successfully from these trying times. In addition, think of an adolescent sitting in the middle of a spider web with hundreds of intersecting silk threads, many of which pose as problems for the developing teen. The problems teens face today interconnect to one another. For example, young adolescents undergoing a family divorce are apt to become depressed and may start to use substances. And importantly, adverse childhood events that an adolescent could experience may have important ramifications in their adult life. Exposures to such events in early adolescence have been more strongly associated with later adverse outcomes than exposures earlier in childhood.

It is important to note that there is some disagreement on the definition of adolescence. Although the World Health Organization defines adolescence as the period between 10 and 19 years, some authorities believe that adolescence begins with the first stages of pubertal development, which may be as early as 8 years. Others contend that adolescence should be between 12 and 21 years, and still others consider adolescence to end at age 25, when the brain's growth is completed. As might be expected, the many hundreds of research studies referenced in this book vary in how they define the age of adolescence.

Issues impacting adolescents continue, and new issues will present in the future. This book should be an informative resource for faculty, clinicians, and students in medicine, nursing, social work, sociology, and psychology. It also should be useful for teachers, counselors, coaches, and clergy. And of course, parents will find this book helpful in understanding and helping their teens as they progress through adolescence.

PART I
BIOLOGICAL ISSUES

1
Sleep

Introduction

Good quality and quantity of sleep are of the utmost importance for the development of adolescents. However, epidemiological studies have found that large numbers of adolescents are not obtaining sufficient sleep. Most of these studies are based on self-reports; when sleep is objectively measured by actigraphy (device that measures sleep), the sleep durations are even shorter.[1] While sleep problems may affect teens of all socioeconomic, racial, or ethnic backgrounds, disparities in sleep have been well documented in financially disadvantaged adolescents, as well as those identifying as racial or ethnic minorities. Older adolescents who work after school, socialize in the evening, or strive for academic excellence are also at increased risk for sleep deprivation.

There is a sizeable body of research that has found that adolescents with sleep issues have worse outcomes for physical, mental, social, and academic performance than their peers who obtain appropriate sleep.[2-5] These diminished outcomes may present with disease, mental health disorders, social disturbances, and academic issues. Good-quality sleep of appropriate length is needed for adequate physical growth and neurological development. In adolescents, changes in the pattern of sleep may signal a medical, mental, or social problem. For example, an adolescent who begins to have difficulty falling or staying asleep and frequent awakenings may be developing a mood disorder, such as depression, or be experiencing cyberbullying.

There are a number of other issues that may impact a teen's sleep. It is well known that the use of electronic media by adolescents, including computers, smartphones, and tablets, has a profound effect on sleep. These devices emit more blue light than white incandescent bulbs, and blue light modifies the biological clock. Blue light suppresses the release of melatonin, which may trigger a delayed onset of sleep. Coupled with early school opening times, this may cause adolescents to suffer from drowsiness and academic and behavioral problems.

In recent decades, sleep issues in adolescents have become more of a problem. Since the 1990s, sleep duration for adolescents has dramatically decreased.[6] Using nationally representative multicohort data from over 270,000 teens, a study found that their self-reported sleep duration had diminished from 1991 to 2012.[7] While the National Sleep Foundation recommends that teens between the ages of 14 and 17 years sleep 8 to 10 hours per night, most adolescents sleep fewer than 7 hours each night. All teens should sleep at least 8 hours per night; for the age group of 18 to 25 years, the recommendation is 7 to 9 hours.[8]

It is important not to underestimate the need for sleep in adolescents. Appropriate amounts of sleep are necessary to regulate teen cognition, physiological systems, and behavioral outcomes.[9] There are a number of physical and mental morbidities associated with the lack of restorative sleep. Further, there are myriad biological, psychological, and social factors that may affect the adolescent's ability to achieve restorative sleep.

The Biological Basis of Sleep

According to Mary Carskadon in Rhode Island, two processes regulate sleep. The first, known as the circadian rhythm, originates in the suprachiasmatic nucleus of the hypothalamus, located in the undersurface of the brain. Think of it as the brain's "clock" as it helps regulate 24 hours of arousal and sleep. The second process is sleep-wake pressure or the growing pressure to sleep as the time awake increases. The origin of sleep-wake pressure is unknown. These two processes work interactively to regulate sleep.[10]

Andrade and colleagues from Brazil determined that adolescent sleep patterns changed during puberty. During physical development in adolescence, there are changes in sleep onset, wakeup time, and duration of sleep. When compared to weekdays, adolescent sleep patterns on weekends resulted in sleep starting an hour later, waking up 3 hours later, and sleeping for 1 to 1.5 hours longer.[11] These changes of the circadian delay have been seen in other mammals including rats, mice, and the Rhesus monkey.[12] According to a technical report from the American Academy of Pediatrics, a reversal of this weekend delay for the onset of sleep may be a marker for the "biological" end of adolescence.[13]

These changes in sleep physiology result in the delayed sleep-wake phase disorder (DSPD). During adolescence, the amount of time needed for restorative sleep is stable or increases. But, due to the phase delay in the circadian timing system, the need for onset of sleep ("I feel sleepy") is later in the day. As a result, the adolescent obtains fewer hours of sleep when the need is greatest.[14] However, many social systems, such as schools, have not altered their opening and closing times. In a study of students transitioning from grade 9 to 10, a 65-minute earlier opening time resulted in less than half of the students obtaining 7 or more hours of sleep per night; this caused significant daytime sleepiness.[15,16]

In adolescents, insufficient sleep is associated with a number of problems but most significantly, safety. There have been a number of different studies on motor vehicle crashes and teens. In one Kentucky study, researchers examined the sleep habits and motor vehicle crash rates for adolescents in one county school district before and after the implementation of a 1-hour delay in school starting times. The researchers learned that after the delay in school opening times, the students slept longer and the teen crash rate decreased by 16.5 percent despite a 7.8 percent increase in teen crash rates statewide.[17]

A few years later, researchers published a study on teen crash rates in neighboring cities in Virginia. In one county, where the high schools opened 75 to 80 minutes earlier than those in the other county, researchers compared the crash rates for teens between the ages of 16 and 18 years. When compared to the city with the later opening time, the city with the earlier opening time had a significantly elevated crash rate during the school commute.[18] These studies present a compelling argument for later school openings for adolescents—a preventive measure that may be implemented by local governments.

Epidemiology

Sleep disorders are commonly seen in adolescents, but they are frequently unrecognized. Insomnia is the most prevalent sleep disorder in adolescents with a current prevalence rate of 9.4 percent in those ages 13 to 16 years old, although some studies report up to 39 percent prevalence. As many as 35 percent of adolescents report some insomnia during a single month, with the prevalence being more common in females. There is a peak prevalence for obstructive sleep apnea during adolescence that is associated with weight gain.

The prevalence of sleep disorders is not uncommon in adolescents with psychiatric morbidities. Sleep disruptions are often seen in adolescents with anxiety, and nightmares are frequently a symptom of posttraumatic stress disorder (PTSD). A majority of adolescents with depression may have a sleep disturbance including early morning awakenings, insomnia, or increased need for sleep.[19]

Etiologies of Sleep Problems in Adolescents

A number of factors may trigger sleep problems in adolescents. These range from conditions or situations throughout the biopsychosocial spectrum to the current ongoing political fighting. Although the biological or disease states are somewhat limited, there are numerous mental health concerns that may interfere with sleep, and the most widespread impacts are social in nature.

Biopsychosocial Issues and Sleep

Biological Issues and Sleep

Idiopathic Hypersomnia
As the name suggests, idiopathic hypersomnia has no clear etiology. Patients with this disorder have a normal or increased need for sleep, and adolescents may complain of chronic and excessive daytime sleepiness where sleep may occur unintentionally and at inappropriate times. Naps may be 1 hour or longer. The medication modafinil may be useful for treatment.

Narcolepsy
Narcolepsy is a medical condition in which people have periodic or daily profound needs for sleep. Because it is caused by a loss of hypocretin-secreting neurons in the lateral hypothalamus, it is believed to be an autoimmune disorder. Medications include methylphenidate, modafinil, and armodafinil.

Obesity

A short sleep duration is a risk factor for obesity in adolescents since it increases energy usage as well as increases hunger, appetite, and food intake. This may lead to night eating, reduced physical activity, and a more sedentary lifestyle. As a result, a reduced insulin sensitivity could also increase the risk for type 2 diabetes.[20]

As the prevalence of obesity (a body mass index [BMI] of 30 or more or a BMI at 95 percent or higher) rises in adolescents, so does the likelihood that teens with obesity will suffer from obstructive sleep apnea.[21] This condition, which affects the upper airway and results from enlarged the tonsils and adenoids, may lead to sleep-disordered breathing, occasional apneic spells, and habitual snoring. As a result, teens with sleep apnea tend to suffer from daytime fatigue and drowsiness. The first line of treatment may be a tonsillectomy. The use of a continuous positive airway pressure (CPAP) machine may be the second line. Used at night, a CPAP machine keeps the patient's airway open, relieving some of the obstructions to breathing.

Stress

Unlike anxiety, which is a psychiatric problem, stress is a normal physiologic reaction. All people develop a stress response early in life. Dewald and associates conducted a study on stress and sleep in the Netherlands. Using actigraphy, the researchers compared sleep quality in teens during low-stress weeks and high-stress exam weeks. The cohort consisted of 175 teens with a mean age of 15.1 years, and the study continued for 3 weeks. When compared to the low-stress weeks, the researchers found that the teens' sleep was more fragmented, that is, restless, during the high-stress exam weeks. The importance of this study is that stress has a negative effect on adolescents' sleep fragmentation, especially for those who have chronic reduction in their sleep duration.[22]

There is other evidence of stress affecting sleep. According to the Swedish researcher Akerstedt, stress causes increased psychological and physiological activity that activates the hypothalamic-pituitary axis. The resulting insomnia leads to further stress in a vicious cycle incompatible with normal sleep. Additionally, high work strain and a lack of social support networks may likewise lead to sleep issues.[23] And there is evidence that adolescents who report higher levels of family stress perceive lower sleep quality.[24]

Psychological Issues and Sleep

Anxiety

Anxiety disorders are common in adolescents, with a lifetime prevalence of up to 20 percent. Further, there is strong evidence that children and teens with a diagnosis of anxiety will likely have one or more sleep disorders.[25] Moreover, there is a growing consensus that sleep-related disorders may cause anxiety. Using the National Comorbidity Survey Adolescent Supplement, a nationally representative cross-sectional survey of over 10,000 adolescents between the ages of 13 and 18 years, researchers found associations between sleep patterns and mental health diagnoses from the past year. The average sleep duration was 7.72 hours, mean weeknight bedtime was 22.37 hours, and weekend bedtime delay was 1.81 hours, with oversleep on weekends around 1.17 hours. The researchers found associations with anxiety, mood disorders, suicidality, substance use, and the perception of poor mental and physical health with those who had suboptimal sleep patterns.[26] Another research group studied eight sleep-related problems in 128 children and teens diagnosed with an anxiety disorder. Eighty-eight percent of the youth had at least one sleep-related problem, and the majority of subjects had four or more sleep issues.[27] This is evidence of a robust association between sleep and anxiety in adolescents.

It is important that adolescents have an annual screening for anxiety at their primary care appointments. There are well-accepted treatments for anxiety that may include cognitive behavioral therapy and/or medications such as selective serotonin reuptake inhibitors.

Depression
There appears to be strong evidence of a relationship between sleep disturbances and depression in adolescents. Lovato and Gradisar from Australia conducted a literature search for studies on the association between sleep disturbances and depression in adolescents between the ages of 12 and 20 years. They identified 23 studies that met their criteria, which addressed issues including the role of sleep disturbance in the development of depression and depression and subsequent sleep issues. The researchers learned that the adolescents who were depressed had more wakefulness in bed, including delayed onset of sleep, more awakenings after sleep onset, and worse sleep efficiency (sleep time divided by time in bed). In contrast, most young adults have a sleep efficiency of greater than 90 percent. The researchers suggested that sleep disturbances may be a precursor to depression in adolescents, rather than the converse.[28] Similarly, a team of Finnish researchers investigated the prevalence of sleep disorders in adolescents with major depression. Their cohort consisted of 166 Finnish teens with unipolar depression between the ages of 13 and 19 years who were interviewed and completed a questionnaire. Eighty-three percent of the teens had significantly disturbed sleep, including nonrestorative sleep and insomnia, supporting the work of Lovato and Gradisar.[29]

As with anxiety, all adolescents should be screened annually for depression. Parents who notice sleep problems in their adolescents, including frequent nightmares, should consider the possibility of a mood disorder, and they should express their concern to their child's primary care clinician.[30]

Eating Disorders
The four eating disorders seen in adolescents include anorexia nervosa, bulimia, avoidant-restrictive food intake disorder (ARFID), and binge eating disorder (BED). Anorexia, which usually begins in adolescence, is more commonly seen in females. It is characterized by body image issues and fear of weight gain. Teens with anorexia present with weight loss and changes in their physical examination consistent with malnutrition. Also seen more often in females, people with bulimia binge and purge with vomiting and use laxatives and/or diuretics, though bulimia may or may not cause

weight loss. Seen in both males and females, ARFID tends to begin before adolescence and manifest as children with small appetites and a narrow spectrum of food choices. Finally, people with BED may periodically binge on a large quantity of food in a short period of time but not necessarily exhibit compensatory behavior, such as self-induced vomiting, use of diuretics, or overexercising.

Teens with an eating disorder may or may not have a mood disorder, such as depression, and those who do may experience sleep issues. Similarly, starvation, as in anorexia, may or may not disrupt sleep.[31] Although patients with anorexia report insomnia, there have been no objective measures of their sleep published in recent years.[32] People with bulimia and BED also have not been studied in an objective manner to determine if they experienced sleep issues as a group, and children with ARFID tend not to have a current mood disorder or report frequent sleep issues.

However, some researchers have found that eating disorders may have a general impact on adolescent sleep. In 2016, Tromp and associates from the Netherlands and Australia surveyed 574 individuals between the ages of 18 and 35 years about eating disorders and sleep problems. They found that subjects who screened positive for an eating disorder frequently had sleep disorders, including insomnia, sleep apnea, and sleep poor quality, and reported impaired daytime functioning.[33]

At present, the management of sleep problems is a secondary issue in the treatment of teens with eating disorders. There is no known cause and effect between sleep problems and eating disorders. Still, if an adolescent has an eating disorder, especially BED, then a sleep problem and its related concerns should be addressed. Adolescents with BED may awaken at night to eat, resulting in disturbances in their sleep cycles.

Substance Use

There appears to be a strong bidirectional relationship between sleep and substance abuse in adolescents: sleep disturbances may lead to substance abuse, and substance abuse may lead to sleep disturbances.[34] A number of researchers have noted the potential pathway between ongoing fatigue and self-medication, which may in turn lead to the use of stimulants, alcohol, and/or marijuana.[35] In particular, Tynjälä and associates in Finland found that morning tiredness in adolescents was associated with addictive behavior. They determined that fatigued adolescent males were more likely to abuse alcohol and tobacco, and fatigued adolescent females were more likely to abuse tobacco.[36]

However, adolescents who abuse certain drugs such as amphetamines, methylphenidate, or caffeine may experience some of the side effects of stimulating substances, such as insomnia. Tobacco contains nicotine, which is a stimulant that increases sleep latency, total sleep time, and rapid eye movement (REM) sleep. Adolescents may have difficulty with sleeping and have unusual dreams when withdrawing from marijuana.[37]

There are studies that have determined that circadian rhythm misalignment (as in early school openings and late bedtimes) may be linked to problematic drinking in older adolescents. These studies are preliminary and need to be tested in larger samples of adolescents.[38,39]

Social Issues and Sleep

Social Media

In a study published in 2021, researchers from the Netherlands reported that 98 percent of Dutch adolescents between the ages of 12 and 15 years owned a smartphone and about a third of these teens used the phone all day on social media platforms, such as Facebook, Instagram, and Snapchat. In their longitudinal study, the researchers determined that the teens who were the most frequent and problematic social media users were more likely to have a later bedtime after 1 year elapsed. The researchers suggested that parents need to create rules to prevent their teens from becoming highly involved social media users.[40] Rules could include media-free periods, no use of smartphones or similar technologies 60 minutes before bedtime, and encouragement of physical activities. In addition, parents need to model appropriate use of technology and media usage.

A group from Australia analyzed the use of electronic media and sleep in children. They located 22 papers on the use of the internet, computers, electronic gaming, or smartphones. It became evident that the use of computers or electronic games was associated with shorter sleep duration, higher levels of daytime fatigue, and longer time to sleep onset. They found that electronic media could displace sleep and caused emotional or physiological arousal, and the bright light could delay the circadian rhythm, resulting in sleep issues and impaired daytime functioning.[41]

Researchers from Massachusetts and Rhode Island examined the relationship between parental phone restrictions and duration and timing of sleep in adolescents living in the northeast region of the United States. The researchers were particularly interested in the access to social technology and the particular content viewed. Did these have any influence on sleep? The researchers learned that problematic use of digital technology, problematic internet behaviors, and watching emotional or violent videos were related to later bedtimes and fewer hours of sleep. Parenting rules restricting mobile phone use and postponing smartphone use to a later age were correlated with increased sleep time and earlier bedtimes. The only bedtime behavior that was linked to earlier bedtime was reading books.[42]

Problematic Internet Use

Problematic internet use (PIU) is the inability to control one's use of the internet, leading to negative consequences in daily life that may include physical and mental health consequences as well as avoidance of academic work or social activities.[43] A number of studies have determined that adolescents who have PIU suffer from sleep issues.[44-46] A cross-sectional school-based survey of grades 9 and 10 high school students in a peri-urban area in Nepal confirmed that there was a significant association between PIU and sleep quality. The researchers also observed borderline or PIU in 35 percent of the cohort. At the time of the study, 67 percent had access to a smartphone and 46 percent to a laptop.[47]

Racism and Discrimination

Research studies, which are often cross-sectional in design, have found that ethnic and racial minorities have health disparities related to discrimination, and it appears that sleep may be added to the rather long list.[48] One study used a dataset from a cross-sectional survey of adults in Chicago as well as interviews to demonstrate that Black adults reported racism-related vigilance and sleep difficulties.[49] Findings in other studies are based on self-reports of an association between acts of discrimination and sleep. Researchers from New York, Michigan, and Alabama investigated same-day associations between discrimination and sleep in adolescents ages 13 to 15 years in a large urban northeast area of the United States. The cohort was 41 percent Asian, 22 percent Black, and 37 percent Hispanic youth. The researchers used wrist actigraphy to measure the delay to the onset of sleep (latency) and wake minutes after the onset of sleep (or how many minutes the subjects were awakened during sleep). They learned that on the days when the teens reported discrimination, they fell asleep faster, reported more disturbed sleep, and had next-day feelings of sleepiness and dysfunction.[50]

A research team from California evaluated the association between ethnic discrimination and teens' sleep in a population of Hispanic and Asian adolescents. The adolescents self-reported discrimination, both subtle and overt; sleep quantity and quality; and perceived stress and sense of school belonging. The researchers found that the teens who reported overt discrimination experienced more sleep problems and restlessness. Further, there was a relationship between the reports of subtle discrimination and poorer quantity and quality of sleep. While the researchers believed that the association between discrimination and sleep could be partially a result of stress, they also reported that overt discrimination and microaggressions had independent effects on sleep. A sense of school belonging seemed to be a positive resource for the teens.[51]

LGBTQ
Disturbances in sleep also appear to occur in sexual minority adolescents. Researchers from the University of California, San Francisco studied the association between gay or bisexual sexual identity and sleep problems in a national sample of U.S. early adolescents using cross-sectional data from the Adolescent Brain Cognitive Development Study. In their sample of 8563 adolescents ages 10 to 14 years, 48.8 percent female, 4.4 percent identified as sexual minority. The results indicated that the sexual minority adolescents were at higher risk of overall sleep disturbances, which included an increased chance for trouble falling or staying asleep, compared with their heterosexual peers. The researchers found an association between the sleep problems and depression. In addition, possible family rejection and low family support were supported by their finding that family conflict and less parental monitoring partially mediated the association between sexual minority status and sleep issues. A prevention intervention could include increased mental health services or family support for sexual minority adolescents.[52]

Mortality
After the death of a parent, one in five children is likely to develop a mental health disorder. In the year after their parent's death, children commonly display grief, dysphoria (generalized unhappiness), and distress. Sleep issues may occur as a symptom

of depression following parental death. However, there do not yet appear to be any studies on the relationship between parental death and adolescent sleep. That said, with so many parents dying as a result of the COVID-19 pandemic, this topic will be studied more in the future.[53]

Current Events and Sleep

Climate Change

There is a wide consensus among climatologists and scientific organizations that climate change is occurring because of human activity. After extreme weather events, children are particularly physically and psychologically vulnerable.[54] Climate changes place adolescents at increased risk for mental health problems, such as PTSD, sleep disorders, anxiety, depression, and substance abuse. Although these impacts occur throughout the world, children and teens in developing countries experience the most dramatic effects.[55]

Researchers from South Carolina interviewed adolescents between the ages of 12 and 17 years who lived in Dade County, Florida, during Hurricane Andrew, which occurred in August 1992. The sample of 189 males and 211 females had a mean age of 14.5 years; 44 percent of the youths were Hispanic, 33 percent were Black, and 19 percent were White. About 44 percent of the subjects reported one or more symptoms consistent with PTSD, which may include sleep issues. Six months after the hurricane, it was estimated that the incidence of PTSD rose from 3 percent to 9 percent. The rates for PTSD were highest among Black and Hispanic participants, and most adolescents reported some posttraumatic symptoms. Sleep difficulties were reported overall by 21 percent of the males and 26 percent of the females.[56]

Violence

Since violence rates in lower-class neighborhoods may be up to six times as high as middle-class neighborhoods, life for teens in distressed, impoverished, urban neighborhoods may be dangerous. Violence causes mental distress, posttraumatic stress, and feelings of hopelessness. Researchers used data from the Mobile Youth Survey in Mobile, Alabama, to examine the effect of violence on sleep. The data, from the years 1998 to 2011, included teens between the ages of 10 and 18 years as well as a subset from a sample of 14- and 15-year-old participants. In total, the dataset included more than 12,000 teens. A small subset showed that the average monthly household income from 2005 to 2006 was $400. The researchers learned that exposure to violence had a negative, independent effect on adolescent sleep patterns, especially among females. They also noted that the trajectory for impoverished adolescents was for these sleep problems to decline, particularly in the younger adolescent. Violence impeded the declines, and those teens who felt hopeless had the smallest decline.[57]

In 2016, researchers from Pennsylvania and Alabama evaluated violence and sleep in 252 adolescents in the southeastern United States. The researchers surveyed the community to measure concerns about violence and examined sleep duration and quality using actigraphy and a survey instrument. The researchers learned that in the population studied, greater community violence was linked to lower levels of sleep quality, chiefly among females.[58]

A few years later, researchers in New York and Alabama examined the role that individual difference variables, physiological regulation, and race played in moderating adolescent concerns about violence and sleep. The cohort consisted of 219 teens who were all 18 years old; 55 percent were female, 70 percent were White, and 30 percent were Black. The study included a questionnaire and actigraphy testing. The researchers learned that the Black teens who had less adaptive patterns of regulating physiological arousal had shorter sleep duration and poor quality of sleep, in the context of community violence concerns. This finding was not seen in the White teens. The researchers suggested that coping strategies for managing stress and arousal may be helpful for improving sleep for some youth.[59]

Domestic violence may also contribute to sleep difficulties in adolescents. Researchers in Missouri studied what types of trauma were related to the presence of sleep problems in children and adolescents. They interviewed and completed a battery of measures on a sample of trauma-exposed children and their guardians seeking treatment at a child advocacy center. The children and adolescents ranged between ages 6 and 18, were racially diverse, and had a mean age of 10.88. Twenty-nine percent of the children experienced domestic violence; nightmares and difficulty sleeping were common symptoms. The researchers determined that bad dreams in the study subjects were associated with experienced domestic violence. When interviewing families about sleep difficulties in adolescents, all types of violence should be considered including physical, sexual, and emotional abuse as well as domestic, school, and community violence.[60]

Treatment

Later school start times may be a solution for the prevention of DSPD. If DSPD is diagnosed in an adolescent, then treatment supervised by a clinician can include avoiding bright lights and blue light from computers and smartphones for 30 minutes prior to bedtime. Shifting the bedtime earlier by 15 to 20 minutes each day, use of melatonin in small doses 4 to 6 hours before bedtime, and using early morning bright lights may also be helpful. The bright lights help to shift the circadian rhythm to an earlier time point. That said, a more natural solution would be for later school opening times.[61]

Conclusion

Sleep problems are common during adolescence, and they may be due to a number of biological, psychological, or social issues. Inadequate-quality sleep may result in disparities including increased risks for obesity, mood disorders, suicidal ideation, drowsy driving, and poor academic performance. Parents play an important role in monitoring electronic media use in their children, and clinicians as well as parents should advocate for later school opening times.

References

1   Short MA, Gradisar M, Lack LC, Wright H, Carskadon MA. The discrepancy between acti-graphic and sleep diary measures of sleep in adolescents. *Sleep Med.* 2012;13:378–384.

2   Tarokh L, Saletin JM, Carskadon MA. Sleep in adolescence: physiology, cognition and mental health. *Neurosci Biobehav Rev.* 2016;70:182–188.

3   Cappuccio FP, Taggart FM, Kandala NB, Currie A, Peile E, Stranges S, Miller MA. Meta-analysis of short sleep duration and obesity in children and adults. *Sleep.* 2008;31:619–626.

4   Phillips AJK, Clerx WM, O'Brien CS, et al. Irregular sleep/wake patterns are associated with poorer academic performance and delayed circadian and sleep/wake timing. *Sci Rep.* 2017;7:3216.

5   Cooper R, Di Biase MA, Bei B, Quach, B, Cropley V. Associations of changes in sleep and emotional and behavioral problems from late childhood to early adolescence. *JAMA Psychiatry.* 2023;80:585–596.

6   Goldstein MA. The changing adolescent: a biopsychosocial and behavioral perspective. *Curr Pediatr Rep.* 2020;8:66–68.

7   Keyes K, Maslowsky J, Hamilton A., Schulenberg J. The great sleep recession: changes in sleep duration among US adolescents, 1991–2012. *Pediatrics.* 2015;135:460–468.

8   National Sleep Foundation. How much sleep do you really need? Sleep and You. October 1, 2020.

9   Balbo M, Leproult R, Van Cauter E. Impact of sleep and its disturbances on hypothalamo-pituitary-adrenal axis activity. *Int J Endocrinol.* 2010;Article ID 759234.

10 Carskadon MA. Sleep in adolescents: the perfect storm. *Pediatr Clin North Am.* 2011;58:637–647.

11 Andrade MM, Benedito-Silva A., Domenice S, Arnhold J, Menna-Barrato L. Sleep charac-teristics of adolescents: a longitudinal study. *J Adolesc Health.* 1993;5:401–406.

12 Hagenauer MH, Perryman JI, Lee TM, Carskadon MA. Adolescent changes in the homeo-static and circadian regulation of sleep. *Dev Neurosci.* 2009;31:276–284.

13 Owens J. Adolescent Sleep Working Group and Committee on Adolescence. Insufficient sleep in adolescents and young adults: an update on causes and consequences. *Pediatrics.* 2014;143:e921–e932.

14 Carskadon MA. Sleep in adolescents: the perfect storm. *Pediatr Clin N Am.* 2011;58:637–647.

15 Owens J. Adolescent Sleep Working Group and Committee on Adolescence. Insufficient sleep in adolescent and young adults: an update on causes and consequences. *Pediatrics.* 2014;134:e921–e932.

16 Carskadon MA, Wolfson AR, Acebo C, Tzischinsky O, Seifer R. Adolescent sleep patterns, circadian timing, and sleepiness at a transition to early school days. *Sleep.* 1998;2:871–881.

17 Danner F, Phillips B. Adolescent sleep, school start times, and teen motor vehicle crashes. *J Clin Sleep Med.* 2008;4:533–535.

18 Verona RD, Szklo-Coxe M, Wu A, Dubik M, Zhao Y, Ware J. Dissimilar teen crash rates in two neighboring Virginia cities with different high school start times. *J Clin Sleep Med.* 2011;7:145–151.

19 Trosman I, Ivanenko A. Classification and epidemiology of sleep disorders in children and adolescents. *Child Adolesc Psychiatr Clin N Am.* 2021;30:47–64.

20 Simon SL, Higgins J, Melanson E, Wright KP Jr, Nadeau KJ. A model of adolescent sleep health and risk for type 2 diabetes. *Curr Diab Rep.* 2021;21:4.

21 Verhulst S, Van Gaal L, Debacker W, Desager K. The prevalence, anatomical correlates and treatment of sleep-disordered breathing in obese children and adolescents. *Sleep Med Rev.* 2008;12:339–346.

22 Dewald JF, Meijer AM, Oort FJ, Kerkhof G, Bogels S. Adolescents' sleep in low-stress and high-stress (exam) times: a prospective quasi-experiment. *Behav Sleep Med.* 2014;12:493–506.

23 Akerstedt T. Psychosocial stress and impaired sleep. *Scand J Work Environ Health.* 2006;32:493–501.

24 Bai S, Buxton OM, Master L, Hale L. Daily associations between family interaction quality, stress, and objective sleep in adolescents. *Sleep Health.* 2022;8:69–72.

25 Crowe K, Spiro-Levitt C. Sleep-related problems and pediatric anxiety disorders. *Child Adolesc Psychiatr Clin N Am.* 2010;30:209–224.

26 Zhang J, Paksarian D, Lamers F, Hickle I, He J, Merikangas K. Sleep patterns and mental health correlates in US adolescents. *J Pediatr.* 2017;182:137–143.

27 Alfano CA, Ginsburg GS, Kingery JN. Sleep-related problems among children and adolescents with anxiety disorders. *J Am Acad Child Adolesc Psychiatry.* 2007;46:224–232.

28 Lovato N, Gradisar M. A meta-analysis and model of the relationship between sleep and depression in adolescents: recommendations for future research and clinical practice. *Sleep Med Rev.* 2014;18:521–529.

29 Urrila AS, Karlsson L, Kiviruusu O, Pelkonen M, Strandhold T, Marttunen M. Sleep complaints among adolescent outpatients with major depressive disorder. *Sleep Med.* 2012;13:816–823.

30 Song TH, Wang TT, Zuang YY, et al. Nightmare distress as a risk factor for suicide among adolescents with major depressive disorder. *Nat Sci Sleep.* 2022;14:1687–1697.

31 Lauer CJ, Krieg JC. Sleep in eating disorders. *Sleep Med Rev.* 2004;8:109–118.

32 Allison KC, Spaeth A, Hopkins CM. Sleep and eating disorders. *Curr Psychiatry Rep.* 2016;18: 92

33 Tromp MD, Donners A, Garssen JJ, Verster JC. Sleep, eating disorder symptoms, and daytime functioning. *Nat Sci Sleep.* 2016;8:35–40.

34 Bootzin RR, Stevens SJ. Adolescents, substance abuse, and the treatment of insomnia and daytime sleepiness. *Clin Psychol Rev.* 2005;25:629–644.

35 Gromov I, Gromov D. Sleep and substance use and abuse in adolescents. *Child Adolesc Psychiatr Clin N Am.* 2009;18:929–946.

36 Tynjälä J, Kannas L, Levälahti E. Perceived tiredness among adolescents and its association with sleep habits and use of psychoactive substances. *J Sleep Res.* 1997;6:189–198.

37 Bolla K, Lesage S, Gamaldo C, et al. Sleep disturbance in heavy marijuana users. *Sleep.* 2008;31:901–908.

38 Hasler BP, Soehner AM, Wallace ML, et al. Experimentally imposed circadian misalignment alters the neural response to monetary rewards and response inhibition in healthy adolescents. *Psychol Med.* 2021;17:1–9.

39 Hasler BP, Graves JL, Soehner AM, Wallace ML, Clark DB. Preliminary evidence that circadian alignment predicts neural response to monetary reward in late adolescent drinkers. *Front Neurosci.* 2022;16:803349.

40 van den Eijnden RJJ, Geurts S, Ter Bogt TFM, van der Rijst VG, Koning IM. Social media use and adolescents' sleep: a longitudinal study on the protective role of parental rules regarding internet use before sleep. *Int J Environ Res Public Health.* 2021;18:1346.

41 Cain N, Gradisar M. Electronic media use and sleep in school-aged children and adolescents: a review. *Sleep Med.* 2010;11:735–742.

42 Charmaraman L, Richer AM, Ben-Joseph EP, Klerman EB. Quantity, content, and context matter: associations among social technology use and sleep habits in early adolescents. *J Adolesc Health.* 2021;69:162–165.

43 Spada MM. An overview of problematic internet use. *Addict Behav.* 2014;39:3–6.

44 Chen YL, Gau SS. Sleep problems and internet addiction among children and adolescents: a longitudinal study. *J Sleep Res.* 2016;25:458–465.

45 Çelebioğlu A, Aytekin Özdemir A, Küçükoğlu S, Ayran G. The effect of internet addiction on sleep quality in adolescents. *J Child Adolesc Psychiatr Nurs.* 2020;33:221–228.

46 Demirci K, Akgönül M, Akpinar A. Relationship of smartphone use severity with sleep quality, depression, and anxiety in university students. *J Behav Addict.* 2015;4:85–92.

47 Karki K, Singh DR, Maharjan D, Sushmita KC, Shreesha S, Deependra KT. Internet addiction and sleep quality among adolescents in a peri-urban setting in Nepal: a cross-sectional school-based survey. *PLoS One.* 2021;16:e0246940.

48 Goosby BJ, Cheadle JF, Strong-Bak W, Roth T, Nelson T. Perceived discrimination and adolescent sleep in a community sample. *RSF.* 2018;4:43–61.

49 Hicken MT, Lee H, Ailshire J, Burgard SA, Williams DR. Every shut eye, ain't sleep: The role of racism-related vigilance in racial/ethnic disparities in sleep difficulty. *Race Soc Probl.* 2013;5:100–112.

50 Yip T, Cheon YM, Wang Y, Cham H, Tryon W, El-Sheikh M. Racial disparities in sleep: associations with discrimination among ethnic/racial minority adolescents. *Child Dev.* 2020;91:914–931.

51 Huynh V, Gillen-Oneel C. Discrimination and sleep: the protective role of school belonging. *Youth Soc.* 2016;48:649–672.

52 Nagata JM, Lee CM, Yang JH, et al. Sexual orientation disparities in early adolescent sleep: findings from the adolescent brain cognitive development study. *LGBT Health.* 2023;10:355–363.

53 Dowdney L. Childhood bereavement following parental death. *J Child Psychol Psychiatry.* 2000;41:819–830.

54 Ahdoot, S, Pacheco SE. Council on Environmental Health. Global climate change and children's health. *Pediatrics.* 2015;136:e1468–e1484.

55 Burke SEL, Sanson AV, Van Hoorn J. The psychological effects of climate change on children. *Cur Psychiatry Rep.* 2018;20:35.

56 Garrison CZ, Bryant ES, Addy CL, Spurrier PG, Freedy R, Kilpatrick DG. Posttraumatic stress disorder in adolescents after Hurricane Andrew. *J Am Acad Child Adolesc Psychiatry.* 1995;34:1193–1201.

57 Umlauf MG, Bolland AC, Bolland KA, Tomek S, Bolland J. The effects of age, gender, hopelessness, and exposure to violence on sleep disorder symptoms and daytime sleepiness among adolescents in impoverished neighborhoods. *J Youth Adolesc.* 2015;44:518–542.

58 Bagley EJ, Tu KM, Buckha JA, El-Sheikh M. Community violence concerns and adolescent sleep. *Sleep Health.* 2016;2:57–62.

59 Philbrook LE, Buckhalt JA, El-Sheikh M. Community violence concerns and adolescent sleep: physiological regulation and race as moderators. *J Sleep Res.* 2020;29:e12897.

60 Wamser-Nanney R, Chesher RE. Trauma characteristics and sleep impairment among trauma-exposed children. *Child Abuse Negl.* 2018;76:469–479.

61 Kansagra S. Sleep disorders in adolescents. *Pediatrics.* 2020;145(Suppl 2):S204–S209.

2
Obesity

Introduction

Obesity is a global health issue in adolescents; it is highly prevalent in high-income countries, and its prevalence in low- and middle-income countries is increasing. Adolescents with obesity are likely to continue into adulthood with this condition and will be at risk for cardiometabolic and psychosocial morbidities.[1] Obesity is recognized by the American Medical Association as a chronic disease. It is a medical problem that can increase the risk of other medical conditions in adolescents including sleep apnea, hypertension, liver disease, and type 2 diabetes.

Obesity is defined by the body mass index (BMI), which is calculated by dividing a person's weight in kilograms by the height in meters squared. Adults who have a BMI of 30 or more are described as having obesity; those with a BMI from 25 to 29.9 are overweight. For teens, obesity is defined as a BMI equal to or greater than the gender- and age-specific 95th percentile on the Centers for Disease Control and Prevention growth charts.[2] Adolescents with a BMI equal to or greater than the gender- and age-specific 85th percentile but less than the 95th percentile are considered overweight. However, it is too simplistic to note that obesity is caused by energy intake greater than energy output.

There are a number of genetic and nongenetic factors that increase the risk of excess weight in adolescents. Recently a single gene was reported to be the cause of excessive obesity in a young adolescent.[3] Also, there are a few genetic disorders that lead to obesity in adolescents. An example is Prader-Willi syndrome; while exceedingly rare, it is the most common genetic problem associated with obesity. More often, there appears to be an epigenetic (a nongenetic alteration of the gene function) etiology for childhood obesity.

In some adolescents, the COVID-19 pandemic with remote learning and the discontinuation of many sports activities and increased screen time at home were notable factors in the more recent serious weight gain. Further, the added stress and anxiety from the pandemic could have led to abnormal eating patterns in teens. And the marketing of certain high-calorie food through technology may easily have influenced food preferences.

A systematic review and meta-analysis by researchers in China found that adolescents with obesity had a higher risk for major depression compared to healthy controls.[4] Another less discussed factor for adolescent obesity is the emergence of atypical antipsychotic medications. Since the 1980s, these have greatly benefited adolescents with certain mental health disorders, such as depression. However, a significant side effect of this new generation of medications is weight gain. Coupled with the tendency of adolescents who are depressed to be relatively inactive, these medications may easily cause excessive weight gain.

Other factors may play an important role. Sections of some urban areas offer few options for physical activity and limited availability of healthier foods. In addition, as noted in Chapter 1, there is an association between disrupted sleep and obesity. Also, even before birth, the perinatal environment, which includes the maternal intrauterine hormonal milieu and the mother's nutrition status, may influence the fetus. Of course, the postnatal environment may support further epigenetic changes that foster obesity in children and teens.[5] Researchers from New York studied children of mothers who had delivered either before or after bariatric (weight loss) surgery. They compared children from mothers who delivered a child before surgery and had a mean BMI of 48 to mothers who delivered a child after surgery and had a mean BMI of 31. Thirty-four children were born before the mothers had surgery, and 79 were born after surgery. For the children born before the surgery, the prevalence rate for obesity up to their 18th birthdays was 41.2 percent; for the children born after the surgery and after their mothers had experienced a significant weight loss, the prevalence rate was 17.7 percent. The researchers commented that weight loss for such severely overweight women was a potentially modifiable epigenetic factor in the etiology of obesity for their children.[6]

Researchers in Pennsylvania followed 1336 adolescents beginning when they were 14 years old for 4 years and measured screen time on television/videos and video games and calculated their BMI on self-reported height and weight every 6 months. Increasing screen time was positively associated with changes in BMI at the 50th, 75th, and 90th BMI percentiles but not at the lower BMI percentiles. The researchers concluded that screen time is an important adolescent obesity risk factor, especially among adolescents who are already overweight or have obesity.[7]

It is evident that a combination of biological, psychological, and social factors may promote obesity in adolescents. This results in overwhelming challenges for adolescents and their families, schools, communities, and countries. It is the responsibility of everyone to support healthy weight in this age group.

Complications for Adolescents With Obesity

Adolescents with obesity are at significant risk for biological, psychological, and social problems, making the obesity epidemic of great public health importance.

Medical Complications

Fatty Liver Disease

It is estimated that 36 percent of adolescents with obesity may have fat deposited into their liver tissue, a medical problem known as nonalcoholic fatty liver disease (NAFLD). Since adolescents with obesity often remain obese into adulthood, this is an important finding. NAFLD in adults is known to contribute to the risk of liver cirrhosis and hepatocellular carcinoma; these individuals also have risk for the development of type 2 diabetes, heart disease, and chronic kidney disease. In teens, there is a clear association between excessive weight gain and NAFLD.[8] NAFLD is more common in males with obesity than female adolescents so affected. Healthy eating, physical activity, and appropriate weight loss are some treatment options.

Hypertension
Largely due to the epidemic of obesity in adolescents, the prevalence of hypertension or elevated blood pressure levels in teens has increased during the past few decades. Approximately 30 percent of adolescent males with obesity have prehypertension or hypertension; the number is slightly lower in adolescent females. Untreated hypertension may lead to additional medical problems, including kidney and heart complications. While weight reduction is crucial to management of hypertension in adolescents, increased exercise and a heart healthy diet are helpful. Sometimes, antihypertensive medications may be prescribed.[9]

Premature Menarche
Girls with obesity have a higher likelihood of early pubertal development leading to an early first menstruation (menarche). Further, when compared to girls with a normal BMI, girls with an elevated BMI may develop breasts before the age of 8. Girls who develop earlier than normal may experience psychological issues such as bullying.[10] And some have an early onset of sexual activity, with a high risk of unintended pregnancy.

Sleep Apnea
As noted previously, obstructive sleep apnea (OSA) is a complication of obesity in adolescents. An adolescent who has OSA will have a partial, repeated, and prolonged obstruction of the upper airway during sleep. This causes a disruption of normal breathing, which in turn interrupts normal sleep patterns. Up to 30 percent of teens with obesity have OSA, a disorder that may cause daytime sleepiness and related issues, such as problems with academic achievement. Appropriate weight management and exercise may help adolescents with OSA, and a referral to a sleep specialist may be required. On occasion, a surgical approach is advised that may include procedures on the soft palate, tongue, or nasal septum.[11]

Type 2 Diabetes
Adolescents with obesity may have elevated blood sugar levels. Although some insulin resistance normally occurs during adolescence, the resistance may increase significantly in teens who have obesity and may lead to rising blood sugars. Treatment includes exercise, weight loss, dietary modification, and occasional use of medication.[12]

Psychological Issues

Poor Self-Esteem
Self-esteem is an individual's perception of their self-worth. It may represent the capacity to feel worthy of happiness and the capability to face the challenges of life. Adolescents with low self-esteem may develop physical, psychological, and social

problems, including mood disorders, suicidal thoughts, disordered eating, and substance abuse.

Researchers from Minnesota reviewed 35 studies to determine if self-esteem was related to weight issues in children. Seven of the nine cross-sectional studies found an inverse relationship between self-esteem and obesity in adolescents ages 13 to 18 years. In this age group, there was also an inverse relationship between overall self-esteem, weight, and body esteem.[13] In a population-based study of 6522 U.S. adolescents between the ages of 12 and 16 years, researchers examined characteristics associated with low self-esteem. Among their findings, they learned that low self-esteem was strongly associated with obesity. Moreover, while television time did not support self-esteem, participating in team sports did. Teens who participated in team sports had a lower risk for poor self-esteem.[14]

Depression
It is often asked if adolescents with depression have a higher risk for obesity. Researchers from Texas examined the relationship between depression in teens and obesity. They surveyed 4175 adolescents between the ages of 11 and 17 years at baseline and after 1 year. The researchers found no association between major depression at baseline and obesity at the 1-year follow-up.[15]

Another concern is whether obesity is a trigger for depression. In a 4-year prospective study of 496 adolescent females between the ages of 11 and 15 years, researchers in Minnesota and California interviewed the adolescents for evidence of depression. The teens completed questionnaires and had their height and weight measured at baseline and during three follow-up visits. The prevalence of obesity was 11 percent. Though the researchers did not find an association between obesity and the diagnosis of major depression, there was a consistent relationship between obesity and depressive symptoms.[16] However, in Sweden, researchers studied a nationwide group of 12,507 male and female children and teens with obesity and compared them to 60,063 other children and teens. The study group with obesity had a 9.7 percent prevalence of anxiety and depression compared to 5.0 percent in the comparison group. The researchers observed that obesity was a strong risk factor for both anxiety and depression.[17]

Social Issues

Bullying
Researchers from New York and Mississippi conducted an analysis of 31,770 adolescents ages 10 to 17 years included in the National Survey of Children's Health. Most of the teens were White non-Hispanic, not poor (family income equal to or greater than 185 percent of poverty), and older than 12 years. The researchers wanted to determine if adolescents with higher weights would have a different odds ratio for being a bully victim, perpetrator, or both when compared to adolescents with healthy weights. The adolescents were placed into one of three groups according to their BMIs—healthy weight (BMI greater than 5th percentile and less than 85th percentile), overweight (BMI equal to or greater than 85th percentile and less than 95th percentile), and obese (BMI equal to or greater than 95th percentile). About 71 percent of the teens were a

healthy weight, about 15 percent were overweight, and about 14 percent had obesity. The researchers learned that the adolescents who were overweight or had obesity had greater odds of bullying behavior—both as a perpetrator and as a victim—than adolescents with healthy weights. In addition, those adolescents who were overweight or had obesity who were engaged in bullying behaviors had significantly greater odds of behavioral conduct problems, depression, and difficulty making friends.[18]

Weight Stigma

Unfortunately, in the United States, stigmatization on the basis of weight is often propagated and tolerated—sometimes by clinicians. To learn more about weight stigmatization, researchers from Wisconsin and Missouri conducted semistructured interviews with 12 adolescents with severe obesity and 19 of their parents. Common themes were weight-based bullying and teasing, inappropriate interactions with health care providers, and blame. Both the teens and the parents reported repeated bullying about the teens' weights. Some had uncomfortable interactions with health care providers leading them to feelings of shame, ineptness, and guilt. All of the adolescents described feeling often that they were being criticized by others for weight issues.[19]

Wanting to learn more about their quality of life, researchers from California and Texas conducted a cross-sectional study of 106 male and female children and teens referred to an academic medical center for obesity evaluations. Patients and parents separately completed a quality-of-life inventory. The inventories were compared with a group of healthy weight children and teens as well as children and teens with cancer. In all the measured domains, which included physical, emotional, and social health and school functioning, the children and adolescents with obesity had lower quality-of-life scores than those with healthy weights. In addition, the children and adolescents with obesity had scores that were similar to the children and adolescents with cancer.[20]

Weight stigma is most often seen as victimization, teasing, and bullying. Stigmatization may lead a teen to socially isolate, avoid health care, and create barriers to healthy behaviors. These teens may have adverse academic outcomes and avoid participating in athletics and other physical activities, which may lead to more teasing and bullying.[21] Moreover, there is evidence that youth who are bullied about their weight have an increased vulnerability to anxiety, a mood disorder, or substance use.

Epidemiology

In the National Health and Nutrition Examination Survey 2015–2016, the prevalence of obesity among adolescents ages 12 to 19 years was 20.6 percent, with 20.9 percent among females and 20.2 percent among males. For all children aged 2 to 19 years, the prevalence of obesity from 1999 to 2016 increased from 13.9 percent to 18.5 percent.[22] African American females and Hispanic American males are disproportionately impacted by obesity. In addition, adolescents from low-income communities have a higher prevalence of this disorder.[23] While physical activity helps to prevent obesity, adolescents in the South, those with parents who have a high school education or less, and those with a family income less than 100 percent of the federal poverty level are at highest risk for nonparticipation in organized sports.[24] The prevalence of obesity is now more than three times higher than it was in the 1960s and 1970s.

For children in higher-income countries, there are increased rates of obesity in the lowest socioeconomic groups. In both higher- and lower-income countries, children who live in urban areas are more likely to have obesity.[25] Native American and Alaska Native adolescents have an increased risk for obesity; in the fiscal year 2015, the prevalence rate for obesity in the 12- to 19-year-old Native American and Alaska Native teens was 33.8 percent.[26]

The World Obesity Federation reported that there will be 254 million children and adolescents ages 5 to 19 years living with obesity in 2030, with the highest prevalence in China, India, the United States, Indonesia, and Brazil. In lower- to middle-income countries, children and adolescents of higher socioeconomic status are more likely to be overweight or have obesity, whereas in high-income countries, children and adolescents living in socioeconomic disadvantage are at higher risk.[27]

Biopsychosocial Issues and Obesity

Biological Issues and Obesity

Stress

In adolescents, there is good evidence that chronic stress (persistent or repeated stressors) is obesogenic—supporting the development of obesity. It fosters an increase of energy intake and decreases physical activity and energy expenditure. And it seems to stimulate abdominal obesity or visceral fat accumulation.[28]

It is well known that for many teens, stress is highly associated with cravings for comfort foods. The neuroendocrine system responds to stress in several ways. One of these is the release of cortisol, which acts on a brain reward system, inducing the urge for high-caloric comfort foods. After these foods are consumed, this urge is deactivated possibly through the release of endogenous opioids—opioids that are naturally created by the body. Approaches to stress-related overeating in adolescents could include recognizing patterns of emotional eating and mindfulness to reduce stress levels.[29]

Researchers from Greece conducted a literature review to identify randomized controlled trials on the utility of mindfulness or stress management as a treatment tool for adolescents with obesity. They identified six studies that met their inclusion criteria with specific markers for change in adiposity. Two studies found no significant changes after a 6- to 10-week mindfulness-based treatment program. One study showed lower BMI in the intervention group after a 6-week program of mindful eating. Three programs, which offered mindfulness-based stress reduction, had BMI reduction or improvement of the waist-to-hip ratio in the treatment group and an increase in BMI in the control group.[30]

Psychological Issues and Obesity

Anxiety

When discussing obesity and anxiety in adolescents, two questions readily come to mind. Does an adolescent with anxiety have a higher risk for obesity? Does an adolescent with obesity have a higher risk for anxiety? Researchers from Texas and Vietnam reviewed data from the teen health multiwave study of adolescents completed in the Houston, Texas area. The cohort consisted of 4175 adolescents, and the data included computer-assisted personal interviews and self-administered questionnaires. Using standard field procedures, height and weight measurements were recorded. At baseline, no association was found between overweight and anxiety disorders. However, there was a significant association with obesity only in male adolescents; any anxiety disorder was associated with 46 percent increased odds of obesity. At the same time, obesity and overweight were not related to a future risk of developing an anxiety disorder. The authors suggest that the association between anxiety disorders and obesity is possibly related to neuropeptide Y, which reduces anxiety and stress but is also a stimulant for carbohydrate intake and may lead to abdominal obesity.[31]

Eating Disorders

As discussed in Chapter 6, in adolescents, binge eating disorder (BED) is defined as the consumption of a quantity of food that is larger than most would eat under similar circumstances. It is associated with a loss of control over eating. In adolescents, BED is associated with obesity, and it can lead to physical health consequences from excess weight as well as symptoms of depression and disordered eating. BED tends to begin in late adolescence.[32] In adults, BED has been reported in 25 percent or more of patients with obesity.[33] One systematic review and meta-analysis found BED to be as common in adolescents as anorexia and bulimia.[34] Cognitive behavioral therapy is the first line of treatment; for those adolescents who want pharmacological therapy, selective serotonin reuptake inhibitors (SSRIs) are usually recommended. After SSRIs, medical providers may prescribe topiramate or lisdexamfetamine. However, it is unclear if medication is as effective as cognitive behavioral therapy.[35]

Substance Use

Adolescents who are overweight or obese are vulnerable to health risk behaviors and are more likely to have problems with peer relationships and weight bias and stigma than normal-weight teens. In response to these stresses, the teens may experiment with risky behaviors. Researchers from the National Institutes of Health investigated the relationship between overweight/obesity and adolescent substance use and whether it varied by gender and age. They used results from the U.S. 2005/2006 Health Behavior in School-Age Children survey, which is a nationally representative sample performed every 4 years, to examine the link between overweight/obesity and substance use. The data included information to calculate BMI as well as statistics on the use of tobacco, alcohol, and marijuana. The sample size, which was 7825, was about evenly split between the genders. Most respondents were younger than 15 years and lived in two-parent families. While most of the subjects had a normal weight,

17.8 percent were overweight and 14.3 percent had obesity. The researchers learned that substance use was significantly related to overweight/obesity only in females. Among older females, only those who had obesity had a higher risk of being frequent smokers and drinkers. The researchers theorized that overweight/obesity in females may lead to greater stress, and the females may try to cope with this stress through substance abuse.[36]

Another study from a researcher in California found no relationship between adolescents with obesity and the use of alcohol or cannabis. Further, there was no significant evidence of BMI status and e-cigarette use in males or females.[37]

Social Issues and Obesity

Social Media

It has been demonstrated many times that there is a strong association between screen exposure and obesity in adolescents through the promotion of unhealthy diets and physical inactivity. Social media contains advertisements with high-calorie, low-nutrient foods and beverages, barely mentioning the intake of fruits and vegetables. Adolescents who spend significant amounts of time on screens tend to reduce their physical activity and sleep time, thus promoting weight gain. Studies in communities where screen time was lowered experienced a direct (cause-and-effect) lessening of weight gain in children.[38]

Researchers from Pennsylvania performed a systematic review on the use of social media to influence adolescent food choices. They located six articles that met their criteria. From the studies, the researchers learned that companies use celebrities and influencers to promote unhealthy foods and beverages. Teens who are fans of these well-known people may be swayed by their recommendations. Another tactic is to suggest that most adolescents consume the marketed products. Likewise, on certain social media outlets, posts from adolescent peers may obscure the lack of nutritional value of the foods and beverages.[39]

While social media may clearly promote obesity, could it also encourage weight loss in adolescents with obesity? Researchers from Spain conducted a systematic review on weight loss interventions delivered by social media and found 14 articles that met their criteria. The platforms included Facebook and Twitter, and the study designs consisted of randomized and nonrandomized controlled trials, an online survey, an experimental format, and a descriptive study. It appears that the best results were seen in a randomized controlled study in college students.[40] In that randomized controlled trial, college students with a BMI in the overweight or obese range were assigned to one of three groups: a private Facebook group that informs and encourages weight loss, a separate private Facebook group that informs and encourages weight loss and uses text messaging, and a control nonintervention group. While the students in the control group gained weight, the students in both Facebook groups lost weight, with better results in the group that had text messaging. The researchers commented that using a social media platform and text messaging might be a useful means to encourage weight loss in this population.[41]

Problematic Internet Use

Is it possible that problematic internet use (PIU) may lead to obesity, or is the converse true? To evaluate the association between PIU and BMI, researchers in Turkey created a cohort of 437 youths between the ages of 8 and 17 years, of which 268 had obesity and 169 had normal weight. The researchers determined that 24.6 percent of the youth with obesity had PIU compared to 11.2 percent of the control/healthy group. Thus, there appeared to be a positive relationship, but not cause and effect, between BMI and PIU. Clinicians should consider screening adolescents with obesity for PIU.[42] A similar association was observed in another study from Turkey. Moreover, in this study, the researchers found a relationship between the youth with obesity and less weekly exercise and increased daytime sleepiness.[43] No cause and effect was demonstrated. However, it is probable that adolescents with obesity and PIU have a more sedentary lifestyle, leading to weight issues.

Poverty

Adolescents living in poverty have limited food budgets and food choices. Using data from the National Longitudinal Study of Adolescent to Adult Health, also known as Add Health, researchers from Florida wanted to understand the effects of neighborhood environments and the BMI trajectories in adolescents. Add Health is a large, nationally representative, school-based study of adolescents, their families, and their schools. When this study was published, the cohort included 9115 teens. The researchers learned that teens living in disadvantaged and low-income neighborhoods were surrounded by a system of obesity in which there is risky eating, limited regular physical activity, food deserts, and stress-laden environments. Teens in these neighborhoods had greater BMIs and gained body weight faster than teens who lived in more advantaged neighborhoods.[44]

Building on this, a researcher from Colorado used Add Health data to determine if moving from a disadvantaged neighborhood to a more advantaged neighborhood or from a more advantaged neighborhood to a disadvantaged neighborhood as a teen would have any impact on obesity. The study included four waves of data from 1994 to 2008 with a total of 12,164 participants. The researcher learned that when compared to adolescents who never lived in those neighborhoods, adolescents who consistently lived in poor neighborhoods were more likely to become young adults with obesity. Leaving severe neighborhood poverty diminished the risk of becoming an adult with obesity, while entering a disadvantaged neighborhood increased the risk.[45] Housing voucher programs provide an opportunity for families to escape neighborhood poverty and possibly eliminate or reduce health disparities.[46]

Climate Change

There has been speculation that extreme global warming may lead to a worsening of the obesity epidemic. A researcher from London determined that people living in warmer climates had a small but statistically significant increase in BMI, weight, overweight, and obesity. The researcher proposed that people who live in warmer climates need fewer calories to meet their needs; people in colder climates use body energy to warm cold air and cold food. Citing the worst set of circumstances, in which there is an increase in temperature from global warming by 10.2° F from the years 1961 to 2081, the researchers noted that this may produce an increase of 2.2 pounds or .37 in BMI in each individual, which could bring more individuals into the obesity range.[47]

Researchers from Pennsylvania, Tennessee, and Maryland theorized that increases in atmospheric temperatures from climate change resulted in less physical activity and the use of fewer calories, worsening the obesity epidemic. They also argued that there is a bidirectional relationship between climate change/global warming and obesity. Thus, with climate change there are economic and social disruptions from storms, droughts, and floods. Some people may respond to such serious problems by engaging in less physical activity. And that in turn may result in weight gain. Climate change may impact the growth of healthier foods, such as fruits and vegetables, and that may make them less available and more costly. People may need to eat foods that are more readily available and not as expensive. Individuals who are heavier add to the costs of transportation, thereby creating more greenhouse gases, and they may have diets containing larger amounts of meat, requiring the raising of more cattle, which are a major source of greenhouse gases.[48]

Interventions

Despite the genetic and nongenetic factors that promote weight gain, it occurs when people take in more calories than they utilize. Interventions may occur at multiple levels. For example, at home there should be more time available for healthy eating and physical activity as well as less screen time. Physical activity should be encouraged. In the primary, middle, and high school settings, physical education should be mandatory, and there ought to be strict standards for school meals, especially the elimination of sugar-sweetened beverages (SSBs). In impoverished neighborhoods, there should be more parks and playgrounds with easy access. Health insurance should cover the medical care for adolescents with obesity. With respect to social media, food advertisements and marketing toward adolescents should be prohibited. And finally, at the governmental level, there should be programming and laws to encourage healthier eating and physical activity.[49]

Researchers in Massachusetts examined the effect of decreasing SSBs on body weight in adolescents. They performed a randomized controlled trial on 103 adolescents ages 13 to 18 who regularly consumed SSBs. In the 25-week study, the intervention group received weekly home deliveries of noncaloric beverages, and they were instructed not to drink SSBs. The control group was to continue their usual beverage consumption habits. The researchers determined that the consumption of SSBs decreased by 82 percent in the intervention group, and decreasing SSB consumption had a beneficial effect on body weight, especially for those adolescents who were in the upper baseline BMI range. BMI change differed significantly between the intervention and control groups. This study demonstrated that behaviors at the family level, programming in schools and communities, and policy changes by government may promote better health in adolescents.[50]

The American Academy of Pediatrics has released a clinical practice guideline (CPG) for the evaluation and treatment of children and adolescents with obesity. This is an evidence-based plan that takes into account the adolescent's health status, family, community, and resources for treatment. The plan emphasizes a nonstigmatizing approach, and it also states that there is no evidence to support watchful waiting or unnecessary delay of appropriate treatment for adolescents with obesity. It also recommends that pediatricians and others who deliver care to adolescents ages 12 years and older with obesity offer weight loss medications as an adjunct to healthy behavior and lifestyle treatment. Furthermore, for those adolescents ages 13 and older with a BMI of 35 or higher, the CPG recommends that the pediatric clinician refer these individuals for evaluation for metabolic treatment and bariatric surgery.[51] One medication that can be utilized is a weekly injection of semaglutide. In a double-blind randomized trial, adolescents with overweight or obesity and ages 12 to less than 18 years were administered semaglutide and lifestyle interventions or placebo and lifestyle interventions. The group administered semaglutide had a greater reduction in BMI than those with lifestyle interventions alone.[52] Semaglutide is now approved for use in adolescents ages 12 years and older who have a BMI at or above the 95th percentile for age and gender.

Prevention

The implementation of healthy eating practices and adequate exercise are essential to the prevention of adolescent obesity. Entire family involvement in these practices yields the greatest results. This includes effective education of parents on meal and snack portion sizes as well as proper nutrition and dietary caloric intake requirements for adolescents. Moreover, schools need to mandate physical education activities and offer healthier meals.[53] In addition, since adolescents learn from their parents and families, adult modeling of healthy eating and appropriate exercise is important. This does not necessarily suggest that parents restrict unhealthy food choices, as this could increase the adolescent's craving for such foods and lead to inappropriate weight gain. However, family mealtime with families eating healthy foods together is important.[54]

Conclusion

Adolescent obesity is a worldwide problem with significant negative effects on adolescents' biopsychosocial domains. In particular for adolescents, increased screen time and decreased physical activities have exacerbated the obesity epidemic. Prevention and treatment programs begin at the family level and continue through pediatric clinicians, schools, and communities and should include changes in state and national policies to promote healthier eating and physical activity. A new CPG for pediatric clinicians emphasizes to not have a watch-and-wait attitude for adolescents with obesity. Adolescents should not be blamed for their body size. Societal issues such as marketing junk food to teens, providing vending machines in schools, and having a lack of walkable neighborhoods all contribute to the increasing incidence of obesity in youth.

References

1   Jacobs DR Jr, Woo JG, Sinaiko AR, et al. Childhood cardiovascular risk factors and adult cardiovascular events. *N Engl J Med.* 2022;386:1877–1888.

2   Set 1 Clinical growth charts with 5th and 95th percentiles. Centers for Disease Control and Prevention.Atlanta, GA, December 15, 2022.

3   Kempf E, Landgraf K, Stein R, et al. Aberrant expression of agouti signaling protein (ASIP) as a cause of monogenic severe childhood obesity. *Nat Metab.* 2022;4:1697–1712.

4   Rao WW, Zong QQ, Zhang E, et al. Obesity increases the risk of depression in children and adolescents: results from a systematic review and meta-analysis. *J Affect Disord.* 2020;267:78–85.

5   Huang S, Barlow S, Quiros-Tejeira R, et al. Childhood obesity for pediatric gastroenterologists. *J Pediatr Gastroenterol Nutr.* 2013;56:99–109.

6   Kral JG, Biron S, Simard S, et al. Large maternal weight loss from obesity surgery prevents transmission of obesity to children who were followed for 2 to 18 years. *Pediatrics.* 2006;118:e1644–e1649.

7   Mitchell JA, Rodriguez D, Schmitz KH, Audrain-McGovern J. Greater screen time is associated with adolescent obesity: a longitudinal study of the BMI distribution from ages 14 to 18. *Obesity (Silver Spring).* 2013;3:572–575.

8   Shaunak M, Byrne CD, Davis N, Afolabi P, Faust S, Davies JH. Non-alcoholic fatty liver disease and childhood obesity. *Arch Dis Child.* 2021;106:3–8.

9   Falkner B. Monitoring and management of hypertension with obesity in adolescents. *Integr Blood Press Control.* 2017;10:33–39.

10 Rosenfield R, Lipton RB, Drum ML. Thelarche, pubarche, and menarche attainment in children with normal and elevated body mass index. *Pediatrics.* 2009;123:84–88.

11 Nevin MA. Pediatric obesity, metabolic syndrome, and obstructive sleep apnea syndrome. *Pediatr Ann.* 2013;42:205–210.

12 Aye T, Levitsky L. Type 2 diabetes: an epidemic in childhood. *Curr Opin Pediatr.* 2003;15:411–415.

13 French SA, Story M, Perry CL. Self-esteem and obesity in children and adolescents: a literature review. *Obes Res.* 1995;3:479–490.

14 McClure AC, Tanski SE, Kingsbury J, Gerrard M, Sargent JD. Characteristics associated with low self-esteem among US adolescents. *Acad Pediatr.* 2010;10:238–244.

15 Roberts RE, Duong HT. Does major depression affect risk for adolescent obesity? *J Affect Disord.* 2015;186:162–167.

16 Boutelle KN, Hannan P, Fulkerson JA, Crow SJ, Stice E. Obesity as a prospective predictor of depression in adolescent females. *Health Psychol.* 2010;29:293–298.

17 Lindberg L, Hagman E, Danielsson P, Marcus C, Persson M. Anxiety and depression in children and adolescents with obesity: a nationwide study in Sweden. *BMC Med.* 2020;18:30.

18 Rupp K, McCoy SM. Bullying perpetration and victimization among adolescents with overweight and obesity in a nationally representative sample. *Child Obes.* 2019;15:323–330.

19 Roberts KJ, Polfuss ML, Marstron EC, Davis RL. Experiences of weight stigma in adolescents with severe obesity and their families. *J Adv Nurs.* 2021;10:4184–4194.

20 Schwimmer JB, Burwinkle TM, Varni JW. Health-related quality of life of severely obese children and adolescents. *JAMA.* 2003;289:1813–1819.

21 Pont SJ, Puhl R, Cook SR, Slusser W. Stigma experienced by children and adolescents with obesity. *Pediatrics.* 2017;140:e20173034.

22 Hales CM, Carroll MD, Fryar CD, Ogden CL. Prevalence of obesity among adults and youth: United States 2015–2016. *NCHS Data Brief.* 2017;288:1–8.

23 Johnson VR, Cao M, Czepiel KS, Mushannen T, Nolen L, Standford FC. Strategies in the management of adolescent obesity. *Curr Pediatr Rep.* 2020;8:56–65.

24 Black LI, Terlizzi EP, Vahratian A. Organized sports participation among children aged 6–17 years: United States, 2020. *NCHS Data Brief.* 2022;441:1–8. PMID: 35969661.

25 Güngör NK. Overweight and obesity in children and adolescents. *J Clin Res Pediatr Endocrinol.* 2014;6:129–143.

26 Bullock A, Sheff K, Moore K, Manson S. Obesity and overweight in American Indian and Alaska Native children. *Am J Public Health.* 2017;107:1502–1507.

27 Jebeile H, Kelly AS, O'Malley G, Baur LA. Obesity in children and adolescents: epidemiology, causes, assessment, and management. *Lancet Diabetes Endocrinol.* 2022;10:351–365.

28 DeVriendt T, Moreno LA, De Henauw S. Chronic stress and obesity in adolescents: scientific evidence and methodological issues for epidemiological research. *Nutr Metab Cardiovasc Dis.* 2009;19:511–519.

29 Sato AF, Fahrenkamp AJ. From bench to bedside: understanding stress-obesity research within the context of translation to improve pediatric behavioral weight management. *Pediatr Clin North Am.* 2016;63:401–423.

30 Paltoglou G, Chrousos GP, Bacopoulou F. Stress management as an effective complementary therapeutic strategy for weight loss in children and adolescents with obesity: a systematic review of randomized controlled trials. *Children (Basel).* 2021;8:670.

31 Roberts RE, Duong HT. Do anxiety disorders play a role in adolescent obesity? *Ann Behav Med.* 2016;50:613–621.

32 Bohon C. Binge eating disorder in children and adolescents. *Child Adolesc Psychiatr Clin N Am.* 2019;28:549–555.

33 Pull C. Binge eating disorder. *Curr Opin Psychiatry.* 2004;17:43–48.

34 Kjeldbjerg ML, Clausen L. Prevalence of binge-eating disorder among children and adolescents: a systematic review and meta-analysis. *Eur Child Adolesc Psychiatry.* 2023;32:549–574.

35 Eddy K, Lawson EA, Goldstein MA. *Approach to Eating Disorders. Primary Care Medicine.* 8th ed. Wolters Kluwer; 2021.

36 Farhat T, Iannotti RJ, Simons-Morton BG. Overweight, obesity, youth, and health-risk behaviors. *Am J Prev Med.* 2010;38:258–267.

37 Lanza HI. Weighing the risk: developmental pathways and processes underlying obesity to substance use in adolescence. *J Res Adolesc.* 2022;32:337–354.

38 Robinson TN, Banda JA, Hale L, et al. Screen media exposure and obesity in children and adolescents. *Pediatrics.* 2017;140(Suppl 2):S97–S101.

39 Kucharczuk AJ, Oliver TL, Dowdell EB. Social media's influence on adolescents' food choices: a mixed studies systematic literature review. *Appetite.* 2022;168:105765.

40 Lozano-Chacon B, Suarez-Lledo V, Alvarez-Galvez J. Use and effectiveness of social-media-delivered weight loss interventions among teenagers and young adults: a systematic review. *Int Environ Res Public Health.* 2021;18:8493.

41 Napolitano MA, Hayes S, Bennett GG, Ives AK, Foster GD. Using Facebook and text messaging to deliver a weight loss program to college students. *Obesity (Silver Spring).* 2013;21:25–31.

42 Bozkurt H, Özer S, Sahin S, Sönmezgöz E. Internet use patterns and internet addiction in children and adolescents with obesity. *Pediatr Obes.* 2018;13:301–306.

43 Eliacik K, Bolat N, Koçyigit C, et al. Internet addiction, sleep and health-related life quality among obese individuals: a comparison study of the growing problems in adolescent health. *Eat Weight Disord.* 2016;21:709–717.

44 Burdette AM, Needham BL. Neighborhood environment and body mass index trajectories from adolescence to adulthood. *J Adolesc Health.* 2012;50:30–37.

45 Lippert AM. Stuck in unhealthy places: how entering, exiting, and remaining in poor and nonpoor neighborhoods is associated with obesity during the transition to adulthood. *J Health Soc Behav.* 2016;57:1–21.

46 Darrah J, DeLuca S. Living here has changed my whole perspective: how escaping inner-city poverty shapes neighborhood and housing choice. *J Policy Anal Manage.* 2014;33:350–384.

47 Kanazawa S. Does global warming contribute to the obesity epidemic? *Environ Res.* 2020;182:108962.

48 Koch CA, Sharda P, Patel J, Gubbi S, Bansal R, Bartel MJ. Climate change and obesity. *Horm Metab Res.* 2021;53:575–587.

49 Ebbeling CB, Pawlak DB, Ludwig DS. Childhood obesity: public-health crisis, common sense cure. *Lancet.* 2002;360:473–482.

50 Ebbeling CB, Feldman HA, Osganian SK, Chomitz VR, Ellenbogen SJ, Ludwig DS. Effects of decreasing sugar-sweetened beverage consumption on body weight in adolescents: a randomized, controlled pilot study. *Pediatrics.* 2006;117:673–680.

51 Hampl SE, Hassink SG, Skinner AC, et al. Clinical practice guideline for the evaluation and treatment of children and adolescents with obesity. *Pediatrics.* 2023;151:e2022060640.

52 Weghuber D, Barrett T, Barrientos-Pérez M, et al. Once-weekly semaglutide in adolescents with obesity. *N Engl J Med.* 2022;387:2245–2257.

53 Sanyaolu A, Okorie C, Qi X, Locke J, Rehman S. Childhood and adolescent obesity in the United States: a public health concern. *Glob Pediatr Health.* 2019;6:2333794X19891305.

54 Srivastav P, Broadbent S, Vaishali K, Nayak B, Bhat HV. Prevention of adolescent obesity: the global picture and an Indian perspective. *Diabetes Metab Syndr.* 2020;14:1195–1204.

3
Stress

Introduction

Imagine that you are living thousands of years ago hunting alone and searching for food for your family. Suddenly, a wild boar charges toward you. The long tusks of this grunting 300-pound beast are pointed directly at your abdomen. Within seconds, you must decide whether to run away as quickly as possible or stay and fight. Your heart begins to race, your breathing escalates, your perspiration flows, and your muscles tense. Realizing you lack the wherewithal to tackle such a creature, you turn and run as fast as you can to your cave, arriving only seconds before the boar.

This is an example of a fight-or-flight response, where the body automatically reacts to acute stress or danger, first described in the early 20th century by Walter Cannon, a physiologist from Harvard Medical School. Everyone needs to be able to respond to the various forms of acute stress, such as illness, injury, or impending peril, yet chronic toxic stress in adolescents may lead to related health issues including depression, anxiety, posttraumatic stress disorder (PTSD), substance use disorder, and personality issues.

When an individual perceives a physical or psychological stressor, the body's stress system may be activated. There are two main components to this stress system. The sympathetic-adreno-medullary axis produces the hormones noradrenaline and norepinephrine, and the hypothalamus-pituitary-adrenal (HPA) axis produces glucocorticoids, such as cortisol. A stress reaction may start in seconds and continue for several days, enabling a quick and ongoing response to the stressor. A physical stressor, such as a new burn, or a psychological stressor, such as a sudden severe thunderstorm, will often elicit a reaction from the sympathetic system, causing a rapid rise in epinephrine and norepinephrine. By raising blood pressure, pulse rate, and muscle tension, these hormones prepare the body for a fight-or-flight response. Stressors may also activate the HPA axis, producing steroids that travel throughout the body and brain.

While the body's reaction to acute stress may be lifesaving, the response to chronic stress may negatively impact health. Chronic stress includes such traumatic childhood experiences as parental death, abuse, neglect, and hunger. Chronic stress, especially in early life and during more sensitive and formative times like adolescence, may cause permanent change in epigenetic, endocrine, neural, immune, and inflammatory functions and disrupt the proper development of certain structures in the brain. This is a risk factor for some psychiatric diseases including major depression in adolescence and adulthood.[1]

Adolescence is also an integral period for rapid brain development. It is believed that the adolescent brain is more susceptible to stressors and the concomitant exposure to high levels of glucocorticoids. This developmental period is associated with heightened basal and stress-induced activity of the HPA axis. During the teen years, glucocorticoid receptors are high in the prefrontal cortex, which helps to modulate cognitive and emotional processes. As a result, chronic stress with resultant elevated glucocorticoids from stimulation of the HPA axis may affect the prefrontal cortex and its functions, including judgment. For example, it is believed that chronic stress in adolescence increases the susceptibility to drug abuse during that developmental period. There is also the possibility that heightened HPA reactivity during adolescence may increase the sensitivity to the onset of stress-related mental disorders.[2]

Chronic stress in adolescence comes in many forms. It may include physical and psychological abuse, personal or parental physical or mental illness, and physical or emotional neglect. There is good evidence from human studies that teens who are exposed to chronic stress may have changes in their neuroanatomical and neuro-endocrine systems, including anatomical and functional changes in the prefrontal cortex, amygdala, and hippocampus as well as issues with corticolimbic circuits that are critical for executive function, reward processing, and emotion regulation.[3-5] These anatomical and functional changes may increase the adolescent's susceptibility to stress-induced neural and behavioral dysfunction including such issues as substance use disorder and depression.[6]

Epidemiology

Stress is part of the daily life of every adolescent. The vast majority of adolescents learn healthy responses to acute stresses such as minor injury, illness, sudden noise, term papers, and tests as part of everyday life. For most teens, daily acute stress reactions should not lead to serious medical problems, including posttraumatic stress issues.

In response to stressful situations, some adolescents develop PTSD. Since adolescence is a time in life when teens have an increased risk of potentially traumatic experiences (PTEs), researchers from Massachusetts wanted to learn more about the exposure of adolescents to PTE and the development of PTSD. The researchers examined data from the National Comorbidity Survey Replication Adolescent Supplement, a national survey of adolescents ages 13 to 17. The study group included 6483 adolescent-parent pairs. The adolescents were interviewed with measures for past-year *Diagnostic and Statistical Manual of Mental Disorders*, fourth edition disorders. Those who reported a PTE had further questioning.

The data indicated that 61.8 percent of the adolescents had suffered at least one lifetime PTE, and the lifetime prevalence of PTSD was 4.7 percent. The predictors of PTSD after a PTE included female gender, prior PTE exposure, and preexisting fear and distress disorders. The authors suggested that interventions to prevent PTSD in PTE-exposed youth should target victims of interpersonal violence who have preexisting fear and distress disorders.[7]

Stress is part of everyday life for all adolescents. But there are significant interrelationships between stress and other psychosocial and current events.

Psychosocial Issues and Stress

Psychological Issues and Stress

Anxiety

It has been repeatedly demonstrated that stressful life experiences are a major cause of anxiety disorders in adolescents. Adolescence is a period of dynamic brain development; during this time, there is a maturation of certain centers of the brain, including the prefrontal cortex, which directs impulse control, focusing, emotional regulation, and planning for the future. During the teen years, the neural circuitry in the brain involving anxiety management is still under development, and this circuitry is rich in corticosteroid receptors. Therefore, the adolescent brain may have a heightened sensitivity to stress hormones, such as steroids. Using adolescent mice as models for the experimental and control groups, researchers from Canada exposed them to chronic mild stress. In this animal model, the stress disrupted the development of the prefrontal cortex.[8] Dealing with repeated stressful life events takes a toll on the body's stress system. When the system reaches its limit, the body may develop an affective disorder, such as anxiety.

How does this information on stress relate to adolescents? In the United States alone, millions of adolescents live in poverty. Poverty is an adverse childhood experience, a chronic stressor that has significant effects on the developing brain. The specific stressors from poverty may include neighborhood noise, cramped housing and limited privacy, household conflict and chaos, violence, inadequate educational opportunities, reduced access to healthful foods, and food insecurity. Studies have found that impoverished children may have changes in brain development in infancy where total gray matter volumes could be half a standard deviation smaller than those infants who are above the poverty line. These reductions were particularly large in brain areas involved in executive functions.[9,10] In addition, studies have demonstrated that children living in poverty have elevated levels of cortisol and other stress markers. It is believed that the effects of glucocorticoid activity due to stress may influence the activity and development of brain structures and neural circuitry involving the stress response as well as executive function abilities. Executive function is essential for self-regulation, and these abilities are found in the prefrontal cortex.[11]

The Western Australian Pregnancy Cohort Study provided a unique opportunity to assess family stress from the beginning of pregnancy to 17 years after birth, and subsequent anxiety and depression during adulthood. In this prospective cohort study of 2868 births, which started in 1989, the researchers designed measures for stress, anxiety, and depression. In one group, termed the ascending trajectory, the subjects had little early life stress but increasing stress from ages 10 to 15 years. Followed into adulthood, when compared to those who had low or reduced stress over their lifetimes, the subjects in the ascending trajectory were more likely to have anxiety and depression.[12]

Depression

It is believed that early stress from adverse childhood events, such as abuse, increases the risk that adolescents will develop depression. Studies have found that structural brain changes in children who have experienced early abuse and depression may emerge as a consequence of abnormalities in the development of the prefrontal cortex. By directly affecting the development of the prefrontal cortex, exposure to stress during the teen years may trigger depression.[13]

Depression is considered to be a stress-related disorder. In adolescents, stressful life events increase the likelihood of depression, possibly as a result of the ongoing maturation of certain brain centers such as the prefrontal cortex. These maturational changes occur in conjunction with intense social interactions, especially in females, which at least partially explains why female teens have significantly higher rates of depression than their male counterparts. There is also a familial predisposition to a depressive response to stressful life events, and specific genes may well play a strong role. Further, some believe that a blunted hormonal response through the HPA axis to stressful life events may account for depression, particularly in females.[14]

Substance Use

Researchers from North Carolina and Texas wanted to determine if the use of alcohol during adolescence was associated with an alcohol use disorder in adulthood. They followed a cohort of 330 adolescents who had a high or low family history of depression. In addition, there were periodic questionnaires regarding alcohol use and stress, and functional magnetic resonance imaging tests were performed. Thirty-two adolescents were identified as early initiators of alcohol. When compared to the teens who either did not drink alcohol or drank low levels of alcohol, the teens who drank larger amounts of alcohol had baseline levels of stressful life events that were significantly higher. Statistically, the early initiators were 15.3 times more likely to have a full drink, 9.1 times more likely to be intoxicated, and 6.7 times more likely to develop an alcohol use disorder by age 19 compared to late initiators. The researchers concluded that higher levels of stress were an important factor in the early alcohol initiator group.[15]

Hoping to learn more about the role that stress plays in the use and misuse of cannabis (marijuana), researchers from Connecticut conducted a comprehensive and exhaustive literature review of papers published over a 50-year period. The researchers determined that people often used cannabis to cope with the stresses of life, such as family dysfunction and negative life events. A subset of people who experienced greater life stresses were more vulnerable and sought cannabis for coping. So it is not unusual for adolescents, who are anxious from social pressures, to begin to use cannabis. That is why parents, teachers, and community and religious leaders should become more aware of the stressors that teens face. Likewise, they should implement strategies to prevent cannabis misuse and provide early identification and referral to treatment.[16]

Does stress affect adolescents' use of other substances? Researchers from Korea used data from the 2018 Korea Youth Risk Behavior Survey to understand the associations between stress and tobacco, e-cigarette use, and heated tobacco products. In the survey, 60,060 students between the ages of 12 and 18 years answered questions about perceived stress, physical activity, internet use, and tobacco use. The researchers learned that there was a link between high levels of perceived stress and the use of any tobacco product and that perceived stress was often related to increased HPA axis reactivity and a craving for nicotine. The researchers commented that adolescents in

Korea faced extreme academic stress and studied long hours to obtain high academic achievement, possibly an explanation for their use of substances.[17]

Social Issues and Stress

Social Media

Social media platforms provide some benefits to adolescents, but there are negative aspects to their use. Studies have shown that the more time one spends on a site, the lower the quality of life for the user. Interactions with some sites appear to reduce self-esteem, enhance cognitive overload, and foster feelings of distress. When they view the profiles of attractive users, some teens may feel worse about their bodies. Without a doubt, these negative feelings create stress for adolescents.[18]

In 2016, researchers from the Netherlands and Belgium surveyed 402 adolescents to determine the relationship between their fear of missing out (FOMO) and their perceived stress from the use of Facebook. Using a structural equation model, the researchers learned that the adolescents' increased need to belong and to be popular was related to an increased use of Facebook, while FOMO mediated or brought about these relationships. The researchers also found that FOMO from Facebook usage increased stress among the surveyed teens. Stress was particularly evident among those who thought they were unpopular on Facebook, with 25 percent of the adolescents who reported not being popular on Facebook experiencing high to extremely high stress.[19]

Similar to FOMO, digital stress is stress that is caused by negative interactions in emails, texts, chat rooms, and various types of forums. Digital stress may include the user feeling overwhelmed by excessive notifications or another user's expectations, responses, or judgments, as well as relational pressures. Researchers from North Carolina and Rhode Island investigated the pressure adolescents feel to meet social media demands, with respect to being available and winning approval of their peers. The cohort consisted of 1680 adolescents who completed a survey at baseline and at a 1-year follow-up. Regardless of race or ethnicity, nearly half of the teens reported experiencing digital distress. And digital stress was associated longitudinally with increases in depressive symptoms.[20]

It is evident to almost everyone that teens and young adults are frequent users of mobile phones. While it is clear that these phones enable young people to easily and readily communicate, researchers in Sweden wanted to learn if such easy access to phones had any negative consequences. The cohort consisted of 4156 subjects between the ages of 20 and 24 years who were followed over 1 year with data obtained from questionnaires. A section of the questionnaire focused on accessibility stress and asked, "To what extent do you perceive accessibility via mobile phone stressful?" The researchers found links between the need for availability via mobile phones and current stress in both males and females, and the high use of the phones was also associated with stress for both genders. The researchers learned that by the end of the study, 24-hour accessibility by mobile phone was stressful to both men and women. In addition, 10 percent of the males and 19 percent of the females reported current stress.[21]

Poverty

Social disadvantage may lead to disparities in health care. Poorer living conditions and riskier health behaviors place greater stress on people throughout their lives, probably beginning before they are even born. Low socioeconomic status (SES) and minority race/ethnicity are associated with chronic stress. Researchers from Massachusetts evaluated adolescents who were socially disadvantaged because of SES or race/ethnicity. The cohort consisted of 1209 non-Hispanic Black and White students in grades 7 to 12 from a midwestern school district, who completed questionnaires. The students' parents also provided information for an SES determination. The researchers learned that stress was higher among Black students, students from lower-SES families, and students who perceived that they were from lower-SES families. The researchers concluded that social disadvantage was associated with increased stress, regardless of whether the disadvantage was due to SES or race.[22]

Is social disadvantage associated with greater exposure to negative life events? Researchers from Pennsylvania examined the relationship between measures of SES, ethnicity, and exposure to life events in adolescents. The cohort consisted of 148 teens with a majority of adolescents identified as Black and female. The teens completed a questionnaire that contained both positive and negative events. Among the positive events was an outstanding personal achievement; among the negative events was the death of a parent. After analyzing the data, the researchers found that the teens who were Black or had fewer SES resources had a higher risk of exposure to stressful life events. Black adolescents reported significantly more discrete life events, which were either negative or ambiguous/not positive. However, rather than ethnicity, the SES of a family appears to be the strongest determination of the incidence of negative events in the life of a teen.[23]

Since this could inform preventive efforts, it is important to understand which factors impact the HPA response to stress. Several researchers wanted to learn if teens who experienced poverty would have a less than normal HPA response to stress. They also wanted to determine if deeper and longer periods of time in poverty were related to evidence of inappropriate cortisol activity. The cohort consisted of 229 teens of Mexican origin with a mean age of 17.15 years. The teens had magnetic resonance imaging done while playing cyberball, a virtual ball-toss game designed to elicit feelings of ostracism, social exclusion, and rejection. Salivary cortisol was obtained at baseline and several times during the imaging. From the testing, the researchers learned that HPA suppression resulting in inappropriate cortisol activity was evident in the youths who lived in deep poverty until the age of 16 years. After undergoing the stressor, the adolescents from more economically secure families had typical cortisol increases. The researchers suggested that efforts to increase family income may promote healthier HPA functioning. A stress response that is blunted may indicate a future mental health issue in the areas of emotion, attention, and behavior that in turn may manifest themselves as substance use disorder, bipolar disease, or borderline personality.[24]

Racism/Discrimination

It is believed that children become aware of stereotypes related to skin color around the middle of childhood. By around the age of 10, they can recognize overt and covert discrimination.[25,26] When they reach adolescence, youth are aware of their own identity and how they are viewed by other races and ethnic groups. To determine whether adolescents' perception of racial/ethnic discrimination was linked to their socioeconomic distress, researchers from Texas and Michigan conducted a broad internet literature search using several different search engines and identified 16,516 abstracts for review. After initial analyses, 76 studies were reviewed for a meta-analysis of the association between discrimination and socioemotional distress in adolescents. Fifty-eight studies had data on internalizing symptoms such as anxiety, loneliness, stress, and somatic problems. The strongest correlations were between discrimination and depression and internalizing symptoms. The researchers concluded that racial/ethnic discrimination was consistently linked to poorer youth adjustment across socioemotional, academic, and behavior domains.[27]

Stress related to racism has been identified as a unique source of concern for Black teens in America. In response to environmental demands and stressors, cortisol is released continuously. Chronic stress may result in aberrations to the normal diurnal and reactivity patterns of cortisol and can lead to physiological dysregulation of the HPA axis. Researchers based in North Carolina wanted to learn more about racism-related stress responses for Black teens. The cohort consisted of 446 Black adolescents between the ages of 14 and 17 years who lived throughout the United States. The evaluated measures included anticipatory racism-related stress, racism, and racial identity studied through individual, institutional, and cultural racism. The researchers learned that Black teens encountered more racism across individuals, institutions, and cultures and reported more stress from current and future racism. And at each of the three levels of racism, they had anticipatory racism-related stress.[28]

Because of the toll from racism, researchers have focused on finding mechanisms that may lessen the negative effects of discrimination and promote positive outcomes, regardless of the levels of discrimination. One such method is ethnic racial identity (ERI). Both protective and supportive, ERI is a composite of connectedness, beliefs, and practices associated with an individual's ethnic heritage. Researchers from Illinois studied the effect of ERI on stress through an evaluation of salivary cortisol; they hypothesized that it had a positive effect on the HPA axis. The cohort consisted of 1482 adolescents starting at age 12 and continuing for 20 years; the subjects were 59 percent Black and 49 percent female. They were assessed for racial discrimination, ERI, salivary cortisol, and demographics including gender, race/ethnicity, parent education, and family income. For the final subset of 112 Black and White subjects, the researchers found that significant changes occurred in the ERI during adolescence and early adulthood. Some of these changes were associated with adult cortisol regulation, primarily contributing to normalization of low cortisol levels for Black participants. This study appears to provide some evidence that stronger ethnic ties may help to diminish the effects of racism for adolescents, thus presumably reducing the stress effects from this form of discrimination.[29]

Mortality

Early life stress (ELS) has been shown to be a risk factor for major depression in adolescents. Researchers based in Vancouver wanted to determine which types of stress increased this risk. As a result, the researchers performed a meta-analysis of 62 journal articles that had four common characteristics: ELS measurements, diagnosis of major depression before the age of 18 years, a nondepressed control group, and a clinical interview to diagnose depression. Statistical analysis demonstrated that the subjects who experienced death, abuse of any type, or domestic violence were more likely to develop depression by adolescence than those who did not experience the stressor. The degree of depression appeared to be a function of the different forms of ELS. While the death of a family member seemed to have a medium effect, emotional abuse had a modestly higher one. Others have found that loss through death was closely related to the onset of depression.[30] Box 3.1 lists the types of ELS.

The loss of a parent at any age is traumatic, but it is especially devastating during the teen years. Adolescents are undergoing major biological, mental, and social changes, and the death of a parent significantly impacts their lives. The death of a teen's parent increases the risk for medical and psychiatric illnesses and suicide during adulthood. This places an increased importance on the role of the remaining parent, as well as the social support network.

Researchers from South Africa investigated interventions that may help teens better adjust to the death of a parent. They used a qualitative design in which 12 subjects between the ages of 19 and 26 years participated in semistructured interviews. All of the subjects had lost a parent between ages 12 and 21. The researchers identified five core areas of assistance for these teens: family support, social networks, religion, coherence, and exercise/journal writing. Family support, including the remaining parent, partner of the remaining parent, and extended family, had significant and helpful roles. Social networks through friends and the community were also notable for providing emotional and distractive support. Religion, as a coping mechanism, was an important resource and for some subjects a means to continue communicating with the deceased parent. Still another coping mechanism was a strong sense of coherence when the subjects felt that they had the capability to adjust to and continue with life, most consistent with resilience. The final support area included exercise, journal writing, and having tangible reminders of the lost parent.[31]

Box 3.1 Early Life Stressors

Death of a family member
Domestic violence
Emotional abuse
Illness/injury
Natural disaster
Physical abuse
Poverty
Sexual abuse

Permission obtained from Elsevier. From LeMoult J, Humphreys KL, Tracy A, Hoffmeister JA, Ip E, Gotlib IH. Meta-analysis: exposure to early life stress and risk for depression in childhood and adolescence. *J Am Acad Child Adolesc Psychiatry.* 2020 Jul;59(7):842–855. doi:10.1016/j.jaac.2019.10.011. Epub 2019 Oct 30. PMID: 31676392.

The death of nonfamily members is another stressor for teens. Among Black teens in particular, there is emerging evidence that exposure to police-related deaths has negative physical, mental, and educational consequences. When compared to White male youths, Black male youths are more likely to have unwarranted police stops and/ or unjustified use of nonlethal force. For Black youths, news reports of a police-related death of other Black youths may easily be a stressor and a reminder of their vulnerability to discrimination.

Researchers from Ohio and Texas wanted to learn more about the physiological stress response Black youths experience from police-related death. They used data from two studies. The first was the Adolescent Health and Development Context (AHDC), which examined the impact of social and spatial environments on the behavioral and health outcomes of youth aged 11 to 17 years in Franklin County, Ohio. The second, termed the Linking Biological and Social Pathways to Adolescent Health and Wellbeing, analyzed nightly samples of saliva for cortisol in a subsample of the participants in the AHDC. The researchers theorized that the cortisol levels among Black youth would be elevated in the aftermath of a police-related death. The researchers found that exposure to a police-related death of a Black person within the past 30 days was associated with a significant and nontrivial increase in nightly salivary cortisol levels, thus proving a physiological stress reaction. The researchers concluded that police-related deaths influenced the biological functioning of Black adolescent males and had a potential negative consequence for their health. Likewise, higher cumulative exposure to such adverse events over sensitive developmental periods of time, such as adolescence, may negatively impact an individual's health over an entire lifespan.[32]

Violence

The majority of adolescents living in urban areas are exposed directly or indirectly to some type of violence in their neighborhoods. Violence may include witnessing or experiencing robberies, stabbings, or shootings. Following such exposure, there is the potential to develop a mental health problem, such as PTSD. To understand more about the effects of exposure to community violence, researchers from Michigan performed a meta-analysis in which they evaluated over 100 studies. The researchers found that exposure to community violence increased the risk of PTSD and had a moderate effect on acting-out behaviors and externalizing issues. Community violence had a small effect on internalizing issues, including anxiety and depression. Adolescents had a stronger association between exposure and externalizing behaviors than children.[33]

Exposure to violence has short-term and long-term stress-inducing properties that may impact an adolescent's mental health, academic achievement, and overall development. Researchers in California conducted a literature review to discover how teens could protect themselves from the harmful effects of violence. They learned that family factors, such as close and warm parental relationships, seemed to moderate the effects of violence on internalizing symptoms, such as PTSD, anxiety, and depression. A few studies addressed moderators outside the family, including teachers. While teachers may provide some protective effects and support positive functioning, there was no evidence that this relationship helped to prevent depression or PTSD. Within the literature review, seven studies examined the protective factors for externalizing symptoms, including substance use and aggression. The only factor that appeared to moderate the effects of violence was a positive parenting bond. There was no consistent verification that parental monitoring was useful in moderating symptoms related to community violence.[34]

Intervention and Prevention

Mindfulness is a meditation practice that may benefit adolescents in preventing or treating stress. First described by Kabat-Zinn as a method to reduce pain in patients, it is a means to intentionally direct one's attention to present-moment experiences.[35] Subsequently, mindfulness has shown some evidence of efficacy in the treatment of obesity, eating disorders, type 2 diabetes, sleep disturbances, attention-deficit disorder, and psoriasis.[36]

To determine its efficacy, researchers in the United Kingdom performed a meta-analysis of randomized controlled trials (RCTs) of mindfulness interventions in children and adolescents. After a literature search, they studied 17 RCTs with active control groups. They determined that mindfulness-based interventions (MBIs) improved symptoms moderately for those adolescents with depression and to a small extent for those with anxiety/stress compared to the control groups. Nonetheless, the analysis advocated for the use of MBIs for improving mental health in adolescents.[37]

Exercise is also a known stress reducer in adolescents. In a systematic review, researchers found that higher physical activity and fitness levels were associated with attenuated physiological responses (including lower increases in heart rate and cortisol) to a known stressor (the Trier Social Stress Test). This suggested that adolescents who have regular exercise and resulting increased cardiorespiratory fitness may moderate their bodily response to a stressful experience.[38]

And finally, after controlling for physical activity and SES, researchers in New York and North Dakota performed a cross-sectional study of 68 adolescents to determine the association between percentage of neighborhood park area and perceived stress. The researchers utilized objective measures of park area and adolescents' physical activity, and they determined that the percentage of park area significantly predicted perceived stress among adolescents. An inverse association existed between perceived stress and park access in adolescents. The authors suggested that both male and female adolescents may be similarly protected by neighborhood green space.[39]

Conclusion

Stress happens to every adolescent, but excessive psychosocial stress is associated with multiple health issues, including anxiety and depression as well as impairment of executive functions. Excessive stress can be associated with poverty, racism, violence, and death of a loved one. Availability of resources such as parks, having a regular exercise routine, or even engaging in mindfulness may be helpful in reducing stress for adolescents.

References

1   Godoy LD, Rossignoli MT, Delfino-Pereira P, Garcia-Cairasco N, de Lima Umeoka EH. A comprehensive overview on stress neurobiology: basic concepts and clinical implications. *Front Behav Neurosci.* 2018;12:127.

2   Lupien SJ, McEwen BS, Gunnar MR, Heim C. Effects of stress throughout the lifespan on the brain, behaviour and cognition. *Nat Rev Neurosci.* 2009;10:434–445.

3   Hanson JL, Chung MK, Avants B, et al. Early stress is associated with alterations in the orbitofrontal cortex: a tensor-based morphometry investigation of brain structure and behavioral risk. *J Neurosci.* 2010;30:7466–7472.

4   Hanson JL, Chung MK, Avants BB, et al. Structural variations in prefrontal cortex mediate the relationship between early childhood stress and spatial working memory. *J Neurosci.* 2012;6:7917–7925.

5   Herringa RJ, Birn RM, Ruttle PL, et al. Childhood maltreatment is associated with altered fear circuitry and increased internalizing symptoms by late adolescence. *Proc Natl Acad Sci U S A.* 2013;110:19119–19124.

6   Sheth C, McGlade E, Yurgelun-Todd D. Chronic stress in adolescents and its neurobiological and psychopathological consequences: an RDoC prospective. *Chronic Stress (Thousand Oaks).* 2017;1:2470547017715645.

7   McLaughlin KA, Koenen KC, Hill ED, et al. Trauma exposure and posttraumatic stress disorder in a national sample of adolescents. *J Am Ac Child Adolesc Psychiatry.* 2013;52:815–830.

8   McCormick CM, Green MR. From the stressed adolescent to the anxious and depressed adult: investigations in rodent models. *Neuroscience.* 2013;249:242–257.

9   Hair NL, Hanson JL, Wolfe BL, Pollak SD. Association of child poverty, brain development, and academic achievement. *JAMA Pediatr.* 2015;169:822–829.

10 Noble KG, Houston SM, Brito NH, et al. Family income, parental education and brain structure in children and adolescents. *Nat Neurosci.* 2015;18:773–778.

11 Blair C, Raver CC. Poverty, stress, and brain development: new directions for preventing and intervention. *Acad Pediatr.* 2016;16:S30–S36.

12 Herbison E, Allen K, Robinson M, Newnham, Pennell C. The impact of life stress on adult depression and anxiety is dependent on gender and timing of exposure. *Dev Psychopathol.* 2017;29:1443–1454.

13 Anderson SL, Teicher MH. Stress, sensitive periods and maturational events in adolescent depression. *Trends Neurosci.* 2008;31:183–191.

14 Oldehinkel AJ, Bouma EM. Sensitivity to the depressogenic effects of stress and HPA-axis reactivity in adolescence: a review of gender differences. *Neurosci Biobehav Rev.* 2011;35:1757–1770.

15 Elsayed NM, Kim MM, Fields KM, Olvera RL, Hariri AR, Williamson DE. Trajectories of alcohol initiation and use during adolescence: the role of stress and amygdala reactivity. *J Am Acad Child Adolesc Psychiatry.* 2018;57:550–560.

16 Hyman SM, Sinha R. Stress-related factors in cannabis use and misuse: implications for prevention and treatment. *J Subst Abuse Treat.* 2009;36:400–413.

17 Lee A, Lee KS, Park H. Association of the use of a heated tobacco product with perceived stress, physical activity, and internet use in Korean adolescents: a 2018 national survey. *Int J Environ Res Public Health.* 2019;16:965.

18 Fox J, Moreland JJ. The dark side of social networking sites: an exploration of the relational and psychological stressors associated with Facebook use and affordances. *Comput Human Behav.* 2015;45:168–176.

19 Beyes I, Frison E, Eggermont S. 'I don't want to miss a thing': adolescents fear of missing out and its relationship to adolescents social needs, Facebook use, and Facebook related stress. *Comput Human Behav.* 2016;64:1–8.

20 Nick EA, Kilic Z, Nesi J, Telzer EH, Lindquist KA, Prinstein MJ. Adolescent digital stress: frequencies, correlates, and longitudinal association with depressive symptoms. *J Adolesc Health*. 2022;70:336–339.

21 Thomée S, Härenstam A, Hagberg M. Mobile phone use and stress, sleep disturbances, and symptoms of depression among young adults—a prospective cohort study. *BMC Public Health*. 2011;11:66.

22 Goodman E, McEwen BS, Dolan LM, Schafer-Kalkhoff TS, Adler NE. Social disadvantage and adolescent stress. *J Adolesc Health*. 2005;37:484–492.

23 Brady SS, Matthews KA. The influence of socioeconomic status and ethnicity on adolescents' exposure to stressful life events. *J Pediatr Psychol*. 2002;27:575–583.

24 Johnson LE, Parra LA, Ugarte E, et al. Patterns of poverty across adolescence predict salivary cortisol stress responses in Mexican-origin youths. *Psychoneuroendocrinology*. 2021 Oct;132:105340.

25 McKown C, Weinstein RS. The development and consequences of stereotype consciousness in middle childhood. *Child Dev*. 2003;74:498–515.

26 Verkuyten M. Perceived discrimination and self-esteem among ethnic minority adolescents. *J Soc Psychol*. 1998;138:479–493.

27 Benner AD, Wang Y, Shen Y, Boyle A, Polk R, Cheng Y. Racial/ethnic discrimination and well-being during adolescence: a meta-analytic review. *Am Psychol*. 2018;73:855–883.

28 Hope EC, Brinkman M, Hoggard LS, et al. Black adolescents' anticipatory stress responses to multilevel racism: the role of racial identity. *Am J Orthopsychiatry*. 2021;91:487–498.

29 Adam EK, Hittner EF, Thomas SE, Villaume SC, Nwafor EE. Racial discrimination and ethnic racial identity in adolescence as modulators of HPA axis activity. *Dev Psychopathol*. 2020;32:1669–1684.

30 LeMoult J, Humphreys KL, Tracy A, et al. Meta-analysis: exposure to early life stress and risk of depression in childhood and adolescence. *J Am Acad Child Adolesc Psychiatry*. 2020;59:842–855.

31 Ludik D, Greeff AP. Exploring factors that help adolescents adjust and continue with life after the death of a parent. *Omega*. 2022;84:964–984.

32 Browning CR, Tarrence J, LaPlant E, et al. Exposure to police-related death and physiological stress among urban black youth. *Psychoneuroendocrinology*. 2021;125:104884.

33 Fowler PJ, Tompsett CJ, Braciszewski JM, Jacques-Tiura A, Baltes BB. Community violence: a meta-analysis on the effect of exposure and mental health outcomes of children and adolescents. *Dev Psychopathol*. 2009;21:227–259.

34 Ozer EJ, Lavi I, Douglas L, Wolf JP. Protective factors for youth exposed to violence in their communities: a review of family, school, and community moderators. *J Clinical Child Adolesc Psychol*. 2017;46:353–378.

35 Kabat-Zinn J. An outpatient program in behavioral medicine for chronic pain patients based on the practice of mindfulness meditation: theoretical considerations and preliminary results. *Gen Hosp Psychiatry*. 1982;4:33–47.

36 Ludwig DS, Kabat-Zinn J. Mindfulness in medicine. *JAMA*. 2008;300:1350–1352.

37 Dunning DL, Griffiths K, Kuyken W, et al. Research review: the effects of mindfulness-based interventions on cognition and mental health in children and adolescents—a meta-analysis of randomized controlled trials. *J Child Psychol Psychiatry*. 2019;60:244–258.

38 Mücke M, Ludyga S, Colledge F, Gerber M. Influence of regular physical activity and fitness on stress reactivity as measured with the trier social stress test protocol: a systematic review. *Sports Med*. 2018;48:2607–2622.

39 Feda DM, Seelbinder A, Baek S, Raka S, Yin L, Roemmich JN. Neighbourhood parks and reduction in stress among adolescents: results from Buffalo, New York. *Indoor Build Environ*. 2015;24:631–639.

PART II
PSYCHOLOGICAL ISSUES

4
Anxiety

Introduction

Adolescents today face many stressors that were not common even a generation ago. It is apparent now that teens do experience panic attacks, insomnia, and obsessive thinking from issues like the global climate crisis, social media, or immigration crises. These emerging concerns, when added to the known biopsychosocial issues of adolescence, could negatively affect adolescent mental health, leading to an anxiety disorder, depression, and/or substance abuse disorder.[1]

Normal everyday anxiety should be short-lived and resolve on its own. Adolescents with an anxiety disorder may have worries that they are unable to stop or control. Anxiety that is more serious is persistent and excessive and results in the impairment of daily activities. For example, if an adolescent avoids attending school because of issues with academics, teachers, students, or other concerns, they may have an anxiety disorder. Other adolescents might manifest their anxiety through explosive behavioral issues, maladjusted eating patterns, or even suicidal behaviors.

Even though everyone experiences some anxiety, researchers have yet to determine exactly why certain teens develop an anxiety disorder. While there is no one factor at the root of anxiety disorder, there are known biological, psychological, and social factors that interact to trigger these disorders.

There is good research demonstrating that genetic factors play an important role in determining which children will have a problem with anxiety. Hettema and associates from Virginia conducted a review and meta-analysis of studies on the epidemiology of anxiety disorder. They found that generalized anxiety disorder aggregates in families. And two large-scale twin studies determined that generalized anxiety disorder has a familial genetic risk.[2]

Among the largest of such work is a Swedish study of 2508 twins that suggested that a gene associated with anxiety and depression is awakened during adolescence. Beginning their study at puberty and during certain time intervals, the researchers examined genetic and environmental risk factors related to anxiety and depression in a cohort of twins between the ages of 8 and 20 years. They felt that the best model to describe the results was that of genetic innovation, where new genes that were previously not affecting symptoms of anxiety and depression became active and/or where genes that impacted these symptoms earlier in development then declined in their influence later in development.[3]

In some adolescents, neurobiological factors may be linked to the onset of anxiety disorders. Imbalances between elevated amygdala activity and other brain networks such as the ventral prefrontal cortex seen during adolescence may activate an anxiety disorder. Researchers at the National Institutes of Health used neuroimaging and genetic analysis to learn more about the functional anatomy and genetic composition of anxiety and stress responses. They learned that a low expression version of the serotonin transporter gene 5-HTT was associated with anxiety and with greater amygdala reaction to emotion. Also, low activity of the catechol-O-methyltransferase (COMT) gene is correlated with anxiety. The effect of this gene is additive to the 5-HTT variant. They concluded that the functional variants of these two genes impact brain functions involved in stress and anxiety.[4]

It is generally believed that there is no single gene that directs the onset of anxiety. Rather, it may well be the cumulative effect of many genes that make an individual more vulnerable to an anxiety disorder.

Some environmental factors are important in the etiology of anxiety disorders. In a twin study of adolescent monozygotic (one egg) and dizygotic (two eggs) twins, researchers based in Canada found a "social contagion" of anxiety between one teen and the other regardless of gender or zygosity. However, this only occurred in same-sex twins of either gender.[5]

Moreover, children of parent(s) who have an anxiety disorder are at increased risk of developing one themselves. There is strong evidence that children who have a parent or parents with anxiety disorders have two to three times the risk.[6] To determine if the transmission of anxiety from parents to children is sex specific, investigators from Canada conducted a cross-sectional study of 398 offspring with a mean age of 11.1 years and their parents. After conducting semistructured interviews, the researchers learned that anxiety disorders in the same-sex parent were associated with increased rates of anxiety disorders in the same-sex offspring. However, anxiety disorders in the opposite-sex parent were not associated with higher odds for the opposite-sex child. The researchers believed that parent modeling might have placed their offspring at higher risk.[7] And children of a parent with obsessive-compulsive disorder are more likely to develop emotional and behavioral problems.[8]

Whether they realize it or not, parents are role models. Parents who are overprotective, anxious, or possibly overly critical may increase the risk of anxiety disorders in children. Ignoring a child's wish to explore, express, or show independent behaviors may cause that child to feel they have no control. Feelings of inhibition may emerge. And parents who view the outside world as a dangerous place may promote anxiety in children. While observing and experiencing life, children learn psychological information that is integral to their development. Researchers from Germany studied 1015 mother-child dyads over 10 years starting at a baseline age of 14 to 17 years for the child. Anxiety disorders and depression were assessed repeatedly. The results indicated that low child autonomy increased the risk for anxiety and depression.[9]

If parents display anxious behaviors, their children may well model these actions. Researchers from Johns Hopkins University investigated the impact of parental modeling of anxious behaviors and thoughts on the level of anxiety in their children. They recruited 25 families from the Baltimore area; each of these families had a child between the ages of 8 and 12 years, two parents, and no history of a diagnosed psychiatric condition. One of the parents was trained to stage anxious and relaxed demeanors concerning an upcoming spelling test. The researchers learned that regardless of the parent gender, the children endorsed the higher level of anxiety and were more likely to want to avoid the spelling test when they were in the anxious environment than when they were in the relaxed one. Fathers had a stronger impact on the subject's anxiety and cognitions. This study highlighted the importance of parental modeling and the environment on the etiology of anxiety in adolescents. For clinicians counseling families, the role of parental modeling and anxiety in children is a subject that should be discussed.[10]

In 2022, the U.S. Preventive Services Task Force recommended that all children and adolescents from ages 8 to 18 be screened for anxiety. The report noted that an anxiety disorder in this age group is associated with an increased likelihood of depression or an anxiety disorder in adulthood.[11]

Epidemiology

Anxiety is the most common mental health disorder found in adolescents. In a study published in 2010, Merikangas and colleagues at the National Institute of Mental Health used the National Comorbidity Survey Adolescent Supplement (NCS-A) to evaluate the lifetime prevalence of mental disorders in adolescents in the United States. The NCS-A is a nationally representative face-to-face survey of 10,123 adolescents who ranged in age from 13 to 18 years. The survey assessed mental health issues by using a modified version of the World Health Organization Composite International Diagnostic Interview. The researchers learned that the lifetime prevalence of anxiety was 31.9 percent, making anxiety the most common mental health condition. A notable 50 percent of the participants had the onset of anxiety by age 6, with the prevalence increasing during adolescence. Female adolescents were more likely than males to be anxious. Since the prevalence of anxiety was so high even before puberty, early interventions may be appropriate for higher-risk children before the onset of adolescence.[12]

While there were no similar studies during the COVID-19 pandemic, Chinese researchers performed a cross-sectional study of Chinese adolescents affected by the COVID-19 outbreak. With the assistance of an online instrument that included an assessment for generalized anxiety disorder (GAD-7), they surveyed 8079 subjects. The study was performed in March 2020, and the students ranged in age from 12 to 18 years and resided in China. Of the males surveyed, 36.2 percent had symptoms of anxiety, and 38.4 percent of the females had similar symptomatology. As the age of the surveyed subjects increased, so did the prevalence of anxiety. Unlike the Merikangas study, this study was cross-sectional rather than the lifetime prevalence, and it was performed online with the respondents using the validated GAD-7 instrument. Nonetheless, it does provide important information about the prevalence of anxiety during the pandemic in China.[13]

Psychosocial Issues and Anxiety

Psychological Issues and Anxiety

Eating Disorders
Anorexia Nervosa
Anxiety is often comorbid with anorexia nervosa in adolescents. Both adolescent patients and their parent(s) have a higher prevalence of anxiety, suggesting genetic or

environmental factors may be involved. Researchers from Denmark wanted to learn if children, teens, and young adults with severe anxiety disorders were at increased risk for anorexia. The study followed a cohort of subjects born between 1988 and 2006 for a minimum of 6 years ending in 2012. The subjects ranged in age from 6 to 24 years. Although there were more than 1.6 million subjects in the cohort, 5065 were identified as having an outpatient or inpatient diagnosis of anorexia nervosa between 1994 and 2012. Of these, 93.3 percent were females; 3.7 percent had a previous diagnosis of a specific anxiety disorder. The researchers learned that the risk of anorexia in people with a severe anxiety disorder is 1.83 times that of the risk in the general population. The highest risk was found in subjects who had been diagnosed with the obsessive-compulsive form of anxiety. The researchers commented that there may be a shared genetic susceptibility for anorexia nervosa and an anxiety disorder, although there may also be common environmental risk factors for both. Parents of adolescents with an anxiety disorder as well as clinicians who care for teens should have a heightened awareness for the onset of an eating disorder.[14]

Researchers in California worked to learn if parents of young adults with anorexia nervosa had a higher risk of generalized anxiety disorder. They enrolled 152 young adult women with at least a 5-year history of anorexia and 181 female subjects without any history of psychiatric illness. At least one parent of each subject was interviewed. The lifetime prevalence of generalized anxiety disorder in the parent of a patient with anorexia was 17.1 compared to 5.3 in those parents whose daughters did not have psychiatric illness. This difference was statistically significant ($p = .0001$).[15]

Avoidant-Restrictive Food Intake Disorder

Anxiety disorders are also more frequently seen in avoidant-restrictive food intake disorder (ARFID), which is an eating disorder characterized by an intake of a limited number of foods or types of foods, a sensitivity to the texture of food, or a general lack of interest in food or eating. It usually begins in early childhood, years before adolescence, in children as young as 2 years. ARFID may cause growth and nutritional problems as well as social issues. More often seen in male adolescents, some people with ARFID avoid entire food groups, such as fruits and vegetables. No etiology has been identified.[16]

Researchers from Wyoming, Massachusetts, and Switzerland wanted to learn which psychiatric diagnoses tended to co-occur with ARFID. Their cohort consisted of 74 males and females between the ages of 9 and 22 years. Using interviews, the researchers determined that 45 percent of the subjects had a concurrent psychiatric diagnosis. Thirty-five percent had a current diagnosis of anxiety, obsessive-compulsive disorder, or trauma-related disorders, and 24 percent had generalized anxiety disorder. The researchers noted that those subjects who feared that they would have adverse reactions or consequences from eating had a higher likelihood of having a comorbid anxiety disorder.[17]

A group of Canadian researchers determined psychiatric comorbidities in 26 patients admitted to a clinic specializing in ARFID. The median age was 13.9 years (range 9.5 to 17.5). They diagnosed general anxiety in 73 percent and obsessive-compulsive disorder in 15.4 percent. Of particular note, autism was seen in 23.1 percent.[18]

Substance Use

Substance use disorders have a documented link to social anxiety disorder in adolescents. Adolescents with social anxiety disorder issues are fearful about one or more social situations they believe will expose them to scrutiny. Such anxiety, which persists for at least 6 months, is so powerful that it often prevents the teen from participating in everyday activities; the anxiety is completely out of proportion to reality. The teen has intense fear from social interactions, such as meeting unfamiliar people, eating outside the home, or giving a speech. Teens who are shy or have some discomfort with social situations may be mentally healthy and do not necessarily have social anxiety disorder, a mental health diagnosis.

Researchers from Québec, Canada, wanted to learn if social anxiety and shyness traits in adolescents were precursors to the abuse of tobacco, alcohol, and marijuana. They located and reviewed 50 relevant studies. Most of the studies showed a negative association between social anxiety and shyness and the use of tobacco, alcohol, and marijuana. Still, there were some positive associations with tobacco and marijuana in those teens with social anxiety disorder. The results with alcohol were inconclusive. While all adolescents should be screened for substance use, those with social anxiety disorder should have systematic screening for substance use disorders. Similar to other anxiety disorders, the causes of social anxiety disorder are multifactorial—genetic, biological, social, and environmental.[19]

Suicidality

It is an incredibly important question: are adolescents with an anxiety disorder more likely to have suicidal ideation or attempt suicide? To estimate the lifetime prevalence of suicidal behaviors and document a history of prior mental health disorders, researchers from Massachusetts performed face-to-face interviews with 6483 adolescents between the ages of 13 and 18 years. Suicidal ideation was noted in 12.1 percent of the respondents; suicide plans were documented in 4.0 percent; actual suicide attempts were noted in 4.1 percent. A diagnosis of generalized anxiety disorder was noted in 9.2 percent of those who had a suicide attempt, which was statistically significant when compared to those with no history of a suicide attempt. Of note, 75.7 percent of the subjects who reported a suicide attempt had a history of major depressive disorder. While the results are concerning, the diagnosis of generalized anxiety disorder was the least frequent in those teens with suicidal issues, and anxiety is not necessarily a precursor to suicidal attempts in adolescents.[20]

Social Issues

Social Media

There appears to be a positive association between social media use and anxiety in adolescents and young adults. But is social media the real culprit for rising mental health problems in adolescents and young adults? Research findings on the relationship between social media use and anxiety have been mixed. One group of investigators in Scotland performed a cross-sectional study of 467 adolescents between the ages of 11 and 17 years, conducted in the classroom. Anxiety was assessed using the

Hospital Anxiety and Depression Scale. The results noted an association between nighttime-specific social media use, emotional investment in the media, and higher levels of anxiety in the subjects. The researchers commented that the timing of the use of social media—at bedtime and during the night—may be a central factor that needs further investigation.[21]

Meanwhile, researchers from Connecticut used a web-based, cross-sectional survey on social media and anxiety symptoms on 563 young adults between the ages of 18 and 22 years (mean age 20.0) to determine the impact of time spent using social media on anxiety symptoms and severity in young adults. In this nationally representative study, the genders were equally divided. Anxiety symptoms were measured with the Beck Anxiety Inventory-Trait and the Overall Anxiety Severity and Impairment Scale. Participants reported using social media an average of 6.63 hours per day. And the higher daily use of social media was correlated with increased symptoms of anxiety/stress and a greater likelihood of having an anxiety disorder.[22]

Researchers in Canada performed a longitudinal study of screen time and anxiety. Using data from the Co-Venture Trial, they studied 3826 seventh graders annually from 7th through 10th grade. Screen time included the use of computers, cell phones, social media, television, and other computer activities. The Brief Symptom Inventory anxiety subscale was used to measure anxiety. The researchers learned that when total screen time increased during a specific year, anxiety symptoms worsened within that exact same year.[23]

An 8-year longitudinal study from researchers at Brigham Young University addressed how social media impacted the mental health of adolescents over time. The cohort consisted of 500 adolescents between the ages of 13 and 20 years; they were all recruited from one city and were studied annually for 8 years, beginning in 2009. The researchers documented the daily time that the subjects spent on social media, and anxiety was measured with the Spence Child Anxiety Inventory. The researchers determined that the time spent on social media networks was moderately related to anxiety and depression. However, when an individual adolescent spent more time on social media than their own typical average, this did not increase the associations with anxiety or depression 1 year later.[24]

Problematic Internet Use
While the internet is a great resource for adolescents to communicate with one another, it is also easily abused. Uncontrollable use of the internet, also known as problematic internet use (PIU), has been compared by some researchers to other addictions like gambling and may cause psychological issues such as anxiety. To learn more about PIU and psychopathology, researchers from several countries in Europe as well as the United States performed a cross-sectional study of school-based adolescents from 11 countries. They had a representative sample of 11,356 adolescents with majority female participants around 15 years of age. PIU was assessed using the eight-item Young's Diagnostic Questionnaire. From the answers on this questionnaire, the researchers placed the adolescents into one of three groups: adaptive internet user, maladaptive internet user, and pathological internet user. The Zung Self-Rating Anxiety Scale, which is a 20-item assessment, was used to measure anxiety. In the adaptive internet user group, which made up 82.4 percent of the cohort,

5 percent had anxiety; in the maladaptive internet group, which was 13.4 percent of the cohort, 16.4 percent had anxiety; and in the pathological internet group, which was 4.2 percent of the cohort, 27.6 percent reported moderate to severe anxiety. It is not clear if adolescents who had preexisting anxiety gravitated to PIU or if PIU resulted in anxiety. Moreover, there were significant and strong correlations between PIU and anxiety ($p < .001$). In any case, if an adolescent is deemed to be using the internet in a problematic way, then these adolescents should be provided with psychological evaluations and possible treatment at the family, clinical, and public health levels.[25]

Poverty
It is well known that there is an association between poverty and mental illness. But another aspect is less well known. Does the adversity and stress associated with poverty increase the risk of mental illness, or is a person with mental illness at higher risk for falling into a state of poverty? The Great Smokey Mountain Study, conducted by researchers at Duke University, may provide some clues. Compiled using a longitudinal design, the study examined the development of psychiatric disorders in urban and rural youth. The cohort consisted of 1420 subjects aged 9, 11, and 13 years; all were given annual psychiatric assessments for 8 years. Midway into the study, 14 percent of the study families moved out of poverty, while 53 percent remained poor. Thirty-four percent of the cohort were never poor. The researchers found that the children who experienced poverty had more psychiatric symptoms than the children who were never poor. However, for those who left poverty, levels of anxiety and depression were unaffected by the economic changes in their lives. This suggested that anxiety in adolescents may result from conditions created by poverty, but there are other factors that are involved in promoting anxiety.[26]

To determine additional factors influencing anxiety promotion in adolescents from impoverished households, researchers in Australia wanted to determine if exposure to poverty during early childhood would increase the risk of anxiety and depression during adolescence or young adulthood. They recruited 2609 women during their early pregnancy months and then studied their children when they were 14 and 21 years old. The investigators recorded family income and used the Youth Self-Report to assess levels of anxiety at age 14 and the Young Adult Self-Report to evaluate the levels at age 21. At some time during the study, about half of the subjects experienced poverty. The subjects who had multiple experiences of family poverty had a 3.2 times risk of being anxious at both age 14 and age 21. The cumulative effects of exposure to family poverty had the most consistent effect on adolescent and young adult anxiety and depression.[27]

Researchers from Ohio investigated the association between material hardship during early childhood and anxiety and depression at age 15. They used data from the Fragile Families and Child Wellbeing Study, which included 4898 children born in 20 large U.S. cities between 1998 and 2000. Follow-up surveys were conducted at ages 1, 3, 5, 9, and 15. The surveys oversampled low-income families and mothers who were unmarried when the child was born. The researchers learned that material hardship such as lack of food, housing, or medical care at age 15 significantly predicted youth anxiety at that age. Those who were higher above the poverty line had reductions in anxiety symptoms. And experiencing material hardship during childhood was positively and significantly related to anxiety and depression at age 15.[28]

Racism/Discrimination

Racism has detrimental effects on the biopsychosocial functioning of adolescents and may seriously impair the well-being of this age group. Hoping to further understand the associations between racism and mental health, researchers in Australia and the United Kingdom conducted a systematic review and identified 121 studies that met their criteria. The studies usually had a cross-sectional design and included teens between the ages of 12 and 18 years; the most frequent groups studies identified Black, Hispanic, and Asian populations. Ninety-six studies reported negative mental health outcomes from racial discrimination. Seven studies addressed the association between racism and anxiety, and 57 studies addressed racism and depression. The researchers found that good personal and ethnic self-esteem reduced issues related to racial discrimination and anxiety. As a result, efforts to improve adolescent personal and ethnic self-esteem may help prevent negative outcomes from racial discrimination.[29]

There are few studies on discrimination among Asian American adolescents. Juang and Alvarez from California examined whether racial and ethnic discrimination in Chinese American adolescents was linked to poor adjustment and anxiety. Their subjects attended two San Francisco high schools that had large numbers of Chinese American students. The study sample of 309 Chinese American adolescents represented 23 percent of that ethnic group in the two high schools. To measure anxiety, the researchers used six items from the Brief Symptom Inventory, and perceived discrimination was measured with these three questions: "How often have you been treated unfairly because you are Asian?" "How often do people dislike you because you are Asian?," and "How often have you seen friends or family be treated unfairly because they are Asian?" The response scale ranged from one to five. In addition, the parents of the subjects answered questions measuring family conflict and cohesion. The researchers learned that the teens who reported greater perceived discrimination had higher levels of anxiety. Though family conflict was not directly linked to anxiety, greater family cohesion was related to less adolescent anxiety. The study demonstrated the importance of family cohesiveness as a moderator against racial discrimination.[30]

Transgender/Gender Dysphoria

Researchers in California and Georgia wanted to learn more about the mental health of transgender and gender nonconforming youth. They performed a review of the electronic medical records of transfeminine and transmasculine children and adolescents. The final adolescent cohort consisted of 427 transfeminine and 655 transmasculine subjects, and each was matched to a cisgender patient. The researchers discovered that 37.2 percent of the transfeminine subjects and 4.6 percent of their matching cisgender subjects had histories of an anxiety disorder. For the transmasculine subjects, anxiety was reported in 38.9 percent compared to 4.5 percent in the cisgender subjects. At least some of the anxiety was caused by dysphoria-distress or being assigned a gender that was not compatible with one's identity. Of note, a history of depressive disorder ranged from 48.5 percent to 61.5 percent in the transgender group.[31]

Using a cross-sectional survey of self-selected subjects rather than a review of longitudinal electronic medical records, researchers from China studied mental health issues of transgender Chinese adolescents. Transgender or gender nonbinary adolescents between the ages of 12 and 18 years completed the seven-item General Anxiety Disorder scale. Study data were collected from 385 respondents. The researchers determined that 148 respondents (38.4 percent) were at risk for an anxiety disorder. It should also be noted that 92.8 percent of the adolescents reported parental abuse and neglect, which may be additional causes for anxiety. These two studies document a high level of anxiety in transgender adolescents, especially in comparison to cisgender individuals.[32]

Violence

Violence in any form may have mental health morbidities for teens. Between the years 2000 and (January) 2020, approximately 240,000 children and teens experienced gun violence in school, and about 60 percent of the school shootings occurred in high schools. In the short term, most adolescents who are directly or indirectly involved in a school shooting incident will have an acute stress reaction that includes anxiety. In the long term, some may develop posttraumatic stress disorder (PTSD), a type of anxiety disorder. It is believed that a school shooting may be more traumatizing than a natural or man-made disaster.

Although about one-third of the people who witness a school shooting develop an acute stress disorder, most will demonstrate stress symptoms, and some may turn to suicide, as with the two adolescent survivors who died by suicide after the 2018 Stoneman Douglas High School shooting in Parkland, Florida. While teens will generally return to their normative state months after an incident, some adolescents may exhibit PTSD symptoms including anxiety, flashbacks, nightmares, irritability, and mood issues. It is also not uncommon for some adolescents to manifest anxiety through psychosomatic symptoms such as headaches.

After a mass shooting, adolescents who have witnessed the violence should quickly have a screening assessment of their mental health requirements and risk factors for further issues. This includes an evaluation of their prior trauma exposure, mental health history, anxiety, sensitivity, and conduct problems. If an adolescent is flagged by this screening, then a more thorough and complete evaluation should be quickly scheduled. A treatment plan needs to be implemented; it should include therapy that addresses the symptoms, builds resilience, promotes safety and social support, and instills hope. The adolescent's parents should be involved in the treatment.[33]

Violence due to war can also affect adolescents. Researchers from Georgia and Israel wanted to learn more about the long-term impact of the rocket attacks on Israeli adolescents. As a result, they recruited 362 high school students who lived in the southern part of Israel and followed them from 2008 to 2011 with annual assessments (wave 1, wave 2, wave 3, and wave 4) for anxiety and violence. Measurements included a scale for exposure to rocket attacks, and anxiety was quantified using a seven-item scale based on the Hebrew version of the State Anxiety Survey. The researchers learned that rocket attacks were associated with adolescent feelings of anxiety during all four waves, but especially during wave 1. The researchers noted that over time, stress from the rocket attacks created strong influences on the amounts of violence committed by the adolescents. Adolescents who witnessed terroristic violence were likely to have internalizing symptoms including anxiety. Their distress from these symptoms would likely be expressed through violence.[34]

Immigration

Concerns about immigration may also trigger anxiety in adolescents, especially so in the Hispanic population. Researchers from California and Arizona examined the relationship between immigration policy concerns and health issues in Hispanic adolescents from immigrant families. As previously noted in the chapter on sleep, there is a correlation between the degree of fear about policy concerns and poor sleep quality. In the same study of adolescents in the Salinas Valley region of California, 397 (96.4 percent) of the subjects had at least one parent who was an immigrant, and a significant number of the parents were undocumented. When the adolescents turned 16 years old, the teens self-reported their immigration policy concerns by completing the Perceived Immigration Policy Effects Scale (PIPES) instrument. They self-reported anxiety scores using the Behavioral Assessment System for Children subscale. The researchers found that teens who had high total PIPES scores had higher levels of self-reported anxiety and were significantly more likely to report anxiety that was clinically significant or at the at-risk level. The results were obtained during the first year after the 2016 election of President Donald Trump, and the researchers concluded that anxiety levels among this adolescent population increased significantly after that election.[35]

In another study of Hispanic adolescents, a group of researchers from Texas, Rhode Island, and Washington, DC administered surveys during the 2018–2019 school year to 306 first- and second-generation students in 11 high schools in Texas and Rhode Island. More than half of the students were first generation, and about half lived in each of the two states. Included in the survey were measures of clinical anxiety, immigration enforcement fear, and perceived discrimination. The researchers determined that 64 percent of the Hispanic adolescents appeared to be suffering from an anxiety disorder, a rate about nine times higher than the rate in the general adolescent population at that time. Immigration enforcement fear and discrimination were factors that contributed to the high levels of anxiety. Also, the researchers noted that the location of the study sample in Texas was in a county that had the highest deportation rate in the country. At the same time, the Rhode Island study sample was in a region in which state policy restricted cooperation with immigration and customs enforcement. Despite these variances, there were no significant differences in anxiety between the students in the two states. This finding suggested that the then-presidential administration's immigration enforcement policies and rhetoric might have generated a nationwide climate of fear in Hispanic communities.[36]

Prevention of Anxiety in Adolescents

Hoping to learn how to prevent social anxiety in older children and young adolescents, researchers in Norway performed a randomized controlled trial with sixth- through ninth-grade students. This universal prevention program consisted of an intervention group of 801 students and a control group of 638 students who lived in different counties in the central portion of Norway. Students in the intervention group listened to a lecture about anxiety and then worked on a handout designed to increase their skills to cope with situations that might increase anxiety. Measures for both groups included SCARED, a 41-item self-report test to assess panic and various types of anxiety as well as screen for depression and bullying. The assessments were conducted prior to the intervention and 1 year later. To emphasize the importance of their undertaking, the researchers involved the community. School nurses, teachers, parents, community health and welfare workers, and primary care physicians were given psychoeducation about anxiety issues. The results were notable. During the year after the intervention, fewer students in the intervention group than the control group developed significant social anxiety. The researchers commented that their study exemplified an example of an effective community- and school-based intervention that helped to reduce the prevalence and severity of anxiety in the age groups that were studied.[37]

A group of researchers in Germany performed a meta-analytic review on the prevention of anxiety symptoms in adolescents. In this evaluation, they reviewed 29 universal programs as well as those with selected/indicated individuals (adolescents at risk or showing subclinical signs of an anxiety disorder). The research team noted that the selective programs produced larger desirable effects on anxiety than the universal programs even though there were time and cost associated with screening adolescents who may be at risk or having subclinical anxiety. Unfortunately, females seemed to benefit less from these programs than males.

An effective selective program to prevent anxiety in adolescents was initiated by researchers in New York. All Puerto Rican eighth and ninth graders ($N = 418$) at a public school in Brooklyn were screened for behavior problems, of which 110 who were not undergoing mental health treatment were placed in the study. A total of 61 were in the intervention group and 29 in the control group with a mean age of 13.7 years and 55.5 percent female. A hero/heroine intervention was based on adult Puerto Rican role models with the purpose of fostering ethnic identify, self-concept, and adaptive coping behaviors over 19 sessions. The control group had eight 90-minute meetings. The 90-item Symptom Checklist measured symptom distress. The researchers determined that there was a significant reduction in anxiety in the eighth-grade subjects compared to the control group, and they concluded that this program was an effective culturally sensitive modality as a preventive mental health intervention for high-risk Puerto Rican adolescents.[38]

Treatment of Anxiety

Since clinical trials have generally not found a significant difference in efficacy between selective serotonin reuptake inhibitor (SSRI) medication treatment and

---

Box 4.1 Nonmedication Treatments for Anxiety

Acupressure
Acupuncture
Aromatherapy
Exercise
Massage
Meditation
Music
Pets
Reflexology
Relaxation techniques
Tai chi
Yoga

---

cognitive behavioral therapy (CBT), the initial treatment for mild to moderate anxiety disorder in adolescents is generally CBT. For adolescents who do not respond to CBT alone or who have severe anxiety, a combination of CBT and an SSRI may be utilized. Other medications such as venlafaxine, buspirone, tricyclic antidepressants, and benzodiazepines have been suggested as second- or third-line agents. In addition, the treatment plan for adolescents may include classroom-based accommodations. For example, if anxiety interferes with homework completion, then the length of homework could be modified to an amount commensurate with the adolescent's capacity.[39]

There are other treatments for anxiety as listed in Box 4.1. In particular, exercise is an activity that contributes to increased well-being and decreases anxiety in adolescents.[40]

Conclusion

Anxiety is a common symptom in adolescents. If it becomes a mental health disorder, it may impact other psychosocial issues, so there is a recommendation to screen adolescents for anxiety. Current technology, such as social media networks; racism and discrimination; school-related violence; or immigration concerns may trigger anxiety in certain adolescents. When anxiety reaches the level of a mental health disorder (persistent, impairing, and excessive) in an adolescent, then one should see a mental health specialist. Generally, CBT is the first choice for treatment.

References

1 Wu J, Snell G, Samji H. Climate anxiety in young people: a call to action. *Lancet Planetary Health*. 2020;4:e435–e436.
2 Hettema JM, Neale MC, Kendler KS. A review and meta-analysis of the genetic epidemiology of anxiety disorders. *Am J Psychiatry*. 2001;158:1568–1578.

3 Kendler KS, Gardner CO, Lichtenstein P. A developmental twin study of symptoms of anxiety and depression: evidence for genetic innovation and attenuation. *Psychol Med.* 2008;38:1567–1575.

4 Xu K, Ernst M, Goldman D. Imaging genomics applied to anxiety, stress response, and resiliency. *Neuroinformatics.* 2006;4:51–64.

5 Serra Poirier C, Brendgen, Vitaro F, Dionne G, Boivin M. Contagion of anxiety symptoms among adolescent siblings: a twin study. *J Res Adolesc.* 2017;27:65–77.

6 Merikangas KR, Lieb RR, Wittchen HU, Avenevoli S. Family and high-risk studies of social anxiety disorder. *Acta Psychiatr Scand Suppl.* 2003;417:28–37.

7 Pavlova B, Bagnell A, Cumby J, et al. Sex-specific transmission of anxiety disorders from parents to offspring. *JAMA Netw Open.* 2022;5:e2220919.

8 Black DW, Gaffney GR, Schlosser S, Babel J. Children of parents with obsessive-compulsive disorder—a 2-year follow-up study. *Acta Psychiatr Scand.* 2003;107:305–313.

9 Asselmann E, Wittchen HU, Lieb R. The role of the mother-child relationship for anxiety disorders and depression: results from a prospective-longitudinal study in adolescents and their mothers. *Eur Child Adolesc Psychiatry.* 2015;24:451–461.

10 Burstein M, Ginsburg GS. The effect of parental modeling of anxious behaviors and cognitions in school-aged children: an experimental pilot study. *Behav Res Ther.* 2010;48:506–515.

11 US Preventive Services Task Force. Screening for anxiety in children and adolescents: US Preventive Services Task Force recommendation statement. *JAMA.* 2022;328:1438–1444.

12 Merikangas KR, He JP, Burstein M, et al. Lifetime prevalence of mental disorders in U.S. adolescents: results from the national comorbidity survey replication—Adolescent Supplement (NCS-A). *J Am Acad Child Adolesc Psychiatry.* 2010;49:980–989.

13 Zhou SJ, Zhang LG, Wang LL, et al. Prevalence and socio-demographic correlates of psychological health problems in Chinese adolescents during the outbreak of COVID-19. *Eur Child Adolesc Psychiatry.* 2020;29:749–758.

14 Meier SM, Bulik CM, Thornton LM, Mattheisen LM, Mortensen PB, Petersen L. Diagnosed anxiety disorders and the risk of subsequent anorexia nervosa: a Danish population register study. *Eur Eat Disord Rev.* 2015;23:524–530.

15 Strober M, Freeman R, Lampert C, Diamond J. The association of anxiety disorders and obsessive compulsive personality disorder with anorexia nervosa: evidence from a family study with discussion of nosological and neurodevelopmental implications. *Int J Eat Disord.* 2007;40(Suppl):S46–S51.

16 Brigham KS, Manzo LD, Eddy KT, Thomas JJ. Evaluation and treatment of avoidant/restrictive food intake disorder (ARFID) in adolescents. *Curr Pediatr Rep.* 2018;6:107–113.

17 Kambanis PE, Kuhnle MC, Won OBP, et al. Prevalence and correlates of psychiatric comorbidities in children and adolescents with full and subthreshold avoidant/restrictive food intake disorder. *Int J Eat Disord.* 2020;53:256–265.

18 Norris ML, Obeid N, Santos A, et al. Treatment needs and rates of mental health comorbidity in adolescent patients with ARFID. *Front Psychiatry.* 2021;12:680298.

19 Lemyre A, Gauthhier-Légaré A, Bélanger RE. Shyness, social anxiety, social anxiety disorder, and substance use among normative adolescent populations: a systematic review. *Am J Drug Alcohol Abuse.* 2019;45:230–247.

20 Nock MK, Green JG, Hwang I, et al. Prevalence, correlates, and treatment of lifetime suicidal behavior among adolescents: results from the national comorbidity survey replication adolescent supplement. *JAMA Psychiatry.* 2013;70:300–310.

21 Woods HC, Scott H. Sleepyteens: social media use in adolescence is associated with poor sleep quality, anxiety, depression and low self-esteem. *J Adolesc.* 2016;51:41–49.

22 Vannucci A, Flannery KM, Ohannessian CM. Social media use and anxiety in emerging adults. *J Affect Disord.* 2017;207:163–166.

23 Boers E, Afzali H, Conrod P. Temporal associations of screen time and anxiety symptoms among adolescents. *Can J Psychiatry.* 2020;65:206–208.

24 Coyne S, Rogers AA, Zurcher J, et al. Does time spent using social media impact mental health?: An eight year longitudinal study. *Comput Hum Behav.* 2020;104:106160.

25 Kaess M, Durkee T, Brunner R, et al. Pathological internet use among European adolescents: psychopathology and self-destructive behaviours. *Eur Child Adolesc Psychiatry.* 2014;23:1093–1102.

26 Costello EJ, Compton SN, Keeler G, Angold A. Relationships between poverty and psychopathology: a natural experiment. *JAMA.* 2003;290:2023–2029.

27 Najman J, Hayatbakhsh MR, Clavarino A, Bor W, O'Callaghan MJ, Williams G. Family poverty over the early life course and recurrent adolescent and young adult anxiety and depression: a longitudinal study. *Am J Public Health.* 2010;100:1719–1723.

28 Edmonds C, Alcaraz M. Childhood material hardship and adolescent mental health. *Youth Soc.* 2021;53:1231–1254.

29 Priest N, Paradies Y, Trenerry B, Truong, M, Karlsen S, Kelly Y. A systematic review of studies examining the relationship between reported racism and health and wellbeing for Children and young people. *Soc Sci Med.* 2013;95:115–127.

30 Juang LP, Alvarez AA. Discrimination and adjustment among Chinese American adolescents: family conflict and family cohesion as vulnerability and protective factors. *Am J Public Health.* 2010;100:2403–2409.

31 Becerra-Culqui TA, Liu Y, Nash R, et al. Mental health of transgender and gender nonconforming youth compared with their peers. *Pediatrics.* 2018;141:e20173845.

32 Peng K, Zhu X, Gillespie A, et al. Self-reported rates of abuse, neglect, and bullying experienced by transgender and gender-nonbinary adolescents in China. *JAMA Network Open.* 2019;2:e1911058.

33 Cimolai V, Schmitz J, Sood AB. Effects of mass shootings on the mental health of children and adolescents. *Curr Psychiatry Rep.* 2021;23:12.

34 Henrich CC, Shahar G. Effects of exposure to rocket attacks on adolescent distress and violence: a 4-year longitudinal study. *J Am Acad Child Adolesc Psychiatry.* 2013;52:619–627.

35 Eskenazi B, Fahey CA, Kogut K, et al. Association of perceived immigration policy vulnerability with mental and physical health among US-born Latino adolescents in California. *JAMA Pediatr.* 2019;173:744–753.

36 Cardoso JB, Brabeck K, Capps R, et al. Immigration enforcement fear and anxiety in Latinx high school students: the indirect effect of perceived discrimination. *J Adolesc Health.* 2021;68:961–968.

37 Aune T, Stiles TC. Universal-based prevention of syndromal and subsyndromal social anxiety: a randomized controlled study. *J Consul Clin Psychol.* 2009;77:867–879.

38 Malgady RG, Rogler LH, Costantino G. Hero/heroine modeling for Puerto Rican adolescents: a preventive mental health intervention. *J Consult Clin Psychol.* 1990;58:469–474.

39 Connolly SD, Bernstein GA; Work Group on Quality Issues. Practice parameter for the assessment and treatment of children and adolescents with anxiety disorders. *J Am Acad Child Adolesc Psychiatry.* 2007;46:267–283.

40 McMahon EM, Corcoran P, O'Regan G, et al. Physical activity in European adolescents and associations with anxiety, depression and well-being. *Eur Child Adolesc Psychiatry.* 2017;26:111–122.

5

Depression

Introduction

Physical isolation, remote learning, fear, loss of social connections and loved ones, and family financial difficulties all due to the COVID-19 pandemic helped to create a mental health crisis for adolescents. The safety and stability of families had been disrupted. Emergency department visits increased by at least one-third for teens; suicide attempts increased by more than 50 percent for girls between the ages of 12 and 17 years.[1] It is estimated that one in five adolescents had a major depressive disorder during the first year of the pandemic. Less than half of the adolescents who needed treatment received mental health services. Adolescents in racial and ethnic minority groups, especially Latinx, had the lowest treatment rates.[2]

Some groups of adolescents were at higher risk for mental health issues during the pandemic. Native American and Alaska Native youth faced challenges because of their limited access to the internet; it was more difficult for them to remain connected to friends and attend online school. Black youth were more likely to lose a parent or caregiver to COVID-19. Latino youth reported higher rates of loneliness and mental health issues. And Asian American, Native Hawaiian, and Pacific Islander youth described increased stress from harassment and hateful acts and speech.[3]

Prior to the onset of the COVID-19 pandemic, the National Institutes of Health (NIH) published data on the prevalence of depression in adolescents in the United States. According to the NIH, in 2019, in the 12- to 17-year-old age group, 15.7 percent of the adolescents had depression, with the prevalence in females almost three times the rate in males. The 12- to 13-year-old age group had a prevalence of 10.5 percent, and the 16- to 17-year-old age group had a prevalence of 20.1 percent. The highest rates of depression were seen in teens of mixed races/ethnicities. That was followed, respectively, by Hispanic, Asian, White, and, finally, Black adolescents. The data were obtained from the 2021 National Survey on Drug UOse and Health.[4]

Canadian researchers hypothesized that the COVID-19 pandemic had considerably increased the global prevalence of mental illness. They performed a meta-analysis of 29 studies that included 80,879 children and adolescents who reported mental health symptoms. The researchers learned that the prevalence of clinical depression was 25.2 percent. They reported that the loss of peer interactions, social isolation, and limited contact with supportive individuals such as teachers and coaches had taken a toll. Moreover, many children and teens received psychological services in the school setting.[5]

In 2022, the U.S. Preventive Services Task Force recommended that adolescents ages 12 to 18 years be screened for a major depressive disorder. No specific interval between screenings was recommended. The Patient Health Questionnaire-9 (PHQ-9) was mentioned as a screening test.[6]

Box 5.1 THE PHQ-9 Depression Questionnaire (6)

---

1. Do you have little interest or pleasure in doing things?
2. Are you feeling down, depressed, or hopeless?
3. Are you having trouble falling or staying asleep, or sleeping too much?
4. Are you feeling tired or having little energy?
5. Are you having a poor appetite or overeating?
6. Are you feeling bad about yourself, or that you are a failure, or that you have let yourself or your family down?
7. Are you having trouble concentrating on things, such as reading the newspaper or watching television?
8. Are you moving or speaking so slowly that other people could have noticed? Or the opposite, being so fidgety or restless that you have been moving around a lot more than usual?
9. Do you have thoughts that you would be better off dead, or of 1999 hurting yourself in some way?

Citation: Kroenke K, Spitzer RL, Williams JB. The PHQ-9: Validity of a brief depression severity measure. *J Gen Intern Med.* 2001;16:606–613.

Clinicians often use the PHQ-9 as a depression screen (Box 5.1) for adolescents.[7] The questions pertain to the prior 2 weeks, and they are scored on a numerical scale as not at all, several days, more than half of the days, or nearly every day.

There are other factors that may predispose adolescents to depression, including inherited factors and early life stressors.[8] Children of parents who are depressed have a significantly higher risk of developing depression. And there are psychological factors as a result of current events, including violence, that may mediate the onset of depression in teens.

Resilient adolescents who are faced with adversity may be able to fend off depressive thinking. Resilience is a protective factor for adolescents who may be at high risk for depression and is defined as those personal qualities that enable people to thrive in the face of difficulties. Researchers Connor and Davidson at Duke University developed a 25-question resilience scale that characterized the qualities of resilience that may protect against depression. These include a person's ability to adapt to change, the capacity to bounce back after adversity, the readiness to cope with issues, and having a strong sense of purpose in life. Other factors include not being discouraged by failure, embracing challenges, staying focused under pressure, and knowing where to turn for help during a hard time or crisis.[9]

According to researchers from the United Kingdom, some of the factors that protect against the development of depression in adolescents include genetic inheritance, high intelligence, good coping mechanisms, and appropriate emotion regulation capacities.

Adolescents who have more resilience to depression tend to have good-quality interpersonal relationships characterized by warmth, acceptance, and low hostility. Low parental control seems to be as important as peer support.[10]

There are some medical conditions in adolescents that may mimic the symptoms of depression. The most recent addition is long-term COVID. Also, clinicians should consider hypothyroidism, Addison's disease, late-term Lyme disease, mononucleosis, chronic fatigue syndrome, and anemia when evaluating an adolescent with depressive symptoms.[11]

Epidemiology

When does depression usually occur during adolescence? Researchers from Wisconsin and New Zealand investigated the emergence of depression over the course of 10 years in 1037 children from the same birth cohort in New Zealand. They examined the subjects from preadolescence to young adulthood using a structured diagnostic interview five times between ages 11 and 21. The researchers learned that females had a slightly higher prevalence of depression at ages 13 and 15. Significantly higher rates of female depression occurred between ages 15 and 18 years. The peak increases in new cases of depression and overall incidence in both genders occurred between 15 and 18 years.[12]

A team of researchers based in Vermont wanted to understand what caused the dramatic increase in the prevalence of depression in female adolescents. Utilizing the Great Smokey Mountain Study, they followed a representative sample of three cohorts of girls ($n = 630$) ages 9, 11, and 13 years at baseline. The subjects were observed and evaluated from 1993 to 2000 with measures for depression and pubertal development. Included in the study were periodic measurements of the male hormone testosterone and the female hormone estradiol. The researchers found an association between the latter portion of pubertal development and an increased risk for depression. Early pubertal developers had a higher risk of depression than on-time or late developers. Testosterone but not estradiol levels were a significant predictor of depression. The researchers queried if testosterone was an activator of depression or had direct effects within the central nervous system in females.[13]

Hormonal contraception appears to increase the risk of depression in adolescents and young women with attention-deficit/hyperactivity disorder (ADHD). Researchers in Sweden utilized data from five national registries to study approximately 800,000 girls and young women ages 15 to 24 years with and without ADHD. Their study also utilized data on methods of contraception as well as diagnoses of depression. Irrespective of hormonal contraception use, women with ADHD had a more than three times increased risk of developing depression compared to women without ADHD. In addition, women with ADHD utilizing the combined oral contraceptive pill or the progestin-only pill had up to five times the risk of developing depression compared to women who did not have ADHD.[14]

Psychosocial Issues and Depression

Psychological Issues

Anxiety

Anxiety may be a precursor to depression in some adolescents. Researchers from New Zealand performed a longitudinal study of a birth cohort of 1265 children born in mid-1977. During their adolescent years, they were studied annually until the age of 16 years. Then they were studied at age 18 and again at age 21. During their 14- to 16-year check-in, the subjects and their parents were interviewed about the extent of any anxiety disorders. At the 16- to 21-year reviews, sample subjects were asked about their mental health and substance use. The researchers discovered that the adolescents with an anxiety disorder were at increased risk for the subsequent development of major depression as well as drug dependence and educational underachievement during young adulthood. For example, 26 subjects had three or more anxiety disorders between the ages of 14 and 16 years. Of these, 84.6 percent had major depression at the subsequent appointments as older adolescents. This suggested the need for continued surveillance as well as treatment for adolescents who have recurrent anxiety disorders. And there appeared to be a significant risk for adolescents with anxiety to continue as adults with the same mental health issues.[15]

Certain types of anxiety in adolescents may lead to major depression. Researchers at the NIH studied the relationship between adolescent fears and the risk for major depression. They used a cohort of 776 subjects who were children and adolescents in the Children in the Community Study in New York State. During interviews, the researchers assessed the subjects for depressive and anxiety symptoms. The researchers found that a specific fear of darkness in adolescents predicted a future risk for major depression, and they underscored the need to follow adolescents carefully if they had a fear of darkness as well as anxiety.[16]

Eating Disorders

In the past, some clinicians treated patients with anorexia nervosa with antidepressant medications, and this was often ineffective. Researchers in Germany wanted to determine the prevalence of a mood disorder in 101 consecutive female adolescents treated for anorexia in an academic clinical setting. Their mean age was 15.2 years. The subjects and their parent(s) were jointly interviewed. For those adolescents with restrictive anorexia nervosa, 57.7 percent of the patients had a mood disorder, 16.9 percent had an anxiety disorder, 16.9 percent had obsessive-compulsive disorder, and 1.4 percent had a substance use disorder. This study confirmed that a mood disorder, such as depression, is seen in significant numbers in adolescents diagnosed with anorexia.[17]

To determine the prevalence of depression and anxiety in patients with avoidant-restrictive food intake disorder (ARFID), researchers at Massachusetts General Hospital compared patients with ARFID to those with anorexia nervosa. Results could inform treatment strategies. The cohort consisted of 67 patients; the average age of onset was 8.3 years, and 50.8 percent were female. The subjects completed questionnaires in an outpatient setting. The patients with ARFID reported lower levels of depression and anxiety than those with anorexia.[18]

In a retrospective chart review study of 28 children and adolescents with ARFID and under the age of 18 years, Canadian researchers searched for psychiatric comorbidities. The researchers determined that two subjects (7.1 percent) were diagnosed with major depressive disorder, which was not a significant prevalence for depression in patients with ARFID. Most people develop ARFID in early childhood and do not have or develop a mood disorder at that time, so antidepressant medications would not be indicated.[19]

Substance Use

There are two main categories of adolescents who abuse substances and have a mood disorder; those with a mood disorder, such as depression, induced by substance use and those already with a mood disorder like depression who then begin to use substances. Some experts believe that drug use that begins in early adolescence, defined as ages 14 to 16 years, may be tied to a past history of adverse childhood experiences (ACEs). ACEs then set the stage for adolescent depression, which some adolescents attempt to treat by using substances. Studies from treatment centers for adolescents who abuse alcohol have found that up to half of the patients have an affective (mood) disorder, mostly depression. This dual diagnosis makes treatment more complicated because the underlying causes may be difficult to delineate. Researchers based in Michigan wanted to learn how to predict which adolescents with depressive symptoms were also at increased risk for substance abuse. At an academic medical center inpatient psychiatric unit, they studied 103 adolescents with major depression. The mean age of the cohort was 15.3 years, and about two-thirds were female. There were measurements for depression, suicidal ideation and behavior, and social adjustment. Alcohol and substance use were documented. The researchers found a number of warning signs for substance use in female adolescents, including parental conflict, schoolwork difficulties, conduct problems, and a high level of involvement in romantic relationships with males. For males, conduct and academic problems were predictors of substance abuse. While older adolescent males seemed to have an increased risk, that did not appear to be true for older adolescent females.[20]

Adolescents who are depressed may use cannabis for symptom relief. This is particularly true for male adolescents. Although there are anecdotal reports that cannabis does relieve depressive symptomatology in some teens, there is little evidence to support its use as an antidepressant treatment in this group. There is some evidence that the use of cannabis may lead to the onset of depression, and some adolescents may become more depressed after using cannabis.[21]

Researchers based in Canada performed a systematic review and meta-analysis to investigate the association between cannabis use in adolescence and depression, suicidality, and/or anxiety in young adulthood (18 to 22 years). The researchers located 11 studies that met their criteria. From these studies, they learned that cannabis use in adolescents was associated with an increased risk for major depression and suicidality in young adulthood. Further, younger users of cannabis, defined as 14 to 15 years old, were at a significantly higher risk for suicidal behaviors. If they smoked cannabis during adolescence, female adolescents were more susceptible than male adolescents to develop adult depression.[22]

Suicidality

Depression is a major factor in the cause of suicidal behavior in adolescents. Researchers in North Carolina periodically assessed 180 adolescents between the ages of 12 and 19 years for up to 13 years after they were admitted for a psychiatric hospitalization. Although none of the subjects died by suicide, during the course of the study, 46 subjects made 128 suicide attempts. Major depression, dysthymic disorder (persistent depressive symptoms), or a depressive disorder was present in 49.9 percent of the subjects making their first suicide attempt. For the subjects who repeated attempts at suicide, 96 percent had one of those three disorders. The researchers noted that many of the subjects had more than one diagnosis, such as substance abuse, generalized anxiety, or conduct disorder.[23]

A systematic review conducted by researchers located in countries throughout the world determined the psychosocial risk factors for suicidality in adolescents. The researchers located 44 studies that met their criteria. From these studies, they identified three main factors that appeared to increase suicidality among teens. The first, psychological factors, included depression, anxiety, and a history of a previous suicide attempt and substance abuse. The second factor was stressful life events such as family problems and peer conflict. The third was the individual's personality traits, such as impulsive behavior and neuroticism.[24]

Decreasing the risk for depression should also lower the risk for suicidal behavior in adolescents. Researchers from the NIH and Johns Hopkins University wanted to determine which traits promoted resilience, life satisfaction, and optimism and, in so doing, reduced the risk of suicidality. They studied 1904 youth from the NEXT Generation Health Study, in which adolescents were followed over 7 years. At the final wave, the average age was 22.6 years, and 60 percent were female. During the course of the study, measures of suicidality, depression, life satisfaction, and optimism were taken. Both life satisfaction and optimism moderated the association between depressive symptomatology and suicidality. As a result, building adolescent resilience may be a factor in reducing the risk of adolescent depression and suicidality.[25]

Social Media

There are strong and convincing data that there have been significant increases in younger adolescents seeking mental health services and college and university students visiting their schools' counseling services. Some experts believe that at least some of the reasons for such increases are related to the use of electronic communications and social media. During the past decade, the rates of depressive symptoms and suicide have increased in adolescents. Researchers from California and Florida used data from the Monitoring the Future Survey, the Youth Risk Surveillance System, and the Centers for Disease Control and Prevention to evaluate this association. They focused on death by suicide for adolescents ages 13 to 18 years, and they were able to obtain data on depressive symptoms, suicide-related outcomes, measures for electronic and social media use, in-person social interactions, sports pursuits, religiosity, and employment. The researchers discovered that depressive symptoms, suicide-related outcomes, and deaths by suicide increased from 2010 to 2015. The increase in depressive symptoms and suicide-related outcomes was driven almost entirely by female adolescents. Likewise, screen time, especially from social media and smartphones, appeared to have more significant mental health effects on female adolescents. The researchers observed that the teens who devoted more time to nonelectronic pursuits such as homework, in-person social interactions, sports, exercise, reading print media, and attending religious services were less likely to report mental health issues. They also determined that by 2012, about half of all Americans used smartphones, which corresponded to the uptick in mental health issues. By 2015 when their study ended, 92 percent of teens and young adults owned a smartphone and levels of depression had peaked.[26]

Problematic use of social media may also be linked to depression in adolescents. Researchers in Maryland examined 42 studies for the association between depression, suicidality, and the use of social media among adolescents. Social media included emails, texts, blogs, message boards, online dating, games, apps, and social networking sites. All of the subjects were between the ages of 10 and 18 years. From their analyses, the researchers learned that problematic social media use was correlated with depressive symptoms, possibly more often in female adolescents and in those who began using social media at earlier ages. Studies that investigated social comparisons—where adolescents compare themselves to peers—over social media found significant associations between making these comparisons and depression. Individuals tended to make more positive comparisons of themselves over social media, and individuals with low self-esteem were particularly at risk for the negative effects of such comparisons. The researchers also found that body image concerns may be a mediator to negative effects of social media on adolescent mental health. The researchers commented that programming directed to gender and age as well as parental involvement may help prevent the development of depressive symptoms.[27]

Researchers from Washington State were interested in factors from social media use that might be risks for depression in adolescents. They formulated a cohort consisting of 226 participants, with 113 parents and 113 adolescents. The researchers asked each parent and adolescent dyad to complete online surveys about adolescent social media activities. The investigators learned that social media activity, defined as the number of these accounts the adolescents had and their self-reported frequency of social media checking, was positively related to fear of missing out (FOMO) and loneliness. Depression and anxiety were highest among the adolescents whose parents reported that their adolescents had a relatively large number of social media accounts and a relatively high FOMO.[28]

Poverty
Different researchers have found varying results when they have studied the relationship between poverty, a social determinant of health, and the prevalence of adolescent depression. Researchers in Australia used data from a prospective longitudinal study of people born between 1981 and 1984 to determine if family poverty in the early life of a child would predict adolescent and young adult depression. The researchers used data from the Youth Self-Report for the 14-year evaluation and data from the Young Adult Self-Report at the 21-year follow-up. The investigators found no evidence that poverty during the first 6 months of life was related to depression during adolescence. But they found that multiple experiences of family poverty was associated with an estimate of 3.2 times the risk of the subject being depressed at both the 14- and 21-year exams.[29] However, a researcher at the University of Iowa examined the relationship between early childhood poverty, poverty persistence, and current poverty and adolescent depressive symptoms. The results indicated that associations between poverty and depressive symptoms in adolescents were explained by the mother's childhood depression and whether the adolescent had lived with both parents during the first year of life.[30]

Researchers based in Canada conducted a systematic review and meta-analysis to determine if exposure to early life stress was correlated with an increased risk for developing major depression before the age of 18 years. They located 62 journal articles with 44,066 subjects that met their criteria. Several of the studies examined poverty or low socioeconomic status as potential sources of early life stress. The researchers learned that poverty had a very modest effect on the development of adolescent depression—an odds ratio of 1.22. However, they did note that poverty had adverse effects on the health of children, intellectual development, and later achievements. And they commented that early life stresses including sexual, emotional, and physical abuse; death; domestic violence; and natural disasters appeared to have a notable impact in the future development of adolescent depression.[31]

Racism/Discrimination

Racism is associated with poorer mental outcomes, including depression and anxiety, in adolescents. Researchers in Australia conducted a systematic review on the connection between racism and well-being in children and adolescents. They analyzed 153 papers representing 121 studies that met their inclusion criteria. Most of the studies, which were cross-sectional in design and included subjects who were 12 to 18 years, were conducted in the United States. Black, Hispanic, and Asian populations were most frequently included. Of the 72 studies on depression, 79 percent noted an association between reported racial discrimination and depression.[32]

To understand the association of racism and depression over time, researchers in Washington, DC and Baltimore followed 504 Black adolescents from grade 7 to grade 10. Each year, during interviews, the students shared their experiences with racial discrimination and depressive symptoms. Racial discrimination was assessed with the Racism and Life Experiences Scale, and depressive symptoms were measured with the depression subscale of the Baltimore How I Feel—Adolescent Version, Youth Report. The researchers found that Black adolescents who experienced racial discrimination were at increased risk for depressive symptoms 1 year later. The correlation of racism and depressive symptoms was stronger in female adolescents than in male adolescents.[33]

Researchers from Massachusetts hypothesized that youth who faced anticipated and vicarious racial/ethnic discrimination (rather than "first-hand" experiences) had an increased risk of depressive symptoms, major depressive disorder, or suicidal behavior. Their cohort consisted of 1147 youth (50.3 percent female and ranging in age from 9 to 12 years) from the Project on Human Development in Chicago Neighborhoods. The study was cross-sectional in design, and the youth came from 79 different neighborhoods. The racial/ethnic distributions for the subjects were 46.14 percent Hispanic, 34.73 percent Black, 15.01 percent White, and 4.12 percent other. Measurements for self-reported depression, major depression, and suicidal behavior were administered, as were measurements for experienced, anticipated, and vicarious racial and ethnic discrimination. The researchers found an association between experienced and anticipated racial/ethnic discrimination and self-reported depression and major depressive disorder; vicarious racial/ethnic discrimination was not related to the two depressive measures. In addition, the findings demonstrated a strong relationship between experienced, anticipated, or vicarious discrimination and suicidal behavior. The researchers commented that racial and cultural socialization and preparation for bias may support coping skills against the effects of this discrimination.[34]

Transgender/Gender Incongruence

There is a general consensus that transgender youth, when compared to cisgender youth, are at increased risk for mental health disorders. Researchers in Boston studied 106 female-to-male and 74 male-to-female transgender teens and young adults ages 12 to 29 years and matched them to cisgender patient controls at a community-based health center. Electronic medical records were reviewed for physician-diagnosed depression per current *Diagnostic and Statistical Manual of Mental Disorders* criteria. The cohort had an average age of 19.6 years. The transgender group had a notably elevated prevalence of depression—50.6 percent in comparison to 20.6 percent in the cisgender group. The rates were equally high in both the female-to-male and male-to-female transgender groups. The researchers recommended that any adolescent/young adult with gender identity issues be carefully screened for mental health problems.[35]

Researchers from North Carolina wanted to determine if parents recognized the symptoms of depression and anxiety in their transgender and gender diverse (TGD) children, teens, and young adults. They conducted a study in a pediatric gender clinic for patients ages 8 to 22 with a mean age of 14.9 years. Prior to a visit to the clinic, both parents and the subjects completed a questionnaire that assessed for symptoms of depression and anxiety. Approximately half of the TGD subjects had signs of moderate to severe depression and anxiety, and their symptoms tended to be more severe than recognized by their parents. The researchers concluded that there was a need for more interventions to increase parental recognition of their child's mental health.[36]

Researchers from California wanted to learn if parental support for transgender adolescents had any notable impact on the symptoms of depression and quality of life. The transgender adolescents and young adults, who ranged in age from 12 to 24 years, were gender nonconforming; prior to being seen by the medical staff, they had a mental health assessment. Parental support (defined as help, advice, and confidante support), quality of life, and depression were measured with appropriate scales. The researchers learned that the teens who felt a greater perceived burden from being transgender and who felt lower life satisfaction had more depressive symptoms. However, parental support was significantly related to higher life satisfaction, lower perceived burden, and fewer depressive symptoms.[37]

Washington State researchers wanted to learn if mental health concerns changed after children transitioned. Their cohort consisted of 63 children and adolescents who had transitioned, 38 of their siblings, and 63 cisgender children, who were the controls. The children were between the ages of 9 and 14 years. Social transition was defined as the individual using the pronoun associated with their asserted gender in all contexts. Parents and all of the participants answered questions designed to measure depression and anxiety in the subjects. The researchers noted that the transitioned transgender children reported depression and self-worth that did not differ from their matched-control or sibling peers. They did report marginally higher rates of anxiety. These findings suggested that social transition for transgender children may be an effective intervention that helps prevent mental health issues such as depression.[38]

Mortality

The death of a parent is one of the most stressful events that an adolescent may experience; and, sadly, thousands of adolescents have lost a parent or parents to the COVID-19 epidemic and recent wars. Mourning for a parent comes at a time when the adolescent is already undergoing significant physical, mental, and social changes. It is understandable for an adolescent who is mourning the death of a parent to feel depressive symptoms. Researchers in Canada noticed that there has been a paucity of research on parental loss during adolescence. They searched the literature for relevant studies published between 1987 and 2020 and located 36 articles that met their criteria. The researchers determined that depression and anxiety were the most common psychological reactions in adolescents to parental death. One paper observed that adolescents who were particularly passive or dependent were prone to depression if they received low support after the death. Another paper reported higher depression in adolescents who had a poor past relationship with the deceased parent. Teens who had support from immediate and extended family members, extended family friendships, and school-based professionals coped better. Further, the roles played by peers and the school may be more important than family and other types of support.[39]

To learn more about the depressive symptoms that an adolescent may have upon the death of a parent, researchers in Pennsylvania and Ohio interviewed 325 children and adolescents and their surviving parent about 2 months after a parental death. They compared the bereaved children and adolescents to 129 nonbereaved community controls and 110 nonbereaved depressed control subjects.

The data demonstrated that depressive symptoms and depression were a common occurrence in children and adolescents 2 months after a parental death. In particular, bereaved adolescents demonstrated dysphoria (dissatisfaction with life), loss of interest, appetite and sleep changes, slowed speech and cognition, low energy, guilt, decreased concentration, and suicidal thinking at a much higher rate than the nonbereaved control group. If such concerning symptoms are observed, the surviving parent and/or family should seek professional help.[40]

Violence

Adolescents with a history of violence including physical and sexual abuse have a higher risk of developing depression. Researchers from South Carolina studied a subsample of 548 adolescents from the National Survey of Adolescents. During the previous year, each adolescent met the criteria for a major depression diagnosis. The researchers noted that there were differences in depressed teens who had a history of physical and/or sexual abuse and those who did not. Teens with a history of both types of abuse were more likely to be depressed than those without either abuse or only physical abuse. Teens who had a series of abuses for a longer duration had more severe depression. And regardless of abuse history, female adolescents were always more likely to be depressed than their male counterparts.[41]

Physical or sexual abuse by a dating partner is another type of violence that may be experienced by up to 20 percent of female and 9 percent of male adolescents. Researchers from Minnesota wanted to learn if adolescents who had suffered dating violence had a higher risk of depression. They used data from Project EAT, an epidemiologic study of adolescent eating behaviors and weight-related issues that included two waves of data collected in 1999 and 2004. Drawn from middle and high schools in Minnesota, the study included 1516 adolescents (54 percent female); two of the questions asked about physical and sexual violence. A total of 23 (3.1 percent) male and 102 (13.2 percent) female adolescents reported dating violence. The researchers learned that in female adolescents, dating violence was significantly related to high depressive symptoms—though this was not necessarily a cause and effect. In addition, this study did not determine if female adolescents who were depressed were more likely to experience dating violence or if dating violence may trigger depression. However, it is important to underscore that both male and female adolescents who report dating violence should undergo careful screening for mental health issues.[42]

Another major source for adolescent mental health issues is violence associated with mass shootings. In the aftermath of 15 mass shootings, 9 of which took place in high schools or universities, researchers from New York and Massachusetts examined 49 relevant peer-reviewed articles. Posttraumatic stress syndrome was the most frequently reported medical problem related to the shootings; these were noted in 36 of the studies. Major depression was the second most common associated mental health disorder. With the assistance of the Center for Epidemiologic Studies Short Depression Scale, eight studies measured the prevalence of major depressive symptoms in student survivors 2 weeks after the attacks. The highest prevalence of depressive symptoms was 71 percent, which was seen in a combined sample from the Virginia Tech shooting in 2007 and the Northern Illinois University shooting in 2008. Although long-term follow-up was not available, the researchers commented that early postincident mental health support has been found to predict later postincident mental health well-being.[43]

Treatment of Adolescent Depression

Treatment for adolescents with depression includes therapy, medication, or a combination of both. A review of controlled trials determined that cognitive behavioral therapy (CBT) and interpersonal psychotherapy (IPT) were well-established interventions for depressed adolescents with evidence of efficacy found in multiple trials by independent investigative teams.[44] IPT is a therapy that attempts to improve an adolescent's interpersonal relationships and social interactions and focuses on improving these relationships, thereby decreasing their depressive symptoms.

Researchers based in North Carolina and at multiple institutions studied the efficacy of four different treatments for adolescents with depression: placebo, fluoxetine, CBT, and CBT with fluoxetine. When compared to the placebo, the combination of CBT with fluoxetine showed the best results. Fluoxetine was a superior treatment to CBT alone. The combination of medication and therapy was most effective in reducing suicidal ideation.[45]

The first choice for medication is generally one of the selective serotonin reuptake inhibitors (SSRIs). Fluoxetine and escitalopram are approved for use in adolescents, even though other SSRIs and serotonin norepinephrine reuptake inhibitors (SNRIs) such as venlafaxine are used off label for treatment of adolescents with depression. The side effects include sedation, insomnia, headache, or gastrointestinal discomfort.

Occasionally, adolescents may experience activation manifested as insomnia, disinhibition, or restlessness. There is a small risk that some adolescents may have an increased risk for suicidal thinking or behavior including attempted suicide. This necessitates close follow-up of these adolescents by the treating clinician.[46]

About 60 percent of adolescents show improvement with the initial treatment trial by an SSRI. Researchers in Pennsylvania and nationwide studied four different treatment strategies for adolescents who continued to have depression after initial treatment with the SSRI. The strategies included a different SSRI (paroxetine, citalopram, or fluoxetine), a different SSRI and CBT, an SNRI (venlafaxine), or venlafaxine and CBT. The results indicated that CBT and a switch to another antidepressant resulted in a higher clinical response than a medication switch alone. The new medication could be an SSRI or SNRI, but there were fewer adverse effects with a new SSRI.[47]

Researchers in Hong Kong performed a systematic review and meta-analysis to determine the efficacy of physical activity intervention to alleviate symptoms of depression in adolescents. They reviewed 21 studies with 2441 participants with a mean age of 14 years, and 47 percent were male. They determined that physical activity interventions produced greater reductions in depressive symptoms compared to control conditions, especially in subjects older than 13 years and with a mental illness and/or diagnosis of depression.[48]

Prevention

Prevention of depression in adolescents should focus on maximizing protective factors and minimizing risk factors for mental illness. Box 5.2 lists some ways to protect adolescents from depression, and Box 5.3 lists risk factors.

Programming to prevent adolescent depression may be school based. For example, a program in Australia targeted grade 8 students. In the study, 751 students received teacher-administered CBT based on the Problem Solving for Life program, and 749 students served as controls. The students were monitored for depression and dysthymia over a 4-year period. Those students with high and low symptoms for depression initially showed positive short-term benefits after participation in the intervention compared to controls. However, the short-term benefits were no longer noted by the 1-year follow-up.[49]

A family-based intervention appeared to be more effective. Researchers from Tennessee, Vermont, and North Carolina reviewed a family-based intervention for

---

Box 5.2 Protective Factors Against Adolescent Depression

Personal: resilience, strong coping skills, avoidance of substances, emotion regulation skills
Strong relationships: family, adults, peers, school, clergy
Activities: exercise, sports, monitoring of online time and social media sites by parents

Box 5.3 Risk Factors for Adolescent Depression

Personal: gender (female), low self-esteem, negative body image, ineffective coping style, history of physical, emotional, or sexual abuse
Family: parent with depression, broken family, divorce, bereavement
Social: decreased connections, poverty, exposure to violence, cyberbullying, sexual or gender identity issues, racism/discrimination

children between the ages of 9 and 15 years who had parents with depression. The study included 95 mothers, 16 fathers, and 155 children. Fifty-five families received written materials to review, and 56 families participated in an intervention: family group CBT. At 12 months, the family-based intervention group was judged to have better outcomes for the youth.[50]

Another program that also showed efficacy was the Competent Adulthood Transition with Cognitive-behavioral, Humanistic, and Interpersonal Training (CATCH-IT), an internet-based program. This program includes modules using the therapeutic modalities of IPT, CBT, and resilience components. Researchers from Massachusetts and Illinois compared CATCH-IT ($n = 193$) to online health education ($n = 176$) on internalizing symptoms in adolescents between the ages of 13 and 18 years. The researchers found that long-term improvement in depressive symptoms and anxiety was significant for both groups.[51]

Conclusion

Adolescent depression is a common mental health issue, and it is a major factor in the cause of suicidal behavior. Adolescents should be screened periodically for depression, and if the screen is positive, they should be referred to a clinician. There are effective medications and therapies for this health problem, but close monitoring and long-term follow up are important.

References

1 Yard E, Radhakrishnan L, Ballesteros MF, et al. Emergency department visits for suspected suicide attempts among persons aged 12–25 years before and during the COVID-19 pandemic-United States, January 2019–May 2021. *MMWR Morb Mortal Wkly Rep.*2021;70:888–894.
2 Flores MW, Sharp A, Carson NJ, Cook BL. Estimates of major depressive disorder and treatment among adolescents by race and ethnicity. *JAMA Pediatr.* 2023;177:1215–1223.
3 *Protecting Youth Mental Health.* The U.S. Surgeon General's Advisory. Washington, DC; 2021.
4 Substance Abuse and Mental Health Services Administration. Key substance use and mental health indicators in the United jStates: results from the national survey on drug use and health 2022. (HHS Publication No. PEP22-07-01-005, NSDUH Series H-57). Center

for Behavioral health Statisitics and Quality, Substance Abuse and Mental Health Services Administration.

5   Racine N, McArthur BA, Cooke JE, Eircih R, Zhu J, Madigan S. Global prevalence of depression and anxiety symptoms in children and adolescents during COVID-19: a meta-analysis. *JAMA Pediatrics* 2021;175:1142–1150.

6   US Preventive Services Task Force. Screening for depression and suicide risk in children and adolescents: US Preventive Services Task Force Recommendation Statement. *JAMA.* 2022;328:1534–1542.

7   Kroenke K, Spitzer RL, Williams JB. The PHQ-9: Validity of a brief depression severity measure. *J Gen Intern Med.*2001;16:606–613.

8   Lee HY, Kim I, Nam S, Jweong J. Adverse childhood experiences and the associations with depression and anxiety in adolescents. *Child Youth Serv Rev.* 2020;111:104850.

9   Connor KM, Davidson JR. Development of a new resilience scale: the Connor-Davidson resilience scale (CD-RISC). *Depress Anxiety.* 2003;18:76–82.

10 Thapar A, Collishaw S, Pine DS, Thapar AK. Depression in adolescence. *Lancet.* 2012;379:1056–1067.

11 Hazen EP, Goldstein MA, Goldstein MC. *Mental Health Disorders in Adolescents: A Guide for Parents, Teachers, and Professionals.* Rutgers University Press; 2011.

12 Hankin BL, Abramson LY, Moffin TE, et al. Development of depression from preadolescence to young adulthood: emerging gender differences in a 10-year longitudinal study. *J Abnorm Psychol.* 1998;107:128–140.

13 Copeland WE, Worthman C, Shanahan L, Costello EJ, Angold A. Early pubertal timing and testosterone associated with higher levels of adolescent depression in girls. *J Am Acad Child Adolesc Psychiatry.* 2019;58:1197–1206.

14 Lundin C, Wikman A, Wikman P, Kallner HK, Sundstrom-Poromaa I, Skoglund C. Hormonal contraceptive use and risk of depression among young women with attention-deficit/hyperactivity disorder. *J Am Acad Child Adolesc Psychiatry.* 2023;62:665–674.

15 Woodward LJ, Fergusson DM. Life course outcomes of young people with anxiety disorders in adolescence. *J Am Acad Child Adolesc Psychiatry.* 2001;40:1086–1093.

16 Pine DS, Cohen P, Brook J. Adolescent fears as predictors of depression. *Biol Psychiatry.* 2001;50:721–724.

17 Salbach-Andrae H, Lenz K, Simmendinger N, Klinkowski N, Lehmkuhl U, Pfeiffer E. Psychiatric comorbidities among female adolescents with anorexia nervosa. *Child Psychiatry Hum Devel.* 2008;39:261–272.

18 Becker R, Keshishian AC, Liebman RE, Coniglio K, Wang SB, Franko DL. Impact of expanded diagnostic criteria for avoidant/restrictive food intake disorder on clinical comparisons with anorexia nervosa. *Int J Eat Disord.* 2019;52:230–238.

19 Cooney M, Lieberman M, Guimond T, Katzman DK. Clinical and psychological features of children and adolescents diagnosed with avoidant/restrictive food intake disorder in a pediatric tertiary care eating disorder program: a descriptive study. *J Eat Disord.* 2018;6:7.

20 King CA, Ghaziuddin N, McGovern L, Brankd E, Hill EW, Naylor M. Predictors of comorbid alcohol and substance abuse in depressed adolescents. *J Am Acad Child Adolesc Psychiatry.* 1996;35:743–751.

21 Feingold D, Weinstein A. Cannabis and depression. *Adv Exp Med Biol.* 2021;1264:67–80.

22 Gobbi G, Atkin T, Zytynski T, et al. Association of cannabis use in adolescence and risk of depression, anxiety, and suicidality in young adulthood: a systematic review and meta-analysis. *JAMA Psychiatry.* 2019;76:426–434.

23 Goldston DB, Daniel SS, Erkanli A, et al. Psychiatric diagnoses as contemporaneous risk factors for suicide attempts among adolescents and young adults: developmental changes. *J Consult Clin Psychol.* 2009;77:281–290.

24 Carballo JJ, Llorente C, Kehrmann L, et al. Psychological risk factors for suicidality in children and adolescents. *Eur Child Adolesc Psychiatry*. 2020;29:759–776.

25 Yu J, Goldstein RB, Haynie DL, et al. Resilience factors in the association between depressive symptoms and suicidality. *J Adolesc Health*. 2021;69:280–287.

26 Twenge JM, Joiner TE, Rogers ML, Martin GN. Increases in depressive symptoms, suicide-related outcomes, and suicide rates among U.S. adolescents after 2010 and links to increased new media screen time. *Clin Psychol Sci*. 2018;6:3–17.

27 Vidal C, Lhaksampa T, Miller L, Platt R. Social media use and depression in adolescents: a scoping review. *Int Rev Psychiatry*. 2020;32:235–253.

28 Barry CT, Sidoti CL, Briggs SM, Reiter SR, Lindsey RA. Adolescent social media use and mental health from adolescent and parent perspectives. *J Adolesc*. 2017;61:1–11.

29 Najman JM, Hayatbakhsh MR, Clavarino A, Bor W, O'Callaghan MJ, Williams GM. Family poverty over the early life course and recurrent adolescent and young adult anxiety and depression: a longitudinal study. *Am J Public Health*. 2010;100:1719–1723.

30 Butler AC. Poverty and adolescent depressive symptoms. *Am J Orthopsychiatry*. 2014;84:82–94.

31 LeMoult J, Humphreys KL, Tracy A, Hoffmeister JA, Ip E, Gotlib IH. Meta-analysis: exposure to early life stress and risk for depression in childhood and adolescence. *J Am Acad Child Adolesc Psychiatry*. 2020;59:842–855.

32 Priest N, Paradies Y, Trenerry B, Truong M, Karlsen S, Kelly Y. A systematic review of studies examining the relationship between reported racism and health and wellbeing for children and young people. *Soc Sci Med*. 2013;95:115–127.

33 English D, Lambert SF, Ialongo NS. Longitudinal associations between experienced racial discrimination and depressive symptoms in African American adolescents. *Dev Psychol*. 2014;50:1190–1196.

34 Zimmerman GM, Miller-Smith A. The impact of anticipated, vicarious, and experienced racial and ethnic discrimination on depression and suicidal behavior among Chicago youth. *Soc Sci Res*. 2022;101:102623.

35 Reisner SL, Vetters R, Leclerc M, et al. Mental health of transgender youth in care at an adolescent urban community health center: a matched retrospective cohort study. *J Adolesc Health*. 2015;56:274–279.

36 McGuire F, Carl A, Woodcock L, et al. Differences in patient and parent informant reports of depression and anxiety symptoms in a clinical sample of transgender youth and gender diverse youth. *LGBT Health*. 2021;8:404–411.

37 Simons L, Schrager SM, Clark LF, Belzer M, Olson J. Parental support and mental health among transgender adolescents. *J Adolesc Health*. 2013;53:791–793.

38 Durwood L, McLaughlin KA, Olson KR. Mental health and self-worth in socially transitioned transgender youth. *J Am Acad Child Adolesc Psychiatry*. 2017;56:116–123.

39 Farella Guzzo M, Gobbi G. Parental death during adolescence: a review of the literature. *Omega (Westport)*. 2021 Jul 29:302228211033661. doi: 10.1177/00302228211033661.

40 Gray LB, Weiller RA, Fristad M, Weller EB. Depression in children and adolescents two months after the death of a parent. *J Affect Disord*. 2011;135:277–283.

41 Danielson CK, de Arellano MA, Kilpatrick DG, Saunders BE, Resnic HS. Child maltreatment in depressed adolescents: differences in symptomatology based on history of abuse. *Child Maltreat*. 2005;10:37–48.

42 Ackard DM, Eisenberg ME, Neumark-Sztainer D. Long-term impact of adolescent dating violence on the behavioral and psychological health of male and female youth. *J Pediatr*. 2007;151:476–481.

43 Lowe SR, Galea S. The mental health consequences of mass shootings. *Trauma Violence Abuse*. 2017;1:62–82.

44 Weersing VR, Jeffreys M, Do MT, Schwartz LTG, Bolano C. Evidence base update of psychosocial treatments for child and adolescent depression. *J Clin Child Adolesc Psychol.* 2017;46:11–43.

45 March J, Silva S, Petrycki S, et al. Treatment for Adolescents With Depression Study (TADS) Team. Fluoxetine, cognitive-behavioral therapy, and their combination for adolescents with depression: Treatment for Adolescents With Depression Study (TADS) randomized controlled trial. *JAMA.* 2004;292:807–820.

46 Miller L, Campo JV. Depression in adolescents. *N Engl J Med.* 2021 Jul 29;385:445–449.

47 Brent D, Emslie G, Clarke G, et al. Switching to another SSRI or to venlafaxine with or without cognitive behavioral therapy for adolescents with SSRI-resistant depression: the TORDIA randomized controlled trial. *JAMA.* 2008;299:901–913.

48 Recchia F, Bernal JDK, Fong DY, et al. Physical activity interventions to alleviate depressive symptoms in children and adolescents: a systematic review and meta-analysis. *JAMA Pediatr.* 2023;177:132–140.

49 Spence SH, Sheffield JK, Donovan CL. Long-term outcome of a school-based, universal approach to prevention of depression in adolescents. *J Consult Clin Psychol.* 2005;73:160–167.

50 Compas BE, Forehand R, Keller G, et al. Randomized controlled trial of a family cognitive-behavioral preventive intervention for children of depressed parents. *J Consult Clinical Psychol.* 2009;77:1007–1120.

51 Gladstone T, Buchholz KR, Fitzgibbon M, Schiffer L, Lee M, Van Voorhees BW. Randomized clinical trial of an internet-based adolescent depression prevention intervention in primary care: internalizing symptom outcomes. *Int J Environ Res Public Health.* 2020;17:7736.

6
Eating Disorders

Introduction

Eating disorders in adolescents are psychiatric issues that impair physical function-ing. Each is characterized by abnormal eating or weight control activities. Obesity, discussed in Chapter 1, is not an eating disorder. The *Diagnostic and Statistical Manual of Mental Disorders*, fifth edition, list six eating disorders: avoidant-restrictive food intake disorder (ARFID), binge eating disorder, pica, rumination disorder, ano-rexia nervosa, and bulimia nervosa. Although this chapter will focus on anorexia and bulimia that typically begin during adolescence, the remaining four eating disorders may be seen in adolescents.

ARFID typically begins in early childhood. Children with ARFID may have a smaller appetite and a limited repertoire of food. They may avoid all foods in certain groups, such as all fruits. These children tend to be thin, and they may have nutri-tional insufficiencies. As children with ARFID progress through adolescence, their parents may seek medical care because of the social issues that people with ARFID encounter. For example, it may become difficult to eat away from home, an activity that many adolescents enjoy together. Recent research from Sweden of twin pairs ages 6 to 12 years suggested that the heritability of ARFID was high at 79 percent, while nonshared environmental factors played a smaller but significant role at 21 percent.[1]

Binge eating disorder, which is more commonly seen in female adolescents than male adolescents, is characterized by the excessive eating of food during a single meal, far more than one would normally consume. Adolescents with this disorder often eat alone and feel disgusted, guilty, and embarrassed by how much food they consumed. They may not have compensatory behaviors, such as purging, that offset their intake of such large amounts of calories. These teens often have obesity and are beset by problems associated with high weight, such as type 2 diabetes.

Pica, which usually begins in childhood and is rarely seen in adolescents, is the on-going consumption of nonfood substances such as hair, pebbles, soap, and metal. The prevalence of pica is higher in people with intellectual disabilities.

Rumination disorder is characterized by the repeated regurgitation of food that is then chewed and swallowed or spit out. This rare disorder occurs in the absence of other eating disorders or general medical conditions such as gastroesophageal reflux disease.

More common among adolescents are anorexia nervosa and bulimia nervosa. Adolescents with anorexia have a distorted body image. This may include a percep-tion that they are overweight, even when they are not, and/or that their weight and body shape have an undue influence on their self-worth. These teens are fearful of gaining weight and becoming "fat," when they are actually underweight. All adoles-cents diagnosed with anorexia restrict their intake of calories (energy) so that they usually weigh less than 85 percent of their ideal weight, based on their height, gender, and age, and have a distorted body image and a fear of weight gain. In some instances, adolescents who are overweight or considered to have obesity may be diagnosed with anorexia if they have caloric restriction, body image issues, and fear of weight gain. Adolescents may further restrict their caloric intake by purging and/or using laxatives, diuretics, or both. In addition, adolescents may exercise excessively to maintain a low weight or lose more weight. There are two main types of anorexia: binge eating/purging type and restricting type. In one type, the adolescent engages in binge eating and purging regularly during the previous 3 months; in the other subtype, the teen does not engage in these actions during the same period of time.

Because adolescents with anorexia have weights that are below normal, they are at risk for a number of different medical problems and complications. These include low blood pressure, pulse, and body temperature; loss of menstruation; abnormal heart rhythm; electrolyte abnormalities; bone loss; blood count changes; and cognitive problems such as difficulties with memory.

It is well known that genetic and environmental factors may place some adolescents at increased risk for anorexia and that this disorder may aggregate in families. To learn more about the aggregation of anorexia in families, researchers from Denmark and Switzerland turned to a Danish national dataset of all people entering the public mental health system; they identified 2370 children and adolescents with anorexia. For each subject with anorexia, three control individuals without anorexia were identified in another Danish national dataset. As might be expected, the researchers learned that anorexia occurred more often in relatives of the subjects than in the relatives of controls. And there were statistically significant higher proportions of an affective disorder, such as depression, in the mother and siblings of the subjects.[2]

Researchers from many locations but based in North Carolina also examined the inherited or genetic basis of anorexia. Using data from the 1000 Genomes Project, they evaluated 3495 individuals with anorexia and 10,982 controls. From these data, the researchers learned that a significant locus on chromosome 12 was linked to anorexia. They also found significant genetic correlations between anorexia, schizophrenia, neuroticism (a trait disposition for negative affects including anger, anxiety, and emotional instability), and educational attainment. There also was a genetic overlap between anorexia and obsessive-compulsive disorder (OCD).[3]

Although bulimia is a different disorder than anorexia, there are a few similarities. The diagnostic criteria for bulimia include a history of recurrent episodes of binge eating followed by inappropriate behaviors to prevent weight gain. With binge eating, adolescents eat a larger-than-normal amount of food during a 2-hour period of time followed by self-induced vomiting; misuse of laxatives, diuretics, or enemas; and/or excessive exercising. By definition, these actions occur an average of once weekly for 3 months. Adolescents with bulimia have a disproportionate concern about weight and body shape. Medical complications with bulimia are often in the gastrointestinal tract. These include abdominal pain, blood in vomit, gastrointestinal reflux, diarrhea, constipation, irritable bowel syndrome, and rectal prolapse. Stomach acid may cause dental erosions. Adolescents with bulimia may have low potassium levels, and they may develop irregular heart rhythms. Electrolyte disturbances may be quite serious, even fatal.

Adolescents who have a family member diagnosed with bulimia have an increased risk of developing this disorder. It is not clear if the increased risk is a result of genetic, familial, or a combination of factors. There are currently several studies pursuing genome-wide investigations.[4]

Epidemiology of Eating Disorders

Using data from the National Comorbidity Survey Replication Adolescent Supplement, a nationally representative sample of adolescents between the ages of 13 and 18 years, researchers at the National Institutes of Health and several other institutions studied the epidemiology of eating disorders in adolescents. They wanted to estimate the 12-month and lifetime prevalence of eating disorders, examine the sociodemographic and clinical correlates of eating disorders, and describe the level of role impairment and suicidal behaviors. In this cross-sectional study, the adolescents participated in face-to-face interviews, and a parent of each teen completed a self-administered questionnaire. The researchers learned that the lifetime prevalence of anorexia was 0.3 percent equally distributed between the genders, and the median age of onset was 12.3 years. The lifetime prevalence for anorexia was highest for White adolescents at 0.4 percent. In addition, the lifetime prevalence for anorexia increased from 0.1 percent for those adolescents from families with incomes less than 1.5 times the poverty line to 0.4 percent for those at or greater than six times the poverty line. The prevalence rates were similar for urban, metropolitan, and rural youth. About 55 percent of adolescents with anorexia had another psychiatric diagnosis, most often oppositional defiant disorder, and 97.1 percent reported that anorexia impaired their daily lives. With respect to suicidality, 31.4 percent had a history of suicidal ideation, and 8.2 percent reported a suicide attempt. Meanwhile, bulimia had a lifetime prevalence of 0.9 percent, with the prevalence three times more common in female adolescents than in male adolescents. The median age of onset was 12.4 years. The highest lifetime prevalence for bulimia was 1.2 percent, which was found in families whose income was less than 1.5 times the poverty line; as family income increased, the lifetime prevalence was stable, averaging 0.8 percent. As with anorexia, the prevalence rates for bulimia were similar for urban, metropolitan, and rural youth. And adolescents with bulimia tended to have another psychiatric problem, most often an anxiety disorder, and 78 percent reported impairment of their daily lives. The lifetime suicidality measures were higher in all categories of bulimia, with 35.1 percent making at least one attempt at suicide.[5]

To understand trends in the hospitalization of children and adolescents for eating disorders in Ontario, Canada, researchers utilized a population-based, cross-sectional study. They were able to link several databases to identify individuals ages 5 to 17 years who had inpatient admissions for eating disorder diagnoses from 2002 to 2020. The findings included a 139 percent increase in pediatric admissions for eating disorders over the 17-year study period. The most impressive changes were increases found in male patients (416 percent), adolescents ages 12 to 14 years (196 percent), and patients with an eating disorder diagnosis other than anorexia or bulimia. These findings are important since there may be misperceptions about which pediatric patients are at risk for eating disorders, particularly in reference to males and younger adolescents. These misperceptions could lead to delay in diagnosis and treatment.[6]

Understanding the risk factors for the development of eating disorders in adolescents may help to shape prevention programs. Researchers from the Netherlands and New York wanted to learn the risk factors for 2229 preadolescents to develop eating disorders in young adulthood. They used data from the Tracking Adolescents' Individual Lives Survey, a Dutch population-based cohort study that follows preadolescents into young adulthood. Data were derived from age 11 years from subject self-reporting, parent reporting, and a review of the child's health preventive visit information. When the subjects were 19 years, they were screened by eating disorder experts; at ages 22 and 26, eating disorder pathology was measured with a scale. The researchers determined that 49 female subjects and 9 male subjects developed an eating disorder between the ages of 11 and 19 years. Female gender, high weight, and high levels of anxious distress in preadolescence (age 11) were consistently associated with the development of eating pathology in adolescence and young adulthood. (Anxious distress was defined as having at least two of the following: feeling keyed up or tense, unusual restlessness, difficulty concentrating because of worry, fear that something awful is going to happen, and feeling a potential loss of control.) The researchers concluded that generalized anxiety and social phobia were strongly associated with the development of an eating pathology.[7]

It should be mentioned that disordered eating is a global problem among children and adolescents. A group of investigators performed a systematic review and meta-analysis to determine the proportion among children and adolescents of disordered eating using the SCOFF (Sick, Control, One, Fat, Food) tool (a five-question screening measure for eating disorders). They determined from a review of 32 studies involving 16 countries that 22 percent of children and adolescents demonstrated disordered eating.[8]

Biopsychosocial Issues and Eating Disorders

Biological Issues and Eating Disorders

Obesity

Adolescent obesity is a risk factor for the development of an eating disorder. An adolescent who has obesity may have general body dissatisfaction, feel pressure to lose weight, and strive to be thin. Hurtful remarks about weight from friends, family members, or even physicians may trigger the onset of an eating disorder. Parents may easily encourage weight loss in their teen with overweight or obesity, and no one may realize that the weight loss is excessive until the teen has developed an eating disorder. If too much weight is lost, there may be problems with blood pressure, pulse rate, temperature, menstruation, and certain organ systems such as the liver and heart.

Risk for an eating disorder may occur in childhood. Researchers in Italy and Boston conducted a retrospective chart review of 537 adolescent and adult patients at the Italian Dietetic and Nutrition University Center. In this cohort, 118 had a history of an eating disorder and 419 had no such history. The researchers obtained information on the subjects' weight history, dieting behavior, and eating disorders diagnoses from the medical record. From these records, they learned that childhood-onset obesity was associated with a positive history of an eating disorder at a later age ($p < .05$).[9]

Researchers from Pennsylvania and Sweden found further evidence that a child's weight may be a risk factor for later onset of anorexia. They wanted to learn if there were differences in the body mass index (BMI) levels between teens with adolescent-onset anorexia and healthy controls. Their cohort consisted of 51 subjects with a mean age of 16.1 years at their anorexia assessment, which included a physical examination, a review of their growth charts, and an interview with a psychiatrist. Fifty-one matched controls participated in the same evaluation. The researchers found that the subjects who later developed anorexia had, between school grades 1 and 6, higher BMIs than the healthy controls, by an average of 1.42 BMI units.[10]

Additional evidence concerning the risk from being overweight as a child was noted by researchers at the Mayo Clinic and the University of Miami, who reviewed the charts of 170 adolescents with a mean age of 15.3 years seen for an eating disorder evaluation. They discovered that 17 percent of the adolescents had a history of a BMI above the 85th percentile, which defines overweight, and 19 percent had a history of a BMI above the 95th percentile, which defines obesity. Of note, the subjects with a history of overweight or obesity had a more significant drop in BMI at their clinic appointment than the subjects who had a history of normal-range weights/BMI. This indicated that they had delayed access to treatment, possibly because they had a delayed diagnosis.[11]

There is also an association between obesity and bulimia. Researchers in Spain and the United Kingdom studied 1383 female patients with an eating disorder; of these, 551 had bulimia. Their evaluations included a detailed weight history and comprehensive psychological assessments. About 29 percent of the patients had a history of lifetime obesity. Of the patients with bulimia, 33 percent had that history. The researchers observed that children, adolescents, and even adults with obesity have a lifetime risk for an eating disorder such as bulimia.[12]

Stress

Most adolescents with anorexia will recall a specific stressful event that prompted the onset of their eating disorder. Examples of such events include parental divorce, death of a grandparent, transition to middle school or high school, or a significant illness or injury. The COVID-19 pandemic, as a source of stress due to isolation, fear of disease, remote learning, and increases in family issues, has been correlated with a spike in eating disorders among adolescents. Australian researchers interviewed and surveyed 14 female adults who developed eating disorders during their adolescence, when they were gifted and high-achieving students. Each of the subjects reported stressful events before the onset of their disordered eating issues. They all noted academic issues that included academic pressure, possible bullying from teachers, and anxiety about future achievement. The majority had stressful events involving female peers, their families, or physical and body issues.[13]

If all adolescents experience upsetting and emotionally challenging events, why do only a small minority develop an eating disorder? While the answer is not clear, it is almost certainly the result of biopsychological factors. Studies on epigenetics and anorexia may provide a few answers. Researchers in London and Italy examined the literature on stress and eating disorders. They hypothesized that people with anorexia were more likely to have had greater adversity, such as abuse, during their early life, and their mothers probably had higher levels of anxiety during their pregnancies. These events, which may occur during so-called sensitive periods, such as the prenatal period, early childhood, and adolescence, may cause alterations in a person's response to stress. One example the researchers cited was Project Ice Storm, a progressive study that assessed the children of women exposed to severe ice storms during their pregnancies. The children had been studied and epigenetic changes had been documented. At age 13 years, the adolescents demonstrated high scores on the Eating Attitudes Test (EAT-26) consistent with an increased risk for an eating disorder. The researchers created the term "maltreated ecophenotype" to describe the teens who experienced these epigenetic changes and noted that they may be at risk for psychological issues. The researchers commented that there is sound evidence that people with eating disorders have this phenotype, and under certain conditions, such as social stressors or rejection, they may have an abnormal response that prompts an eating disorder.[14]

Psychological Issues and Eating Disorders

Anxiety/Depression

Researchers from Virginia and New Zealand investigated the prevalence of childhood and adult anxiety disorders in adult women with anorexia or bulimia. Are anxiety disorders, in fact, a risk factor for anorexia and bulimia? The cohort consisted of 68 women with anorexia, 116 women with bulimia, 56 women with major depression, and 98 controls. All subjects had structured interviews with trained clinicians. Of the subjects diagnosed with a lifetime anxiety disorder, 90 percent of those with anorexia, 94 percent of those with bulimia, and 71 percent of those with depression reported that the anxiety disorder predated the onset of the eating disorder or depression ($p = .01$). The odds ratio for overanxious disorder (13.4) and OCD (11.8) were significantly elevated for anorexia. With respect to bulimia, the odds ratio was 4.9 for overanxious disorder and 15.5 for social phobia. The researchers commented that a past history of anxiety was a risk factor for a subsequent eating disorder, and the data determined that a history of OCD or social phobia was a risk factor for future eating disorders. Medical providers and others should carefully monitor adolescents with histories of anxiety for the symptoms of an eating disorder.[15]

Hoping to learn more about the temporal relationship between anxiety and eating disorders, researchers from Louisiana and Oregon used data from the Oregon Adolescent Depression Project. It contained assessments of 1709 adolescents from 1987 to 1989 with a mean age of 16.6 years. Subsets of the teens were reevaluated with diagnostic interviews and questionnaires 1 year later, at their 24th birthdays, and at age 30. The researchers determined that OCD, which is a type of anxiety, was a unique predictor for subsequent anorexia. Likewise, they found that adolescents with bulimia were at a subsequent risk for developing social anxiety and panic disorders. Measures to monitor for and/or prevent anorexia should be directed to adolescents with OCD.[16]

It is possible, however, that certain adolescents may have some of the characteristics of anorexia such as a distorted body image or practice weight control measures but do not fulfill all the criteria for anorexia. Researchers in Canada, France, and Ireland wondered if females with subclinical anorexia had a higher risk for an anxiety or mood disorder. They used data from the Longitudinal Study of Kindergarten Children in Quebec, which periodically conducted diagnostic interviews with children/teens from kindergarten to age 16 years. From these data, the researchers learned that the females who had separation anxiety, which generally started in childhood, were at higher risk for subclinical anorexia. Female adolescents with subclinical anorexia should be evaluated for an anxiety or mood disorder, and those with anxiety and mood disorders should be assessed for subclinical eating disorders.[17]

Researchers from France, Switzerland, and Canada compared the frequency of mood disorders in females with anorexia or bulimia to a control group matched for age and gender. The age range of the subjects with anorexia was 15 to 30 years, and the range for those with bulimia was 15 to 40 years. The controls were matched to adolescents and young adults ages 15 to 24 years and to adults ages 25 to 40 years. The researchers determined that the subjects with anorexia and bulimia had significantly more mood disorders; in fact, they had approximately three to four times as many mood disorders as the control subjects. In about one-third of the women with anorexia or bulimia, the onset of major depression preceded the onset of the eating disorder.[18]

Substance Use

In almost every instance, adolescents with anorexia deny using substances such as alcohol, tobacco, marijuana, and other drugs. However, adolescents with bulimia may be at higher risk for substance abuse. Researchers in Spain studied 95 adolescents (95 percent female) aged 12 to 17 years who attended an eating disorders clinic and had a restrictive or purging eating disorder. To establish an eating disorder diagnosis, the clinic performed diagnostic interviews with measures for substance abuse. For the teens who had a restrictive disorder without purging, the researchers learned that 23 percent used alcohol, 16 percent used tobacco, and a small number used marijuana. For the adolescents who purged, as with bulimia (without a history of restriction), 46 percent used alcohol, 54 percent used tobacco, and 23 percent used marijuana. The data clearly indicated a higher risk for substance abuse in those adolescents with bulimia, and that adolescents with anorexia may deny substance use although some are using substances.[19]

Fisher and le Grange, researchers from Illinois, provided further evidence that adolescents with bulimia are at high risk for substance abuse. They studied adolescents who were in family-based treatment or individual supportive therapy to treat their bulimia. Their cohort consisted of 80 adolescents with a mean age of 16.1 years; 98 percent were female, and 59 percent were White. They were evaluated for high-risk behaviors, which were defined as behaviors that would predispose the subjects to later co-occurring psychiatric problems. Sixty-six percent had a high-risk alcohol use, 30 percent used illegal drugs, and 42 percent smoked cigarettes. Of note, 48 percent had depression and 25 percent had suicidal behavior. The researchers noted that their findings supported the high risk of substance abuse in adolescents with bulimia, as well as the presence of other psychiatric diagnoses, including depression. Many adolescents use alcohol or marijuana to self-treat depression. Clinicians should be aware that adolescents with bulimia might have a dual diagnosis—bulimia and substance abuse—which may require special treatment or program interventions.[20]

Social Issues and Eating Disorders

Social Media

Social media sites may play a pivotal role in promoting eating disorders in adolescents. At the same time, they may also help to prevent the development of such disorders by fostering user autonomy and the quick formation of interpersonal peer relationships. Characteristics of social media that are attractive to adolescents and relevant to eating disorders include high visual content with little text, carefully selected and curated information such as personal photographs, an interactive nature with peer feedback, lack of moderation, and a strong presence of commercial influences, which may direct specific content to the users based on their previous website views. It is not uncommon for teens to come together in social networks to create pro–eating disorder content. These groups promote the belief that disordered eating is a lifestyle choice rather than a mental health disorder. Teens, especially younger teens and those who are invested in their online appearance, are the most vulnerable to this misleading information. In addition to peer feedback, social media may also use social comparisons to promote eating disorders.[21]

Photo-based online platforms such as Instagram and TikTok have highly visual content that could easily support distorted eating. Hoping to learn more about these sites, researchers in Australia used a cross-sectional design to examine the relationship between social media use, activities on social media (such as taking selfies), valuation of body shape, body weight, body dissatisfaction, and dietary restraint. The cohort consisted of 101 females in grade 7, with a mean age of 13.1 years. The researchers measured social media exposure, photo activities including selfies, photo manipulation, questions on body image, dietary restraint, and internalization of the thin ideal. The researchers learned that the subjects who engaged in more social media–related selfie activities had higher levels of body-related and eating concerns. They significantly overvalued their body shape and weight, had more body dissatisfaction and dietary restraints, and had greater internalization of the thin ideal. The researchers suggested that active media use by young female adolescents might promote these body-related and eating concerns.[22]

Researchers in Australia wanted to learn more about the relationship between social media use and disordered eating in young adolescents. The cohort consisted of 996 private school students in grades 7 and 8 who lived in one of two Australian states; 53.6 percent were female. Data were collected during an eating disorder randomized controlled risk reduction trial. Assessments were made of disordered eating cognitions, disordered eating behaviors, and social media use. The researchers learned that disordered eating behaviors, including skipping meals, eating very little food, and binge eating, were reported by significantly more females than males, with more than half of the females saying they had at least one disordered eating behavior. At the same time, a significantly higher proportion of females had accounts with Instagram and Tumblr, while more males had Facebook. For both male and female adolescents, the frequency in disordered eating behaviors and cognitions increased in proportion to the number of social media accounts. In females, increases in daily time spent on Instagram and Snapchat were associated with higher disordered eating behaviors. The findings demonstrated that social media use, especially those platforms with a strong emphasis on image posting and viewing, was directly correlated with eating behaviors and cognitions in young adolescents. Preventive measures, such as increased parental surveillance and control of adolescent media usage, should be considered.[23]

Peer influence may have positive or negative effects on eating behaviors in adolescents. Researchers from New York performed a scoping review to determine how the social media use of peers influenced adolescent eating behaviors. They located six articles that met their criteria. There were a total of 1225 adolescents, aged 10 to 19 years, from the United States, United Kingdom, Sweden, Norway, Denmark, Portugal, Brazil, and Australia. The researchers determined that peer influence may pathologically encourage eating disorders, or it may be useful by promoting healthy eating. The researchers found a few studies in which adolescents provided one another with tips and strategies for anorexic or bulimic eating behaviors and extreme diets.[24]

Adolescents are a key target for corporate marketing as they are still developing and may lack the ability or motivation to counter the content of some advertisements. Researchers from Ireland and the United Kingdom investigated the responses of 151 adolescents, ages 13 to 15 years, to advertisements of unhealthy foods, healthy foods, and nonfood products (technology, games, sports, or cosmetics) in news feeds similar to Facebook. The sources of the three contents were peers, celebrities, or companies. When compared to healthy foods and nonfood products, unhealthy foods resulted in the most positive actions. The adolescents were more likely to share unhealthy food posts with their peers, and if their peers had unhealthy foods in their posts, they rated them with greater positivity. The adolescents spent more time viewing the unhealthy posts and recalled and recognized a larger number of unhealthy foods. Celebrities also had an important influence on unhealthy food choices.[25]

Given the importance adolescents place on peer interaction, social media may be used to support those with or without eating disorders. Researchers in the United Kingdom described an online discussion that appeared to provide such support. The forum was depicted as a safe space, with peer support for recovery and prevention, friendship, and forum moderation. Unfortunately, social media sites that promote healthy eating and body image are much less available than those promoting disordered eating.[26]

Researchers in the United Kingdom performed a scoping review of the literature to determine the relationship between social media usage, body image, and eating disorders in individuals ages 10 to 24 years. They examined 50 studies from 17 countries and determined that the usage of social media by individuals in this age group led to body image concerns, eating disorders and/or disordered eating, and poor mental health. The researchers concluded that social media usage is a risk factor for the development of eating disorders, and that this risk is present not only in Western countries but also in Asia.[27]

Problematic Internet Use

To determine if problematic internet use (PIU) had any correlation with eating disorders in students, researchers from Spain performed a systematic review and found 12 studies that met their criteria for the review, and 10 were included in a meta-analysis. The study sample consisted of 16,520 students from Turkey, Spain, China, the United States, Colombia, Egypt, and Taiwan. The majority were college students, and the sample size ranged from 314 to 2365. The researchers discovered that PIU was linked to anorexia, bulimia, and binge eating disorder. To reduce the risk of developing these problems, when adolescents begin using social media, parents should consider setting time limits and other interventions to prevent PIU.[28]

Racism/Discrimination

Researchers from multiple countries analyzed cross-sectional data from the Adolescent Brain Cognitive Development Study of 11,075 individuals ages 9 to 12 who were racially diverse. The data indicated that 4.7 percent of the individuals reported racial or ethnic discrimination. In addition, 1.1 percent met the criteria for binge eating disorders. The researchers concluded that children and adolescents who have experienced racial or ethnic discrimination, especially when this has been perpetrated by other students, had higher odds of having behaviors consistent with binge eating disorder.[29]

Transgender/Gender Incongruence

Adolescents with gender dysphoria often have body image issues, making it more difficult for clinicians to establish a diagnosis of anorexia or bulimia. Disordered eating may begin when a trans adolescent wants to lose weight to reduce breast size and suppress menstruation. The criteria to diagnose anorexia are most appropriate for cisgender females. Canadian clinicians described two of the first adolescents with gender dysphoria to have anorexia. The first patient was a 16-year-old biological male who had a history of food restriction and body image distortion, both of which led to significant weight loss and a diagnosis of anorexia. Subsequently, 1 year after his initial assessment, he asked to transition to female. At that time, his weight was stable, and he had stopped restricting food intake. The second case was a 13-year-old biological female with a history of food restriction, body image issues, anxiety and depression, parental divorce, and sexual abuse. During treatment, the patient expressed interest in transitioning to male and later began to dress in clothing typically worn by males. These two cases illustrate the importance of inquiring about gender issues when an adolescent presents with an eating disorder as well as monitoring for gender dysphoria during initial presentation and treatment.[30]

Further investigation on eating disorder issues and adolescents with gender dysphoria was performed by several researchers from Missouri who examined the associations of gender identity and sexual orientation with self-reported eating disorder diagnoses in college students. Using data from the National College Health Assessment, they had a cohort of 289,024 with a mean age of 20 years. The data showed that 479 (0.17 percent) identified as transgender, 5977 as cisgender gay males, 91,599 as cisgender heterosexual males, 9445 as cisgender lesbian females, and 176,467 as cisgender heterosexual females. The remaining were unsure males (1662) and unsure females (3395). In the entire sample, 4384 (1.52 percent) reported having been diagnosed with an eating disorder during the past year. In the sample, 8054 noted that they induced vomiting or used laxatives during the past month and 10,085 used diet pills as compensatory behavior, also during the previous month. The researchers found that the transgender students had higher rates of compensatory eating behaviors, and, when compared to the heterosexual female students, both the transgender students and the gay males had an increased rate of a self-reported eating disorder diagnosis during the previous year. These findings underscored the need to design appropriate targeted prevention and intervention efforts for this college-age population.[31]

Researchers in Boston wanted to determine the incidence of disordered weight management measures in transgender youth in high school. The researchers used data from 67 transgender, 1117 cisgender male, and 1289 cisgender female high school students, with a mean age of 16 years, from the 2013 Massachusetts Youth Health Survey. Most of the subjects had a BMI in the normal range. The researchers determined that when compared to cisgender males, transgender youth had significantly higher odds of fasting greater than 24 hours, as well as using diet pills and laxatives in the past 30 days to lose or maintain their weight. Moreover, during their lifetime, transgender adolescents had higher odds of using nonprescriptive steroids (for body building) than male cisgender subjects. These findings again confirmed that transgender youth in this study of high school age were likely to have unsafe disordered eating.[32]

Researchers in Connecticut, New Zealand, and Canada evaluated the risk and protective factors linked to disordered eating in transgender youth. They conducted an online survey of 923 transgender Canadian youth between the ages of 14 and 25 years. There were measures for harassment, bullying, and discrimination, and a history of violence that they termed "enacted stigma." Protective factors included connectedness to school, family, and friends, and social supports. The researchers noted that nearly half of the subjects between the ages of 14 and 18 years and more than a third of the subjects between the ages of 19 and 25 years engaged in disordered eating behaviors including binge eating, fasting, and/or using pills, laxatives, or vomiting to lose weight. The transgender youth who experienced enacted stigma had higher odds of disordered eating behaviors. However, those who had more family and school connectedness, caring friends, and social support had lower odds of disordered eating during the past year. These findings supported the important roles of family, schools, friends, and social supports in mitigating the effects of enacted stigma toward transgender youth.[33]

Violence

Abusive experiences during dating relationships may disrupt normal developmental processes in adolescents, including body image, that could lead to disordered eating behaviors. Researchers from Minnesota investigated the potential association between date-related violence and disordered eating in female victims. Using data from the Minnesota Student Survey (1998), the study included 81,247 students from 9th to 12th grade. Assessments included date violence, date rape, disordered eating behaviors, and suicide. Among the female adolescents, 4.2 percent reported date violence, as did 2.6 percent of the male adolescents. Of these, 1.4 percent of the females and 1.2 percent of the males indicated that the violence was rape. Although it occurs in both sexes, the female adolescents had a significantly higher rate of disordered eating behaviors, such as binge eating, fasting, or taking diet pills and vomiting ($p < .00001$). Those with a history of date violence or rape or both demonstrated a significant increase in disordered eating, including binge eating, fasting, skipping meals, taking diet pills or laxatives, and vomiting, for either sex. The researchers hypothesized that adolescents who have experienced date-related violence may have a disruption in their normal developmental processes with respect to their body image, which may lead to disordered eating beliefs and/or behaviors.[34]

Researchers from North Carolina, Sweden, and the United Kingdom wanted to learn if childhood, preadolescent bullying may be an etiological factor in the development of adolescent disordered eating. Using data from the prospective Great Smokey Mountain Study, they assembled information from 1420 subjects between the ages of 9 and 25 years. Assessments included childhood bullying and symptoms of eating disorders. The researchers learned that children who were bullied were at increased risk for developing the symptoms of anorexia and bulimia when they become adolescents. Bullies were at increased risk for the symptoms of bulimia. Surprisingly, there was a lack of evidence for any sex-specific associations, and the increased risk for eating issues did not extend into young adulthood—19 years and older.[35]

Weight-related peer teasing in younger adolescents appears to be a risk factor for disordered eating. While bullying refers to intimidation of a weaker person, teasing occurs when an adolescent makes fun of someone in a form that is playful or irritating. Researchers in Australia wanted to determine if this peer teasing may trigger a genetic and/or environmental risk for disordered eating in the victim. They analyzed data from 411 families with female adolescents who were twins. Slightly more than half were monozygotic ("identical"), and the remainder were dizygotic, except for seven pairs with unknown zygosity. During three waves, beginning around ages 14 to 17 years, the twins were interviewed, and the parents completed questionnaires and provided information needed to calculate the BMI levels of the twins. The twins were assessed with an eating disorder protocol and were asked about weight-related peer teasing. In the first wave, peer teasing was significantly correlated with symptoms of disordered eating and higher BMI. As levels of peer teasing increased, both genetic and environmental factors promoted distorted eating, though the genetic factors exerted more influence than the environmental ones. The researchers advised the development of targeted weight-related peer-teasing prevention programs for younger adolescents.[36]

Prevention

During the COVID-19 pandemic, there was concern about the increasing number of adolescents presenting with restrictive eating disorders, especially among females. No specific preventive programs were identified that were effective.[37] Based on research findings, preventive measures might include ensuring children and adolescents have weights in the normal range for their BMI. In addition, they should be screened for anxiety on a periodic basis and referred for treatment if indicated. Bullying in any form as well as weight- or appearance-based teasing must be discouraged. Adolescents should be educated on media literacy, and their social media viewing should be monitored. Importantly, parents, teachers, coaches, and clinicians should be very careful when commenting on the shape and body weight of adolescents, particularly for those who may be at risk for a potential eating disorder.

Treatment

The treatment of adolescents with eating disorders is usually complex and lengthy, necessitating a team approach that includes a primary care clinician, therapist, nutritionist, and possibly a psychiatrist as appropriate. Levels of care include outpatient, intensive outpatient, partial hospitalization, residential, and inpatient hospitalization, if the adolescent is medically unstable. Unlike other psychiatric illnesses, because there is a high likelihood for medical complications from anorexia and less so from bulimia, these adolescents need periodic medical assessments during treatment. Although focused individual therapy is useful for eating disorders, family-based treatment is a highly effective management tool for anorexia.[38-42] Bulimia tends to be treated with cognitive behavioral therapy and antidepressants such as sertraline.[43]

Conclusion

Factors that place adolescents at increased risk for eating disorders include overweight/obesity, anxiety, bullying and weight-based teasing, female gender, and use of social media, particularly those sites that focus on appearance and are highly visual. Adolescents diagnosed with an eating disorder should be referred to a multidisciplinary team for treatment. In general, earlier diagnosis and treatment lead to improved long-term outcomes.

References

1   Dinkler L, Wronski ML, Lichtenstein P, et al. Etiology of the broad avoidant restrictive food intake disorder phenotype in Swedish twins aged 6 to 12 years. *JAMA Psychiatr.* 2023;80:260–269.
2   Steinhausen HC, Jakobsen H, Helenius D, Munk-Jørgensen P, Strober M. A nation-wide study of the family aggregation and risk factors in anorexia nervosa over the generations. *Int J Eat Disord.* 2015;48:1–8.
3   Duncan, L, Yilmaz Z, Gaspar H, et al. Significant locus and metabolic genetic correlations revealed in genome-wide association study of anorexia nervosa. *Am J Psychiatry.* 2017;74:850–858.
4   Watson H, Palmos AB, Hunjan A, Baker JH, Yilmaz Z, Davies H. Genetics of eating disorders in the genome-wide era. *Psychol Med.* 2021;51:2287–2297.
5   Swanson SA, Crow SJ, Le Grange D, Swendsen J, Merikangas KR. Prevalence and correlates of eating disorders in adolescents. Results from the national comorbidity survey replication adolescent supplement. *Arch Gen Psychiatry.* 2011;68:714–723.

6   Smith S, Charach A, To T, Toulany A, Fung K, Saunders N. Pediatric patients hospitalized with eating disorders in Ontario, Canada, over time. *JAMA Netw Open.* 2023;6:e2346012.

7   van Eeden AE, Oldehinkel AJ, van Hoeken D, Hoek HW. Risk factors in preadolescent boys and girls for the development of eating pathology in young adulthood. *Int J Eat Disord.* 2021;54:1147–1159.

8   López-Gil JF, García-Hermoso A, Smith L, et al. Global proportion of disordered eating in children and adolescents: a systematic review and meta-analysis. *JAMA Pediatr.* 2023;177:363–372.

9   Cena H, Stanford FC, Ochner L, et al. Association of history of childhood-onset obesity and dieting with eating disorders. *Eat Disord.* 2017;25:216–229.

10 Berkowitz SA, Witt AA, Gillberg C, Rastam M, Wentz E, Lowe MR. Childhood body mass index in adolescent-onset anorexia nervosa. *Int J Eat Disord.* 2016;49:1002–1009.

11 Lebow J, Sim LA, Kransdorf LN. Prevalence of a history of overweight and obesity in adolescents with restrictive eating disorders. *J Adolesc Health.* 2015;56:19–24.

12 Villarejo C, Fernández-Aranda F, Jiménez-Murcia S, et al. Lifetime obesity in patients with eating disorders: increasing prevalence, clinical and personality correlates. *Eur Eat Disord Rev.* 2012;20:250–254.

13 Krafchek J, Kronborg L. Stressful life events experienced by academically high-achieving females before the onset of disordered eating. *Roeper Rev.* 2018;40:245–254.

14 Chami CM, Monteleone AM, Treasure J, Monteleone P. Stress hormones and eating disorders. *Mol Cell Endocrinol.* 2019;497:110349.

15 Bulik JM, Sullivan PF, Fear JL, Joyce PR. Eating disorders and antecedent anxiety disorders: a controlled study. *Acta Psychiatr Scand.* 1997;96:101–107.

16 Buckner JD, Silgado J, Lewinsohn PM. Delineation of differential temporal relations between specific eating and anxiety disorders. *J Psychiatr Res.* 2010;44:781–787.

17 Touchette E, Henegar A, Godart NT, et al. Subclinical eating disorders and their comorbidity with mood and anxiety disorders in adolescent girls. *Psychiatry Res.* 2011;185:185–192.

18 Godart N, Radon L, Curt F, et al. Mood disorders in eating disorder patients: prevalence and chronology of onset. *J Affect Disord.* 2015;185:115–122.

19 Castro-Fornieles J, Diaz R, Goti J, et al. Prevalence and factors related to substance use among adolescents with eating disorders. *Eur Addict Res.* 2010;16:61–68.

20 Fisher S, le Grange D. Comorbidity and high-risk behaviors in treatment-seeking adolescents with bulimia nervosa. *Int J Eat Disord.* 2007;40:751–753.

21 Saul J, Rodgers RF, Saul M. Adolescent eating disorder risk and the social online world: an update. *Child Adolesc Psychiatr Clin N Am.* 2022;31:167–177.

22 McLean SA, Paxton SJ, Wertheim EH, Masters J. Photoshopping the selfie: self photo editing and photo investment are associated with body dissatisfaction in adolescent girls. *Int J Eat Disord.* 2015;48:1132–1140.

23 Wilksch SM, O'Shea A, Ho P, Byrne S, Wade TD. The relationship between social media use and disordered eating in young adolescents. *Int J Eat Disord.* 2020;53:96–106.

24 Chung A, Vieira D, Donley T, Tan N, Jean-Louis G, Gouley KK. Adolescent peer influence on eating behaviors via social media: scooping review. *J Med Internet Res.* 2021;23:e19697.

25 Murphy G, Corcoran C, Tatlow-Golden M, Boyland E, Rooney B. See, like, share, remember: adolescents' responses to unhealthy-, healthy-, and non-food advertising in social media. *Int J Environ Res Public Health.* 2020;17:2181.

26 Kendal S, Kirk S, Elvey R, Catchpole R, Pryjmachuk S. How a moderated online discussion forum facilitates support for young people with eating disorders. *Health Expect.* 2017;20:98–111.

27 Dane A, Bhatia K. The social media diet: a scoping review to investigate the association between social media, body image and eating disorders amongst young people. *PLOS Glob Public Health*. 2023;3:e0001091.

28 Hinojo-Lucena FJ, Aznar-Díaz I, Cáceres-Reche MP, Trujillo-Torres JM, Romero-Rodriguez JM. Problematic internet use as a predictor of eating disorders in students: a systematic review and meta-analysis study. *Nutrients*. 2019;11:2151.

29 Raney JH, Al-Shoaibi AA, Shao IY, et al. Racial discrimination is associated with binge-eating disorder in early adolescents: a cross-sectional analysis. *J Eat Disord*. 2023;11:139.

30 Couturier J, Pindiprolu B, Finlay S, Johnson N. Anorexia nervosa and gender dysphoria in two adolescents. *Int J Eat Disord*. 2015;48:151–155.

31 Diemer EW, Grant JD, Munn-Chernoff MA, Patterson DA, Duncan AE. Gender identity, sexual orientation, and eating-related pathology in a national sample of college students. *J Adolesc Health*. 2015;57:144–149.

32 Guss CE, Williams DN, Reisner SL, Austin SB, Katz-Wise S. Disordered weight management behaviors, nonprescription steroid use, and weight perception in transgender youth. *J Adolesc Health*. 2017;60:17–22.

33 Watson RJ, Veale JF, Saewye EM. Disordered eating behaviors among transgender youth: probability profiles from risk and protective factors. *Int J Eat Disord*. 2017;50:515–522.

34 Ackard DM, Neumark-Sztainer D. Date violence and date rape among adolescents: associations with disordered eating behaviors and psychological health. *Child Abuse Negl*. 2002;26:455–473.

35 Copeland W, Bulik CM, Zucker N, Wolke D, Lereya ST, Costello EJ. Does childhood bullying predict eating disorder symptoms? A prospective, longitudinal analysis. *Int J Eat Disord*. 2015;48:141–149.

36 Fairweather-Schmidt AK, Wade TD. Weight-related peer-teasing moderates genetic and environmental risk and disordered eating: twin study. *Br J Psychiatry*. 2017;210:350–355.

37 Pellegrini D, Grennan L, Bhatnagar N, McVey G, Couturier J. Virtual prevention of eating disorders in children, adolescents, and emerging adults: a scoping review. *J Eat Disord*. 2022 Jul 6;10(1):94.

38 Society for Adolescent Health and Medicine, Golden NH, Katzman DK, Sawyer SM, et al. Position paper of the Society for Adolescent Health and Medicine: medical management of restrictive eating disorders in adolescents and young adults. *J Adolesc Health*. 2015;56:121–125.

39 Rome ES, Strandjord SE. Eating disorders. *Pediatr Rev*. 2016;37:323–136.

40 Brigham KS, Manzo LD, Eddy KT, Thomas JJ. Evaluation and treatment of avoidant/restrictive food intake disorder (ARFID) in adolescents. *Curr Pediatr Rep*. 2018;6:107–113.

41 Crone C, Fochtmann LJ, Attia E, et al. The American Psychiatric Association practice guideline for the treatment of patients with eating disorders. *Am J Psychiatry*. 2023;180:167–171.

42 Goldstein MA, Dechant EJ, Beresin EV. Eating disorders. *Pediatr Rev*. 2011;32:508–521.

43 Lock J, Le Grange D, Agras WS, Moye A, Bryson W, Jo B. Randomized clinical trial comparing family-based treatment with adolescent-focused individual therapy for adolescents with anorexia nervosa. *Arch Gen Psychiatry*. 2010;67:1025–1032.

7

Substance Use

Introduction

Adolescence is a high-risk developmental period for the use of substances. In the United States, adolescent substance use is a major public health problem. In 2019, 4777 adolescents and young adults between the ages of 15 and 24 years died from drug overdoses. Most were male, and 3391 of the deaths were caused by heroin or illegal opioids, some of which were contaminated with fentanyl. Benzodiazepines accounted for 727 deaths, and prescription opioids for 672. There were no deaths reported for marijuana alone.[1]

During adolescence, the vast majority of youth try alcohol, and about half experiment with an illicit drug. Many adolescents suffer biopsychosocial problems because of their substance use. Some of these problems include motor vehicle accidents, legal issues, and an increased risk for unwanted pregnancy and/or sexually transmitted infections.

Adolescents may be at risk when prescribed opioids or obtain these medications illicitly. Researchers at the Centers for Disease Control and Prevention reviewed overdose deaths by opioid type for adolescents ages 15 to 19 years old in 2010 and 2016. They found that the percentage of deaths involving prescription opioids that also involved illicit opioids including heroin or fentanyl was 5.5 percent in 2010 and 25.0 percent in 2016. Importantly, adolescent prescription opioid overdose deaths frequently involved illicit opioids. Adolescents with any nonmedical use of prescription opioids are an important risk group.[2]

Until around the age of 25 years, the adolescent and young adult brain continues to develop. The prefrontal cortex is involved in decision-making, which is based on previous memories and an assessment of rewards. It is also responsive to dopamine, known to play a role in positive responses and pleasure. Adolescents have a strong motivation for pleasurable activities, but their ability to evaluate the risks and benefits of drug use is still under development and may be flawed. As a result, this age group is a key target for abuse of substances, while also often a receptive participant in drug prevention programs.[3]

Many factors place adolescents at risk for substance use. On an individual level, adolescents with attention-deficit disorder, depression, or posttraumatic stress disorder have been shown to be at a higher risk for substance use. On a social level, peer relationships are a very important risk factor, as is a shared interest in abusing drugs or alcohol. As teens seek to be popular and improve their social image, peer pressure is a strong risk factor. Meanwhile, bully perpetrators have an increased risk of increased alcohol use, and adolescent gang members have higher rates of alcohol and marijuana use.

On the familial level, the risk factors for adolescent substance use include a history of child abuse and neglect. Such abuse and neglect may overstimulate the amygdala, causing it to produce excess amounts of dopamine, suppressing the function of the prefrontal cortex, specifically judgment. Moreover, witnessing domestic abuse and violence as a child may increase the risk for adolescent substance use to two or three times the usual rate.[4] The example set by parents is even more powerful than genetic influence, as teens who are exposed to substance abuse in the home are at very high risk of developing substance abuse disorder problems.[5]

Researchers in Virginia and California wanted to learn more about how genetic and environmental factors influence the use of alcohol, nicotine, and marijuana in adolescents. They turned to the Virginia Twin Registry and formed a randomly selected cohort that contained 1796 male twins with a mean age of 40.3 years. Detailed interviews enabled the researchers to obtain granular information about substance use from age 9 years through midadulthood. Zygosity was determined by self-reporting, photographs, and DNA studies. The researchers learned that in early adolescence both family and environmental influences, such as peers and the community, strongly impacted the use of alcohol, nicotine, and marijuana by teens. As adolescents and young adults matured, the effects of family and environment diminished, and by the age of 35 years they had disappeared for nicotine and marijuana and by the age of 40 years for alcohol. While genetic factors had no apparent influence on the use of these substances in early adolescence, genetics grew in importance as the subjects aged. The researchers hypothesized that the genetic effects become more apparent after people used the substances, and that genes played a more prominent role as people aged. That is, through genetic influences, people selected an environment that either encouraged or discouraged substance use.[6]

Substances may have adverse effects on the brains of adolescents. In particular, teens who use a heavy amount of marijuana often show changes in their neurocognitive performance and brain functioning. Researchers from Minnesota conducted a longitudinal study on adolescents with cannabis use disorder (CUD), a medical problem characterized by the problematic use of marijuana. The study included 22 subjects with CUD; 36.4 percent were female, and the group had a mean age of 17.0 years. There were 43 healthy controls; 46.5 percent were female, and the mean age was 15.9 years. The researchers determined that while only 2.3 percent of the controls had anxiety, 13.6 percent of those in the CUD group had anxiety. While none of the controls used nicotine, 45.5 percent of the CUD group used nicotine. After a diagnostic screening, measurements were taken of intelligence and executive functioning, and functional magnetic resonance images were administered. The trial continued for 18 months. During this time, the subjects in the control group had increases in resting functional connectivity between the anterior cingulate and superior frontal gyrus, which is normal. On the other hand, the subjects in the CUD group had some loss of connectivity in other areas of the brain known to mediate executive function. Further, those subjects who used high amounts of cannabis had a lower IQ and slower cognitive function.[7] Similar findings were noted by researchers from Minnesota who investigated the effect of cannabis on functioning during adolescence and young adulthood. Their cohort consisted of 3762 twins from three longitudinal studies; evaluations were conducted at six target ages ranging from 11 to 29 years. Measures included cannabis use and outcomes in young adulthood (24 to 29 years)—psychiatric disorders, cognitive ability, socioeconomic outcomes, alcohol and tobacco use, disruptive behavior problems, and academic functioning. The researchers discovered that cannabis use in monozygotic twins, who had shared genetic backgrounds and environments, may have led to impaired academic functioning during high school and downward socioeconomic issues, such as educational attainment, occupational status, and income building, in young adulthood. Adolescents who used high amounts of cannabis had a lower IQ.[8]

Researchers from Minnesota, Michigan, and Pennsylvania examined the reasons 12th-grade high school students had used marijuana. They used data from the Monitoring the Future Survey, which yielded an analytic sample of 39,964 adolescents, 47.6 percent female. The sample had subjects born from 1976 to 2016, and the measures included marijuana usage and reasons for marijuana use. The researchers found that over these decades, the use of marijuana for social and recreational reasons actually declined. The high school seniors who had used marijuana in recent years indicated that they used it to help relax, escape problems, "get through day," and gain insight. The movement toward using marijuana for coping-related reasons might be conducive to long-term use and possible significant side effects.[9]

Epidemiology of Substance Use

Swendsen and his colleagues in France used data from the National Comorbidity Survey Adolescent Supplement to study the use of alcohol and illicit drugs in U.S. adolescents. This nationally representative survey, which was conducted between 2001 and 2004, included diagnostic interviews for 10,123 subjects between the ages of 13 and 18 years and measurements for the lifetime estimates of alcohol and illicit substance use. They found that 1 in 10 adolescents between the ages of 13 and 14 reported the regular use of alcohol, and nearly 6 in 10 noted the regular use or abuse of alcohol at some point in their lives. Males and females had essentially equivalent rates of alcohol use, but males had higher rates of regular use and abuse. When given the opportunity, approximately 40.5 percent of the subjects used illicit drugs, and about 36.6 percent of the drug users met the criteria for substance abuse disorder.[10]

In 2021, the National Institute of Drug Abuse published a graphic, shown in Figure 7.1, that documented illicit drug use reported among adolescents. This graph shows fairly consistent illicit drug use by students from 2011 to 2020 with a decline in 2020–2021, especially in 10th grade students.[11]

Since 1975, the Monitoring the Future Survey has measured national adolescent drug and alcohol use, which provides a more detailed view of adolescent substance use. The survey has collected data on the past month use, past year use, and lifetime use of alcohol, cigarettes, Juul e-cigarettes, marijuana, and other illicit substances. From the survey it is apparent that the COVID-19 pandemic brought a reduction of teen drug use in certain sectors. Alcohol use trended downward, with sharp declines around 2020 to 2021. The lifetime prevalence of use in 12th graders has declined from

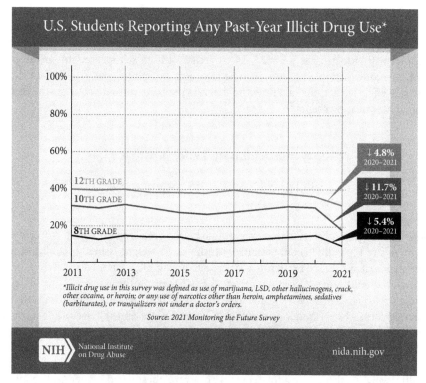

Figure 7.1 U.S. students reporting any past-year illicit drug use.
Source: National Institutes of Health. National Institute on Drug Abuse. 2021 Monitoring the Future Survey.

91.9 percent in 1976 to 54.1 percent in 2021. For marijuana, a sharp decline in 2020 to 2021 is also noted. Cigarette lifetime usage for 12th graders was 75.7 percent in 1976 and 17.8 percent in 2021. In 2019, 12th grader use of Juul was first measured; it was then 33.0 percent; in 2021, it was down to 28.5 percent.[12]

There are reasons for a decline in usage since the beginning of the pandemic. Researchers from Michigan noted that remote learning kept adolescents at home, where they may have had more supervision. Teens were unable to attend their usual gatherings, such as parties, where these substances would be readily available. Sources of substances were harder to find, and peer pressure to use substances diminished in social isolation. Finally, reduced academic and social stress from remote or hybrid learning may have lessened the perceived need to use substances to alleviate that stress.[13] Recent data obtained in 2023 indicated that the trend for adolescents reporting drug use has continued to hold to prepandemic levels.[14]

There has also been a decline in the use of e-cigarettes by adolescents. Until the end of 2019, the use of e-cigarettes in adolescents was steadily increasing, with 28 percent of high school students and 11 percent of middle school students using these products. That was followed by a sharp decline. These changes were promoted by at least two federal government actions. On December 20, 2019, a federal law was enacted that raised the minimum age to purchase tobacco products from 18 to 21 years. And in 2020, the Food and Drug Administration began to enforce the removal of flavored and cartridge-based e-cigarettes from stores; these products are popular with adolescents. In 2022, 14.1 percent of high school students and 3 percent of middle school students reported current e-cigarette use. These data demonstrate effective actions taken by the federal government to discourage the use of e-cigarettes in adolescents.[15]

Biopsychosocial Issues and Substance Use

Biological Issues and Substance Use

Obesity

Both obesity and substance abuse are public health concerns for youth. Adolescents with obesity typically become adults with the same weight issues. In addition, the prevalence of substance use tends to increase during high school and often persists into young adulthood. Using data from the Monitoring the Future Survey of 10th graders conducted in 2008 and 2009, researchers in Ohio, Arkansas, and Utah studied the association between adolescents with excess weight and the use of tobacco, alcohol, and illicit drugs. The survey included questions about body mass index (BMI), subject demographics, and various measures about substance use. The sample was 53 percent female with a mean age of 16.09 years. When compared to the teens with healthy weights, the White adolescents with severe obesity had higher odds of using an illicit substance. Specifically, the White teens with excess weight were more likely than the normal weight teens to experiment with alcohol and marijuana; and this experimentation took place at an earlier age, with them being drunk prior to ninth grade. In contrast, there were few significant findings for Black or Hispanic youth based on their weight. These findings suggested that focused prevention efforts directed to White teens who are overweight or have obesity may help prevent their use of substances.[16]

Researchers from Arkansas, Oklahoma, and Nebraska also investigated the relationship between severe obesity and the use of substances. They used data from the Youth Risk Behavior Surveillance System, which is a cross-sectional survey of a nationally representative sample of high school students. The data included 27,510 students from the 2015 and 2017 surveys. There were measures for alcohol, cigarettes, marijuana and illicit drug use, depressive symptoms, and demographics. After defining severe obesity as a BMI of 35 or higher, the researchers had a final sample of 1223 adolescents with this disorder. When data for both genders were combined, the researchers learned that 86.4 percent were nonusers, 7.1 percent were mild users, 2.4 percent were moderate users, and 4.1 percent were heavy users of substances. Those abstaining from the use of any substances had the poorest mental health. The researchers theorized that using substances helped the adolescents with severe obesity cope with an environment that they perceived as being hostile to individuals with obesity. And they advised that substance abuse prevention programs be targeted at adolescents with severe obesity.[17]

Psychological Issues and Substance Use

Suicidality and Self-Harm

To learn more about the association between substance abuse and suicidal issues in adolescents, researchers in Massachusetts and Italy performed a systematic review, and they located 17 papers that met their criteria. The researchers found that there was a high incidence of attempted and completed suicides in adolescents with substance abuse disorders. While there was no consensus on the cause, three themes emerged. First, substance abuse may cause a breakdown in personal relationships and an increase in suicide risk. Second, substance abuse triggers mood changes that could lead to suicidal ideation or depression and a suicide attempt. Third, substance abuse is intoxicating, which causes impaired judgment and suicide risk. The researchers concluded that there is a frequent association between substance abuse and suicidal behavior in adolescents.[18]

Since there is an association between adolescents who abuse substances and suicidal behaviors, researchers from North Dakota, Minnesota, Illinois, and Canada questioned which substances or other factors placed adolescents at increased risk for suicidal ideation or suicide attempts. They examined data from the Youth Behavioral Survey, which contained information on 11,328 teens from both public and private schools that was collected during the 2017 academic year throughout the United States. The surveyed students were in grades 9 through 12. The researchers calculated the adjusted odds ratio for suicidal ideation (with males at 1.00). Users of cigarettes or marijuana had an odds ratio of 1.71; targets of electronic bullying, 2.19, or physical bullying, 2.49; and victims of sexual violence, 1.81. All were statistically significant at $p < .001$. Students who used alcohol showed no increased risk of suicidal ideation, while playing on a sports team appeared to be protective, with an odds ratio of 0.72. Meanwhile, students who used marijuana and cigarettes had a significantly higher risk of suicide attempts, and victims of bullying or sexual violence had an increased risk for suicide attempts.[19]

Social Issues and Substance Use

Social Media

Among adolescents, the use of electronic media communication (EMC) (telephone, instant messaging, email, and text messages) and social media platforms is almost universal. Unless they have absolutely no access, very few adolescents refrain from using these outlets. Studies have shown an association between this usage and substance use among adolescents. Wanting to investigate the relationship between EMC and adolescent tobacco, alcohol, and marijuana use, researchers in the Netherlands, Germany, and Israel collected data from 5642 Dutch adolescents with a mean age of 14.29 years; 49.2 percent were male. The researchers designed measures for substance abuse, EMC, face-to-face interactions, average classroom substance use, and computer internet usage. The data were collected in a questionnaire completed in their classrooms. The researchers learned that EMC is positively linked to adolescent substance use, especially for alcohol. In addition, adolescents do not use EMC instead of face-to-face interactions; EMC complements their face-to-face interactions. The researchers suggested that adolescents use EMC to send images documenting their use of substances, particularly alcohol. They commented that substance use prevention programs should be structured to address online as well as offline communication and behaviors.[20]

Increasing time spent on social media appears to increase the risk of adolescent heavy drinking. Researchers in Norway examined the association between the amount of time adolescents spend on social media and their risk of episodic heavy drinking (EHD). Social media easily exposes adolescents to advertisements of substances as well as peer-to-peer favorable comments on the use of such substances. The researchers surveyed 851 students in middle and high school; 56.1 percent were male. They devised measures for heavy drinking, demographics, impulsivity, sensation seeking, symptoms of depression, and peer relationship problems. The researchers determined that the more time the adolescents spent on social media, the more frequently they tended to engage in EHD (odds ratio = 1.12, $p = .001$), a finding that remained valid even after controlling for the characteristics measured. The results were consistent with the belief that increasing amounts of time on the internet were associated with a higher likelihood of EHD.[21]

Is it the social media platforms or the connectivity between peers provided by these networks that foster substance use among adolescents? Using data from the 2019 Monitoring the Future Survey, researchers in New York City had a sample of 44,482 students in grades 8, 10, and 12 throughout the contiguous United States, representing approximately 400 public and private schools. A self-administered questionnaire measured the use of entertainment, social media, cell phones, substances, and behavioral issues, including sensation seeking, self-esteem, and depressive affect. Additionally, there were questions about sociodemographics and parental monitoring. The sample was 50.8 percent female, with a mean use of daily social media of 3.06 hours and a standard deviation of 2.90. During the previous 30 days, 15.7 percent of the adolescents used alcohol, 12.6 percent cannabis, 10.6 percent flavored vaping, 4.9 percent cannabis vaping, and 11.2 percent nicotine vaping. The researchers determined that the digital technology that required the interaction with others was associated with an increased risk of using alcohol, cannabis, or vaping. This association was consistent whether the adolescents texted, made phone calls, or participated in video chats. The researchers concluded that it is not the technology itself, but the networks of adolescents that are the social drivers of substance use in this population.[22]

In some cases, however, the platform itself may facilitate increased substance use. Researchers from multiple institutions in the United States studied the relationship between social media use and vaping in adolescents living in Florida. They used data from the 2019 Florida Youth Tobacco Survey with 10,776 subjects in which vaping status was described as experimental or current, and social media use was noted as nondaily or daily in one of four platforms: Facebook, Instagram, Twitter, or Snapchat. Users of these platforms must be at least 13 years old. The researchers determined that all four of the platforms were significantly associated with a vaping status ($p < .001$). Snapchat, in particular, was more consistently associated with experimental or current vaping (adjusted relative risk ratios 2.38 and 5.09). Snapchat allows for peer-to-peer messaging with features that may easily support vaping behavior. Since content on Snapchat disappears after viewing, this makes it more difficult for parents to know if their adolescents are being lured into e-cigarette marketing.[23]

Problematic Internet Use

In adolescents, problematic internet use (PIU) is considered an addictive behavior similar to abuse of substances. Hoping to learn more about the relationship between PIU and substance use in adolescents between the ages of 13 and 18 years, researchers from South Korea and Utah examined data from the Korea Youth Risk Behavior Web-based Survey with 73,238 middle school and high school students. After collecting data in six fields—demographics, smoking, alcohol, drugs, psychiatric illness, and internet use—the researchers learned that 11.9 percent of the subjects were at a potential risk for PIU and 3.0 percent were at a high risk, and these students had an increasing prevalence of alcohol, tobacco, and drug use. The researchers noted that smoking (p = .004) and drug use (p < .001) were potential predictors for high-risk PIU, and they cautioned that students with PIU have a vulnerability for addictive behaviors and should be evaluated for substance abuse disorder.[24]

There is evidence that PIU may be associated with substance use in young adolescents. Researchers from Switzerland examined the association between PIU and substance use in younger adolescents. The 3067 subjects who completed their survey were in their eighth year of school; 50.3 percent were female, and the cohort had a mean age of 14.2 years. The measures included PIU and substance use. The researchers discovered that 360 students, 57.6 percent female, had PIU. Compared to regular users of the internet, those with PIU had a history of current smoking, and during the previous 30 days they misused alcohol, cannabis, and other illegal drugs. Each of the substances used by the PIU group was statistically significant at p < .001. The researchers concluded that young adolescent students with PIU were vulnerable to other addictive behaviors.[25]

Researchers in London, Israel, and Qatar evaluated the ability of the parent/child relationship to offer some protection from substance use for adolescents with PIU. A total of 1613 students from the United Kingdom completed a questionnaire that contained researcher-designed measures for evaluating the parent/child relationship, PIU, substance use, cigarette smoking, bullying and victimization, and cyberbullying and victimization; the students were between the ages of 10 and 16 years, 47 percent female. The researchers confirmed that PIU was a risk factor for substance use in adolescents. However, a good parent/child relationship offered protection against substance use for teens with PIU. Further, the correlation between PIU and substance use was partially promoted by a teen's involvement in traditional bullying and cyberbullying.[26]

Poverty

Although poverty is a risk factor for other issues such as cognitive and psychosocial development, it is generally not a risk factor for substance abuse in adolescence. Researchers at the University of Michigan wanted to learn more about the relationship between familial socioeconomic status (SES) and abuse of substances in young adults. The three SES indicators examined were family income, family wealth, and parental education. The behaviors studied included smoking, drinking, heavy episodic drinking (HED), and marijuana use. To facilitate the analysis, the researchers used data from the Panel Study of Income Dynamics (2011), a nationally representative longitudinal household survey. The Panel Study is composed of approximately 5000 households and 18,000 individuals. In the sample, 97.2 percent of the subjects were ages 17 to 22 years and 51.5 percent were female. Family income and wealth were categorized as bottom or top quartiles. The measures included questions on substance use, as well as the three SES indicators. According to the findings, cigarette smoking was more common in young adults with fewer financial resources, while the use of alcohol, marijuana, and HED were more prevalent in households with greater resources. The researchers also observed a convergence across the three SES indicators of the various substances. For example, marijuana use in young adults tended to increase with family income, wealth, and parental education. In contrast, current smoking tended to decrease as the income, wealth, and parental education increased. The researchers suggested that substance abuse prevention programming should focus on groups that have high risk; thus, for example, an antismoking program would be directed to adolescents from lower-income families.[27]

The life stressors associated with growing up in poverty may presage initiation and escalation of drug use during adolescence. African American adolescents who experience childhood poverty more than any other ethnic group in the United States use drugs less frequently during adolescence than White adolescents. Researchers in Georgia analyzed 385 African American families from impoverished communities in the rural South. With the hypothesis that growing up in poverty was associated with biological stress that would foster substance abuse issues in young adulthood, this prospective study began when the adolescents were 11 years old and continued for 14 years. The researchers believed that supportive parenting would protect the biological stress levels (catecholamines) from rising and result in lower levels of substance use. At the beginning of the study, the average age was 11.7 years, and 53 percent were female adolescents; measures were performed at ages 11 to 13 years and 16 to 18 years. Additional measures assessed parental support and nurturant-involved parenting. Cigarette smoking, alcohol use, heavy drinking, and marijuana were quantified at ages 19 and 25; at age 19, catecholamines were assessed. The data indicated that highly supportive parenting for adolescents living in poverty between the ages of 11 and 18 years was associated with lower catecholamine levels at age 19, while low supportive parenting was associated with rising levels at the same time. Higher catecholamine levels at age 19 years were linked to an increased risk in substance use from ages 19 to 25 years. The researchers concluded that supportive parenting could protect African American youth living in poverty from increasing biological stress during adolescence. An implication of this study is that the presence of a caring, supportive parent is a key protective factor that could prevent children who grow up in poverty from experiencing impaired health profiles in adulthood. A family-centered preventive intervention to enhance supportive parenting could be offered in pediatricians' offices, and this may have stress-buffering effects for adolescents who grow up in poverty.[28]

Transgender/Gender Incongruence

It is well known that gender minority adolescents experience discrimination and are at risk for bullying, which may lead to adverse health risks. Researchers from Massachusetts, New York, and California wanted to determine if gender minority adolescents who experienced bullying also had an increased risk of substance use. They used data from the Teen Health and Technology Study that was collected online from 2010 to 2011 from 5907 U.S. teens between the ages of 13 and 18 years. The measures included gender minority identification, questions on substance use, and bullying experiences. The data identified 11.5 percent of the subjects as gender minority. When compared to the cisgender subjects, gender minority adolescents had a higher rate of ever drinking alcohol, smoking cigarettes, using marijuana, and using any nonmarijuana illicit drug ($p < .0001$). And they were more likely to have experienced bullying during the previous 12 months ($p < .0001$). The researchers commented that bullying mediated the increased odds of substance use in gender minority adolescents. Early interventions to prevent bullying for gender minority teens may be useful to prevent future adverse health risks such as substance abuse or a substance abuse disorder.[29]

To learn more about the disparities that gender minority adolescents may experience, the Centers for Disease Control and Prevention developed gender-related questions for the 2017 Youth Risk Behavior Survey (YRBS). Conducted every other year, the YRBS obtains information from a representative sample of U.S. high school students in grades 9 to 12. The questions were designed to determine the prevalence of transgender students and further understand the violence victimization, substance use, suicide risk, and sexual risk these students might encounter. The data pooled for this analysis had 131,901 students. The researchers learned that 1.8 percent of the students indicated that they were transgender, and when compared to the cisgender students, these students had significantly increased odds for the lifetime use of cigarettes, alcohol, marijuana, cocaine, heroine, methamphetamines, ecstasy, inhalants, and prescription opioid misuse. Moreover, when compared to cisgender students, they had significantly increased odds of violence victimization, suicide, and several areas of sexual risk. The findings affirmed the need for intervention efforts that improve health outcomes and risky behaviors such as substance use for transgender youth.[30]

Researchers from Connecticut, New Zealand, British Columbia, and Boston wanted to understand why transgender youth had an increased risk for using substances. They used a subset of data from the Canadian Trans Youth Health Survey that was compiled online between October 2013 and May 2014; it included 323 adolescents with a mean age of 16.67 years. The researchers developed a 29-question measure for enacted stigma that included such items as physical and sexual abuse, bullying, and harassment. There were also measures for school and family connectedness, perception of friends caring, and substance use. As expected, the researchers found a high rate of substance use in these transgender youth, with about one-quarter smoking cigarettes or marijuana during the previous month. Higher rates of substance use were seen in those who reported a history of high-enacted stigma, while family and school connectedness were protective factors against substance use. The findings demonstrated that the discrimination, harassment, and violence (enacted stigma) directed toward transgender youth were risk factors for their use of substances. Preventive efforts for transgender youth and substance use should account for these risk and protective factors when creating and delivering programs.[31]

Mortality

There is concern about whether the loss of a parent to natural death, accident, or suicide increases the risk of subsequent substance use in adolescents. Researchers at the University of Michigan, Duke University, and the RAND Corporation examined psychiatric symptoms in adolescents and young adults after the death of a parent. Using the Great Smokey Mountain Study, they formed a sample of 172 parent- or parental figure–bereaved youth between the ages of 11 and 21 years. The researchers compared three groups: parent-bereaved youths, bereaved youth resulting from the death of another relative, and youth who were not bereaved. During three waves, parents and their children had psychiatric assessments. The first wave took place shortly after the death; for the nondeath youth, a random wave was selected. Waves were held an average of 18 months apart. The researchers determined that by the second wave, a greater proportion of bereaved youth exhibited substance use problems. This was consistent with previous research which demonstrated that youth had increased risk for substance use 21 months after the death of a parent. The symptoms were generally subclinical, meaning they appeared to be normal variations of behavior. However, there was a notable risk of substance abuse issues in these youth, so screening and prevention programs should be considered for this group.[32]

Since bereaved adolescents appeared to be at higher risk for substance use, research groups attempted to delineate why this risk occurred. Researchers in Israel and Pennsylvania explored the effects of parental bereavement on alcohol and substance use in adolescents. They wanted to learn if the incidence of alcohol and substance issues were higher in this group, and if so, what were the explanations for this elevation. Using data from a longitudinal population-based study conducted between November 2002 and December 2012, the researchers devised a cohort with 235 youth and young adults between the ages of 7 and 25 years whose parent had died suddenly from suicide, an accident, or sudden natural causes. The control group consisted of 178 youth who were not bereaved. The subjects were interviewed and assessed at 9, 21, 33, and 62 months after the death, with parallel timing for the nonbereaved controls. The researchers learned that the bereaved youth had higher rates of alcohol and substance abuse or dependence (ASAD) than the members of the control group (13.6 percent versus 5.6 percent). Though the researchers found that bereaved youth were at increased risk for ASAD over a 5-year period after a parental death, when they controlled for conduct or oppositional defiant disorder and functional impairment, the effect of bereavement was attenuated. This suggested that bereavement may have an overall impact on the functioning of the bereaved youth, leading to the possible development of a disruptive behavior, which in turn promotes ASAD. Interventions could include programming to improve bereaved youth functioning, such as a close and supportive relationship with an adult.[33]

Violence

Children and adolescents who experience violence are at increased risk for substance use. Childhood mistreatment, such as abuse, has been shown to be a risk factor for the early onset of substance use. Male adolescents are more likely to be physically abused, and female adolescents are at increased risk for sexual victimization. Bully perpetration is associated with later alcohol use.[34]

Researchers in Ohio studied the relationship between exposure to violence and early substance use in adolescents who were prenatally subjected to drugs. The longitudinal study examined substance use in high-risk 12-year-old adolescents and attempted to determine if the symptoms of trauma such as anxiety, depression, anger, and posttraumatic stress disorder mediated the relationship between violence and early substance use. The cohort consisted of 297 adolescent-caregiver dyads, and the adolescents had a history of prenatal cocaine/polydrug exposure. Patients were assessed at ages 10, 11, and 12 years. Measures included violence exposure, youth substance use, and trauma symptoms. Violence was evaluated at age 10 years using the Assessment of Liability and Exposure to Substance Use and Antisocial Behavior Scale. This scale is an illustration-based, audio, computer-assisted child self-report interview that measures early manifestations and predictors of substance use and antisocial behaviors.[35] The researchers learned that at age 12 there was a direct relationship between violence exposure and tobacco/illegal drug use in both genders. There was an indirect association between violence exposure and alcohol use in females. The researchers noted that the early screening of adolescents for exposure to violence may result in earlier interventions.[36]

To understand the link between childhood violence and cannabis use and dependence in adolescents, researchers in Mexico performed a systematic review and meta-analysis and located six studies that met their criteria. The studies included 10,843 adolescents of both sexes. The researchers learned that the adolescents who had been victimized physically or sexually or had witnessed violence during childhood were at increased risk of abusing or having a dependence on cannabis during adolescence. The adolescents in the study who had experienced sexual abuse had the highest risk for cannabis use.[37]

Whether performed as a perpetrator or suffered as a victim, bullying is a type of violence. A research group in the Netherlands wanted to learn if bullies or victims of bullying in childhood or adolescence were at risk for later substance use. When compared to their nonbullying peers, would children and adolescents who were bully perpetrators have a higher risk for drug, alcohol, and tobacco use later in life? The researchers hypothesized that these teens would indeed be at increased risk. To test their hypothesis, the researchers conducted a meta-analysis and located 28 publications with 28,477 subjects under the age of 18 years that met their criteria. The researchers learned that children and adolescents who bullied had a higher risk of drug, alcohol, and tobacco use later in life. Additionally, bullying perpetration that occurred during childhood was more strongly linked to later drug, alcohol, and tobacco use than bullying that took place during adolescence. And finally, tobacco use later in life was predicted by bullying victimization. The researchers underscored the importance of bullying prevention programming beginning in childhood.[38]

Treatment

Treatment for adolescents with substance use issues begins with screening. The screening process may identify those teens that need a brief intervention by the clinician or follow-up or a referral to a treatment source.[39] One of the most commonly used screens is the CRAFFT questionnaire, consisting of three screening questions. If the answers to each of the three questions are negative, then no further action is needed. If any answer is positive, then six more questions are answered with recommended dispositions.[40] The Screening to Brief Intervention tool consists of one question on the frequency of using eight types of substances in the past year: tobacco products, alcohol, marijuana, illegal drugs, prescription drugs not prescribed for the subject, over-the-counter medications, inhalants and herbs, or synthetic drugs. The responses include never, once or twice, monthly, weekly, almost daily, and daily. The tool is validated, and the results triage the adolescents into four actionable categories: no past-year substance use, past-year substance use without a substance use disorder (SUD), mild or moderate SUD, and severe SUD. From the results, the clinician is able to direct the patient into appropriate treatment.[41]

On an individual level, a therapist may help the adolescent focus on building insight into the role that substances play in their life. From there, the therapist is able to assist the adolescent in establishing and maintaining abstinence. The skills involved include recognizing the triggers for substance use, managing urges to use, and learning to deal with emotional issues without turning to substances. Cognitive behavioral therapy is one therapeutic modality that may be utilized by the therapist. Comorbid mental health conditions, such as depression, may be treated with medication.

Group therapy exposes the adolescent to others with similar issues. Recognizing that other adolescents struggle with substances and allowing the adolescent to obtain support and advice from peers are helpful. The message from a peer may be heard while the same message from a therapist or parent may not be heeded.

Often, adolescents with a SUD obtain the most effective treatment if the family is involved. The therapist may advise parents on how to manage their adolescent's issues with substances. In addition, since adolescents frequently model behaviors of their parents, it encourages a parent with a SUD, if present, to be treated by another therapist.

In some situations, an adolescent with a SUD needs more intensive treatment than outpatient therapy. When this occurs, inpatient programs may provide that treatment in a safe, structured, and highly supervised environment. These programs are especially suited for those adolescents who have developed a physiological dependence on a substance, as they can be monitored for withdrawal symptoms and the medical consequences of the withdrawal.[42]

By performing a meta-analysis, researchers from Tennessee studied the comparative effectiveness of outpatient treatment of adolescents with a SUD. A literature search identified 45 eligible studies. Adolescents in almost all types of treatment showed reductions in substance use. However, the greatest improvements were found for family therapy and mixed and group counseling. The researchers concluded that family therapy is the treatment with the strongest evidence of comparative effectiveness for adolescents with a SUD.[43]

Prevention

Although it may be difficult to prevent adolescent experimentation with substances, there are protective factors against adolescent substance use. See Table 7.1.

Researchers in New York studied the association between patterns of adolescent use of time and substance usage. They utilized data from the Monitoring the Future Survey with students in grades 8, 10, and 12 from 1991 to 2019. The data were gathered through annual surveys of adolescents, and the measures included the adolescents' time use and substance use. They divided time use into six profiles: working at a paid job and the other five defined by levels of socialization (low/high) and engagement in structured activities such as sports (engaged/disengaged). Those adolescents in the high social/engaged group were further split by levels of unsupervised social activities. While substance use in general had declined over the several decades studied, use was high in those groups with high levels of social time, especially those with low engagement in structured activities, low supervision, or paid employment.[44] These findings are consistent with the protective effects of extracurricular activities and sports against substance use in adolescents.

Researchers from Oregon reviewed programs on the prevention of adolescent substance use. Family-based prevention programs focus on providing education to families, improving the quality of family relations, and teaching key family management skills. The goal is to transform the way parents manage and monitor adolescent behavior. Studies have shown their efficacy in reducing substance use in adolescents. School-based programs targeting substance use may have teachers delivering content on changing attitudes, normative beliefs, and/or resistance skills. These programs may have a small effect on moderating adolescent substance use. Community interventions targeting adolescent access to alcohol and tobacco may also be effective. One program, Reward & Reminder, was a community-based preventive program against sales of tobacco products to adolescents. In this program, underage adolescents would attempt to purchase tobacco products at retailers; if they were in compliance, the retailer would receive a reward card that praised and recognized them for their compliance and their initiative to help prevent youth access to these products. Otherwise, they would receive a reminder card asking them to verify age before selling. Other policy interventions such as restrictions on marketing, economic policies,

Table 7.1 Protective Factors Against Adolescent Substance Use[a]

Domain	Factors
Individual	Resilience, high impulse control and regulation
Parents	Positive role modeling, limit setting, emotional support, enforcement of rules
Peers	Non-substance-using peers
School	Positive role modeling, programming, sports, extracurricular activities
Community	Low availability of substances; zero-tolerance policies

[a] Goldstein MA, ed. *The MassGeneral Hospital for Children Adolescent Medicine Handbook*. 2nd ed. Springer Nature; 2017.

and retail licensing and tax policies may also be effective in curtailing adolescent substance use.[45]

Conclusion

Substance use by adolescents is a major public health problem in the United States that is associated with biopsychosocial issues that include social media use, PIU, and violence. There are multiple levels of care that may provide treatment to adolescents with substance use issues including the primary care clinician. Prevention efforts may include parents, schools, communities, and governmental entities.

References

1   Spencer MR, Minino AM, Warner M. Drug overdose deaths in the United States, 2001–2021. NCHS Data Brief, no 457 Hyattsville, MD: National Center for Health Statistics 2022.
2   Bohm MK, Clayton HB. Nonmedical use of prescription opioids, heroin use, injection drug use, and overdose mortality in U.S. adolescents. *J Stud Alcohol Drugs*. 2020;81:484–488.
3   Garofoli M. Adolescent substance abuse. *Prim Care*. 2020;47:383–394.
4   Whitesell MA, Bachand A, Peel J, Brown M. Familial, social, and individual factors contributing to risk for adolescent substance use. *J Addict*. 2013;2013:579310.
5   Hazen EP, Goldstein M, Goldstein MC. *Mental Health Disorders in Adolescents: A Guide for Parents, Teachers, and Professionals*. Rutgers University Press; 2011.
6   Kendler K, Schmitt E, Aggen SH, Prescott CA. Genetic and environmental influences on alcohol, caffeine, cannabis, and nicotine from early adolescence to middle adulthood. *Arch Gen Psychiatry*. 2008;65:674–682.
7   Camchong J, Lim KO, Kumra S. Adverse effects of cannabis on adolescent brain development: a longitudinal study. *Cereb Cortex*. 2017;27:1922–1930.
8   Schaefer JD. Hamdi NR, Malone SM, et al. Associations between adolescent cannabis use and young-adult functioning in three longitudinal twin studies. *Proc Natl Acad Sci USA*. 2021;118:e2013180118.
9   Patrick ME, Evans-Polce RJ, Kloska DD, Maggs JL. Reasons high school students use marijuana: prevalence and correlations with use across four decades. *J Stud Alcohol Drugs*. 2019;80:15–25.
10 Swendsen J, Burstein M, Case B, et al. Use and abuse of alcohol and illicit drugs in US adolescents: results of the national comorbidity survey—adolescent supplement. *Arch Gen Psychiatry*. 2012;69:390–398.
11 Monitoring the Future 2021 Survey Results. U.S. students reporting any past-year illicit drug use. National Institute on Drug Abuse, National Institutes of Health, December 15, 2021.
12 Johnston LD, Miech RA, O'Malley PM, Bachman JG, Schulenberg JE, Patrick ME. Monitoring the Future national survey results on drug use. 1975–2021: Overview, key findings on adolescent drug use. Ann Arbor: Institue for Social Research, The University of Michigan; 2022.
13 Lundakl L, Cannoy C. COVID-19 and substance use in adolescents. *Pediatr Clin North Am*. 2021;68:977–990.
14 National Institutes of Health. News Release. Reported drug use among adolescents continued to hold below pre-pandemic levels in 2023. December 13, 2023.

15 Cooper M, Park-Lee E, Ren C, Cornelius M, Jamal A, Cullen KA. Notes from the field: e-cigarette use among middle and high school students—United States, 2022. *MMWR Morb Mortal Wkly Rep.* 2022;71:1283–1285.

16 Zeller MH, Becnel J, Reiter-Purtill J, Peugh J, Wu YP. Associations among excess weight status and tobacco, alcohol, and illicit drug use in large national sample of early adolescent youth. *Prev Sci.* 2016;17:483–492.

17 Becnel JN, Giano Z, Williams AL, Merten MJ. Profiles of substance use in adolescents with severe obesity. *Youth Soc.* 2022;54:201–220.

18 Pompili M, Serafini G, Innamorati, M. Substance abuse and suicide risk among adolescents. *Eur Arch Psychiatry Clin Neurosci.* 2012;262:469–485.

19 Labuhn M, LaBore K, Ahmed T, Ahmed R. Trends and instigators among young adolescent suicide in the United States. *Public Health.* 2021;199:51–56.

20 Gommans R, Stevens R, Finne E, Cillessem HN, Boniel-Nissim M, Bogt TFM. Frequent electronic media communication with friends is associated with higher adolescent substance use. *Int J Public Health.* 2015;60:167–177.

21 Brunborg GS, Andreas JB, Kvaavik E. Social media use and episodic heavy drinking among adolescents. *Psychol Rep.* 2017;120:475–490.

22 Kaur N, Rutherford CG, Martins SS, Keyes KM. Associations between digital technology and substance use among U.S. adolescents: results from the 2018 Monitoring the Future Survey. *Drug Alcohol Depend.* 2020;213:108124.

23 Lee J, Tan ASL, Porter L, Young-Wolff KC, Carter-Harris L, Salloum RG. Association between social media use and vaping among Florida adolescents. *Prev Chronic Dis.* 2021;18:E49.

24 Lee YS, Han D, Ki SM, Renshaw PF. Substance abuse precedes internet addiction. *Addict Behav.* 2013;38:2022–2025.

25 Rücker J, Akre C, Berchtold A, Suris JC. Problematic internet use is associated with substance use in young adolescents. *Acta Paediatr.* 2015;104:504–507.

26 Samara M, Massarwi A, El-Asam A, Hammuda S, Smith PK, Morsi H. The mediating role of bullying and victimization on the relationship between problematic internet use and substance abuse among adolescent in the U.K.: the parent-child relationship as a moderator. *Front Psychiatry.* 2021;12:493385.

27 Patrick ME, Wightman P, Schoeni RF, Schulenberg JE. Socioeconomic status and substance use among young adults: a comparison across constructs and drugs. *J Stud Alcohol Drugs.* 2012;73:772–782.

28 Barton AW, Yu T, Brody GH, Ehrlich KB. Childhood poverty, catecholamines, and substance use among African American young adults: the protective effect of supportive parenting. *Prev Med.* 2018;112:1–5.

29 Reisner SL, Greytak EA, Parsons JT, Ybarra M. Gender minority social stress in adolescence: disparities in adolescent bullying and substance use by gender identity. *J of Sex Res.* 2015;52:243–256.

30 Johns MM, Lowry R, Andrzejewski J, et al. Transgender identity and experience of violence victimization, substance use, suicide risk, and sexual risk behaviors among high school students—19 states and large urban school districts. *MMWR Morb Mortal Wkly Rep.* 2019;68:67–71.

31 Watson RJ, Veale JF, Gordon AR, Clark BA, Saewyc EM. Risk and protective factors for transgender youths' substance use. *Prev Med Rep.* 2019;15:100905.

32 Kaplow JB, Saunders J, Angold A, Costello EJ. Psychiatric symptoms in bereaved versus nonbereaved youth and young adults: a longitudinal epidemiological study. *J Am Acad Child Adolesc Psychiatry.* 2010;49:1145–1154.

33 Hamdan S, Melhem NM, Porta G, Song MS, Brent DA. Alcohol and substance abuse in parentally bereaved youth. *J Clin Psychiatry.* 2013;74:828–833.

34 Whitesell M, Bachand A, Peel J, Brown M. Familial, social, and individual factors contrib-uting to risk for adolescent substance use. *J Addict*. 2013;2013: 579310.

35 Ridenour TA, Clark DB, Cottler LB. The illustration-based assessment of liability and ex-posure to substance use and antisocial behavior for children. *Am J Drug Alcohol Abuse*. 2009;35:242–252.

36 Kobulsky JM, Minnes S, Min MO, Singer MI. Violence exposure and early substance use in high-risk adolescents. *J Soc Work Pract Addict*. 2016;16:46–71.

37 Martinez-Mota LG, Jimenez-Rubio G, Hernández-Hernánde OT, Paez-Martinez N. Influence of the type of childhood violence on cannabis abuse and dependence among ado-lescents: a systematic review and meta-analysis. *Adicciones*. 2020;32:63–76.

38 Vrijen C, Wiertsema M, Ackermans MA, van der Ploeg R, Kretschmer T. Childhood and adolescent bullying perpetration and later substance use: a meta-analysis. *Pediatrics*. 2021;147:e2020034751.

39 Jackson P, Yule Am, Wilens T. Adolescent substance use and prevention. In Goldstein MA (Ed.), *The MassGeneral Hospital for Children Adolescent Medicine Handbook* (2nd ed., pp. 259–282). Springer International Publishing; 2017.

40 Knight JR, Sherritt L, Shrier LA, Harris SK, Chang G. Validity of the CRAFFT sub-stance abuse screening test among adolescent clinic patients. *Arch Pediatr Adolesc Med*. 2002;156(6):607–14.

41 Levy S, Weiss R, Sherritt L, et al. An electronic screen for triaging adolescent substance use by risk levels. *JAMA Pediatr*. 2014;168:822–828.

42 Hazen EP, Goldstein MA, Goldstein MC. *Mental Health Disorders in Adolescents: A Guide for Parents, Teachers, and Professionals*. Rutgers University Press; 2011.

43 Tanner-Smith EE, Wilson SJ, Lipsey MW. The comparative effectiveness of outpatient treat-ment for adolescent substance abuse: a meta-analysis. *J Subst Abuse Treat*. 2013;44:145–158.

44 Kreski NT, Cerdá M, Chen Q, et al. Adolescents' use of free time and associations with sub-stance use from 1991 to 2019. *Subst Use Misuse*. 2022;57:1893–1903.

45 Biglan A, Van Ryzin MJ. Behavioral science and the prevention of adolescent substance abuse. *Perspect Behav Sci*. 2019;42:547–563.

8

Suicidality and Self-Harm

Introduction

As the third leading cause of death in youth ages 15 to 19 years in the United States, suicide in adolescents is a public health crisis. Apart from unintentional injuries that account for 37.9 percent of deaths, and homicide which accounted for 20.9% of deaths, intended self-harm (suicide) was the cause of 18.0 percent percent of teen fatalities in 2020.[1] Many, but not all, adolescents who die from suicide have a mental health disorder including depression, oppositional defiant or conduct disorder, attention-deficit/hyperactivity disorder, or bipolar disease.

Suicidal behavior has four components, including completed suicide: suicidal ideation, suicide plan, suicide attempt, and suicide death. Suicidal ideation encompasses both passive thoughts about wanting to be dead and active thoughts about killing oneself without preparatory behavior. A suicide plan arises in adolescents who have been thinking about a suicide attempt including a method, timeframe, and place. A suicide attempt is a nonfatal, self-directed potentially injurious behavior that intends to result in death. Finally, suicide is death caused by a self-directed injurious behavior, with the intent to die.[2] On the other hand, self-harm, which is known in the *Diagnostic and Statistical Manual of Mental Disorder*, fifth edition, as nonsuicidal self-injury (NSSI) is a deliberate and intentional injury to one's body that occurs without the intent of suicide. NSSI may include self-cutting, burning, or self-hitting. Individuals who demonstrate NSSI need further evaluation.[3]

Using the biopsychosocial model as a classification format, the risk factors for suicide in adolescence may be categorized. Biologically, genetics are a key question when it comes to suicide research in adolescents. Recently, researchers from Utah and New Jersey were interested in understanding the genetics of completed suicides. They linked samples from approximately 4500 people who had died from suicide to the genealogical and medical records available on over 8 million people. From this linkage, the researchers were able to identify 43 high-risk extended families with completed suicides. In these families, the researchers located 30 distinct shared genomic segments with 207 genes needing further study. They then determined four gene variants associated with suicide whose roles included gene transcription, brain structure and function, energy supply to nerve synapses, and risk of Alzheimer's disease. Although additional research is needed, the researchers noted that these four variants raised the likelihood that these genes conferred the risk of completed suicide.[4]

There are several other theories on the biological risk factors related to suicide. A researcher in Illinois conducted a review of the literature on adolescent suicide to determine some of these factors. One area of research was the association between low levels of serotonin and suicidal behavior and suicide. Unfortunately, there was no clear evidence to determine if there was a serotonin production issue or an increase in uptake. Other issues included the role of norepinephrine and its metabolites. Norepinephrine is a hormone generated by the sympathetic nervous system that is involved in the fight-or-flight response. Lastly, the researcher raised the possible role of dysfunction in the hypothalamic-pituitary-adrenal (HPA) axis. An abnormal HPA axis in depression is a fairly consistent finding, and in this case, there appears to be a strong relationship between this dysfunction and suicide.[5]

In an attempt to understand the psychological risk factors for suicidality in children and adolescents, researchers in multiple European countries performed a systematic review. The researchers learned that depression is a major psychological risk factor for suicidality in children and adolescents. In fact, major depression is associated with a fivefold higher risk of suicide attempts. But it is also evident that nondepressed adolescents may have symptoms of suicidality. Alcohol misuse was a risk factor for suicidal behavior, even in the absence of depressive symptoms. Other risks for suicidal behavior were the use of tobacco and the abuse of drugs, such as marijuana. The researchers commented that suicidal behavior in adolescents may occur with anxiety disorders, eating disorders, sleep disturbances, and several other mental health conditions. Conditions including bipolar, conduct, and personality disorders are risk factors for suicidal behaviors.

The social risk factors for adolescent suicidality are usually not sufficient reason for a suicide attempt or suicide death in youths. However, for those adolescents who are already at an increased risk, a social risk may precipitate suicidal behavior. Certain stressful life events were considered most impactful, including family conflicts, academic stressors, and trauma. Family conflicts included stress related to parents, physical harm by a parent, and lack of adult support outside the home. Academic stresses included the perception that one's school performance was a failure. Finally, adverse childhood experiences including childhood sexual abuse can lead to a 6.1-fold increase in the odds of a suicide attempt between the ages of 13 and 19 years. Further, victims of bullying have higher rates of suicidal behavior. Identifying these biopsychosocial risk factors enables people to be better informed and implement appropriate screening and prevention programs.[6]

There appears to be a strong relationship between emotional dysregulation and suicidality in adolescents. Emotional dysregulation is an emotional response that does not fit within the accepted range of emotions for a particular event. For example, this might include an adolescent going into a rage after obtaining an average grade on an examination. In adolescents, emotional dysregulation is an independent risk factor for suicidality.[7]

Epidemiology

Shortly after the start of the COVID-19 pandemic, emergency room visits for suspected suicide attempts began to increase among adolescents between the ages of 12 and 17 years, particularly among females. One year later, during the period February 21, 2021, to March 20, 2021, emergency room visits for suspected suicide attempts for females were up by 50.6 percent from the same time period in 2019. Even prior to the pandemic, female adolescents had increasing rates of suicide attempts.[8]

Worldwide, suicide is a leading cause of death among youth and accounts for approximately 8.5 percent of deaths in the age group 15 to 29 years. Suicidal ideation rates in this group range between 19.8 percent and 24.0 percent, with less than that for suicide attempts. Suicidal ideation is rare before age 10 but increases markedly during adolescence. While female adolescents are more likely to attempt suicide, male adolescents are more likely to die by suicide. Generally, older adolescents are more at risk of dying from suicide than younger adolescents. Indigenous youth, including Native American, Alaskan Native, and other Indigenous youth across the world, have a higher risk of suicide death. Risk factors include substance use, poverty, accessibility to lethal means, and loss of cultural identity. In the United States, Black, non-Hispanic adolescents are less likely to experience suicidal ideation. Compared to heterosexual youth, those identifying as LGBTQ have an elevated prevalence of suicidal thoughts and attempts. This may be attributed to the consistently elevated rate of victimization that LGBTQ youth frequently encounter compared to heterosexual youth.[9] Compared to urban areas, youth living in rural areas have double the rates of suicide. This rate apparently is rising faster in rural areas when compared to urban areas.[10]

Using data from the Youth Risk Behavior Survey administered by the Centers for Disease Control and Prevention (CDC), researchers from New York, Ohio, and Missouri studied the trends of suicidal behaviors in high school students during the years 1991 to 2017. Specifically, they were searching for the racial, ethnic, and gender differences in suicidal ideation and behavior. The sample sizes ranged from 10,904 to 16,410. While there were measures for race, Hispanic heritage, and suicidal thoughts and behaviors, there were questions on suicidal ideation, suicide plan, suicide attempts, and injury by attempt. Over the course of the study, there were significant reductions in suicides among females, but not among males. Black participants had a significant increase in reported suicide attempts, while White, Hispanic, Asian American, Pacific Islander, Native American, and Alaska Native participants had a significant decrease. Overall, Black males had a significant increase in rates of injury caused by suicide attempts despite a downward trend for suicidal ideation and suicide plans for all gender, racial, and ethnic groups.[11]

In a separate study also from 2019, the rates of suicide among Black adolescents between the ages of 15 and 19 years increased in 2017 as compared to 2007. The percent change in completed suicides for Black adolescents was higher than for White and Hispanic youth, although each group saw an increase in rates per 100,000 from 2007 to 2017. Though the causes for this are not clear, health disparities, including mental health treatment, racial discrimination, and poverty, could be risk factors.[12] Recently released data documented that suicide rates among persons aged 10 to 24 years increased significantly during 2018–2021 among Black individuals, by 36.6 percent. The reasons for this increase were not specified.[13]

Biopsychosocial Issues and Suicidality/Self-Harm

Biological Issues and Suicidality/Self-Harm

Sleep

Sleep loss may negatively impact adolescent executive functioning, and executive functioning problems may be associated with suicidal behavior. In addition, insufficient sleep has been linked to impaired emotional regulation and heightened emotional reactivity. Other aspects of sleep functioning, including insomnia, short sleep duration, and nightmares, have also been associated with an increased risk for suicide.[14]

Researchers from Japan and California studied the relationship between sleep habits, mental health status, and suicidality in adolescent monozygotic twins, who shared the same genes and environmental influences. The researchers used data from a longitudinal survey of sleep habits and mental health status that was conducted over 3 years in middle and high school students in Tokyo, Japan. The measures included questions on sleep and wake time, suicidality, and demographics. The researchers learned that late bedtimes and short sleep duration predicted subsequent depression and anxiety, including self-injury and suicide risk, and the relationships were statistically significant. The researchers commented that the findings were not a result of the teens' common genes and shared environments. They recommended that prevention efforts could include intervention/education for adolescents with sleep issues.[15]

Researchers from Massachusetts, New York, and Wisconsin further studied the relationship of sleep duration and risk-taking behaviors in adolescents. Using data from the Youth Risk Behavior Survey between 2007 and 2015, the cohort consisted of 67,615 individual surveys; 99 percent were 14 years or older, and 49 percent were female subjects. Each of the four high school grades had approximately the same number of student participants. Only 30 percent noted that they had 8 or 9 hours of sleep each night. The researchers determined that there was an increase in the odds of unsafe behaviors among the adolescents who reported insufficient sleep. The lack of sleep seemed to have the most impact on mood and self-harm. Those adolescents who slept fewer than 6 hours a day were more than three times more likely to have considered suicide, a plan to attempt suicide, or an attempt at suicide, and more than four times as likely to have attempted a suicide that resulted in treatment.[16]

With data from the Shandong Adolescent Behavior and Health Cohort, researchers in China designed a prospective 1-year study to understand the relationship between nightmares and suicidality in adolescents. They sampled 7072 students from middle and high schools in Shandong in grades 7, 8, and 10. The self-administered questionnaire, which was completed in 2015 and also 1 year later, included questions about suicidal behavior, nightmare frequency and distress, insomnia symptoms, sleep duration, and depressive symptoms. The researchers determined that 26.2 percent of the student sample had nightmares at least two times a month. Ten percent noted suicidal ideation, 3.6 percent noted a suicide plan, and 2.7 percent noted a suicide attempt during the 1-year follow-up. During the follow-up, all groups were found to have significant increases in the frequency and distress of nightmares. And with this increase in problematic nightmares came increases in suicidal risks, which were at least partially mediated by depressive symptoms. The researchers commented that assessing and intervening with adolescents who have frequent nightmares and associated depressive symptoms may play a role in preventing adolescent suicide.[17]

Stress

During adolescent development, there is an association between stress from life events and suicidal ideation and behaviors. Some of these stressful events are the result of interpersonal and peer-related issues, and these may increase the potential for suicidality. Researchers in North Carolina and Saudi Arabia investigated the role peers play in promoting suicidality in their friends. Primarily, did a friend's disclosure of distress positively or negatively impact the suicidal ideation of their peers, and did school attachment play a role in this dynamic? The researchers surveyed 702 students between the ages of 15 and 18 years who attended six middle and high schools, both public and private, in Jeddah. A social network portion of the survey had measures for peer mental health and behavior. For this cross-sectional sample, the students named up to six of their closest friends. The researchers discovered that a peer's disclosure of self-harm or depression was positively associated with their friend's suicidal ideation, worse than the peer's own depression. When friends disclosed depression or self-harm, they created an additional stressor on a peer's stress universe that affected their mental health, possibly to the point of higher suicidality. Further, students with the highest level of school attachment and with no friends disclosing depression had a predicted suicidality score of .06, while those with the highest level of school attachment and with all friends having depression had a score of .33. Low school attachment did not appear to moderate the suicidality score. The findings demonstrated that an in-school social network composed of friends with mental distress, particularly self-harm, could act as a stressor. For members of the social network, this stressor could increase youth suicidality.[18]

There may be ways for parents and peers to buffer the stress on adolescents from these interpersonal interactions. Researchers in New York examined the influence of social support on the relationship between life stressors and prospectively assessed suicidal symptoms in adolescent females. The cohort consisted of 550 adolescent females with a mean age of 14.39 years (13.5 to 15.5 years), 80.5 percent non-Hispanic White, from Long Island, New York. The teens completed self-report questionnaires about depressive symptoms and social support during an in-person visit at baseline and at a 9-month phone follow-up. Measures included negative stressful life events, perceived social support, and suicide and dysphoric symptoms. The researchers observed that the adolescents with higher rates of life stress, especially from interpersonal events, reported higher rates of suicidal symptoms. While greater levels of parental support were associated with lower rates of suicidality, the effects of peer support were not as strong as parental support. The researchers concluded that parental support played an important role in protecting adolescents from developing suicidality due to stress.[19]

An approach to stress management in older adolescents and young adults was tested by researchers from the United Kingdom. They conducted a randomized controlled trial of the Mindfulness Skills for Students program, which was offered to University of Cambridge students during the 2015–2016 academic year. The 309 initial students in the experimental group (39 percent male) participated in an 8-week mindfulness course with mental health support, and 307 initial students (35 percent female) were in the control group. Using the Clinical Outcomes in Routine Evaluation Outcome Measure, psychological distress measurements were taken during spring examinations. When compared to the control group, the students who took the program had reduced distress scores during the examination period. Fifty-seven percent of the 214 students in the control group who completed the study had distress scores above an acceptable clinical threshold, but only 37 percent of the 235 students who completed the mindfulness program had distress scores above an accepted clinical threshold. The researchers concluded that mindfulness training could be an effective mental health strategy.[20]

Social Issues and Suicidality/Self-Harm

Social Media

In 2021, U.S. Surgeon General Murthy issued a report on youth mental health in which he expressed concern about the impact social media and other forms of digital technologies were having on the mental health of children and young people in general. During the COVID-19 pandemic, screen use in youth increased from an average of 3.8 hours per day to 7.7 hours per day. Even before the pandemic began, researchers from California and Florida studied several aspects of suicide, such as ideation, plans, attempts, and increases in suicide rates, among U.S. adolescents. They also examined possible causes of adolescent mental health concerns, primarily focusing on their use of leisure time. Using data from the Monitoring the Future Survey and the Youth Risk Behavior Surveillance System, the researchers measured depressive symptoms, suicide-related outcomes, electronic device use, social media use, internet news, TV watching, homework, in-person social interactions, print media, sports and exercise, religious services, paid jobs, demographics, and economic factors. The subjects were between the ages of 13 and 18 years. The researchers learned that suicide-related outcomes, suicide deaths, and depressive symptoms had declined or remained stable among American adolescents before 2010 but had become more prevalent between 2010 and 2015, especially among female adolescents. The researchers observed that during this 5-year period of time, adolescents spent more time on social media and electronic devices, which were activities positively correlated with suicide-related outcomes and depression, and they spent less time on nonscreen activities, including sports and exercise. Other factors, such as the economy, stock market, or unemployment, were not linked to suicide rates.[21]

Researchers at the CDC evaluated the association between a variety of online risk factors, such as depression, and adolescent suicide-related behavior. Using a longitudinal matched case-control study involving a sample from 2600 schools that participated in an online school-based safety-monitoring program, they identified 227 youths who had a severe suicide/self-harm alert. They were monitored using the online safety tools from the software Bark, which warns school administrators if there is a severe suicide/self-harm alert. These tools assessed the students' generated content for suicidal ideation on computers, tablets, and cloud-based accounts. The 227 students identified with such content were matched with 1135 controls for a total of 1362 participants with a mean age of 13.3 years, and majority male. Eight online risk factors were identified: profanity, cyberbullying, depression, low-severity suicide/self-harm, violence, drug related, sexual content, and hate speech. Each risk factor was found to be significantly associated with subsequent severe suicide/self-harm alert. Compared to control subjects, depression had the highest adjusted odds ratio for a subsequent severe suicide/self-harm alert at 1.82. For the youth who displayed five or more of the eight risk factors, the adjusted odds ratio for a severe suicide/self-harm alert was more than 70 times the control (78.64). By identifying online risk factors, the findings of this study may help guide the design of adolescent suicide prevention programs. This study also showed that there is an increasing risk of severe suicide/self-harm alert with each additional type of risk factor.[22]

Despite such proactive measures, between August 2017 and March 2018 in one Ohio county, there were 12 adolescents who died by suicide, forming a suicide cluster. Beginning in April 2018, researchers from the local health department, the Ohio Department of Health, and the CDC conducted an online, anonymous, cross-sectional survey of public school students who attended middle and high schools in the affected county. The researchers examined the association between suicide cluster–related social media and suicidal behaviors. The cohort consisted of 15,083 students from 34 schools (73 percent of the eligible students). The measures included student self-reports of past and current suicidal ideation or attempts and suicide contagion-promoting factors such as postings on social media about the cluster, observing online news related to the cluster, and viewing memorials for victims of the cluster. The researchers found that some of the students who posted suicide cluster–related content to social media were clearly thinking about suicide. Of these students, 22.9 percent reported suicidal ideation and 15.0 percent had a suicide attempt. For students without a history of suicidal ideation or suicide attempt before the suicide cluster, when compared to those students who did not view suicide content, seeing any suicide cluster–related social media posts was significantly associated with increased odds of suicidal ideation and suicide attempt. The researchers concluded that exposure to suicide cluster–related social media was associated with suicidal ideation and attempts during a suicide cluster. The researchers commented that prevention programs aimed at the negative effects of social media in this context were warranted.[23]

Social media is a powerful tool that may foster positive outcomes and healthy behaviors. Online social platforms with supportive communities may help some vulnerable youth. The 2021 Surgeon General's report "Protecting Your Mental Health" listed several ways that technology companies may take responsibility for creating a safe digital environment for youth. These recommendations included developing products that actively safeguard and promote mental health and well-being, measuring the impact that their products have on user health and well-being, and assessing and addressing risk to users at the front end of product development.[24]

Poverty

To design effective adolescent suicide intervention and prevention programs, adolescent suicidality risk factors need to be identified. One area investigated was the role of neighborhoods, especially financially disadvantaged neighborhoods. Researchers from Quebec and Massachusetts examined the relationship between living in an economically disadvantaged neighborhood and suicidal thoughts and attempts in later adolescence. This study controlled for background vulnerabilities as well as other adolescent psychological risks, such as depression, substance abuse, and exposure to suicide. Using data from cycle six of the Canadian National Longitudinal Survey of Children and Youth, the researchers directed their attention to a subset of participants who were 18 to 19 years old. With a total sample of 2776 participants, the study utilized measures including self-reported suicidal behaviors and risk factors. The researchers used Canadian census data to measure poverty, and parental reports obtained in an earlier cycle were used to assess family and individual controls. The researchers learned that the odds of suicidal ideation for the teens from poor neighborhoods were two times higher than the teens from nonpoor neighborhoods, and the odds of attempting suicide were four times higher in the disadvantaged neighborhoods. The researchers concluded that youth living in poor neighborhoods were highly vulnerable and should be provided with suicide intervention and prevention efforts.[25]

Besides neighborhood poverty, community poverty may be a risk factor for adolescents. Using survey data on 7430 adolescents between the ages of 15 and 16 years who were born in 1990 and 1991, researchers in Iceland evaluated the relationship between community poverty and suicidal behavior. The anonymous questionnaires that were completed during school in 2006 included measures for suicidality, household poverty, and community household poverty. The researchers learned that community household poverty increased the risk of adolescent suicidal behavior. According to these researchers, it appeared that in economically disadvantaged communities there is a higher risk for adolescents to associate with other youth who are suicidal. Thus, living in an impoverished community may be a suicidality risk factor for youth.[26]

Researchers in Chicago and Boston wanted to understand the association between pediatric suicide rates (ages 5 to 19 years) and county-level poverty concentration. Using data from the CDC Compressed Mortality File, they conducted a retrospective, cross-sectional study of suicides in U.S. youth from January 1, 2007, to December 31, 2016. During the study period, 20,982 youths majority ages 10 to 19 years died by suicide. Measures included suicide death, methods, annual county poverty concentration, and percentage of the population in the country living below the federal poverty level. The counties were divided into five poverty concentration categories: 0 percent to 4.9 percent, 5.0 percent to 9.9 percent, 10.0 percent to 14.9 percent, 15.0 percent to 19.9 percent, and 20.0 percent or more of the country population living below the federal poverty level. The findings demonstrated that higher county-level concentrations of poverty were associated with increased suicide rates among individuals ages 5 to 19 years. The researchers suggested that this may be a result of toxic levels of stress affecting neurobiological stress-mediated pathways, which may lead to impairment of decision-making, behavioral self-regulation, and mood or impulse control. Further, children living in poor neighborhoods were exposed to more family turmoil, violence, social isolation, and lack of positive peer influences. There is a need for suicide intervention and prevention programs aimed at these risk factors.[27]

Racism/Discrimination

In 2019, the Congressional Black Caucus published *Ring the Alarm: The Crisis of Black Youth Suicide in America*. In that publication, they reported that the suicide rates for Black children and teenagers showed an alarming increase over the previous several years. They wrote that this increase challenged the public perception that Black children do not die by suicide. Their first recommendation was to increase the amount of research into Black youth mental health and suicidal issues through the National Institutes of Health and the National Institute of Mental Health.[28]

A 2021 literature review found relatively few studies on adolescents and racism and suicide. This may be attributed to the design of the studies, which did not focus on Black, Indigenous, and people of color communities and children. Researchers from California and Pennsylvania suggested that people may better understand the inequalities faced by Black adolescents if they spend some time thinking about principles of justice, equity, diversity, and inclusion. Applied to the context of risk factors for suicide, people should consider analyses of adverse childhood experiences, social determinants of health, geography, and socioeconomic status. Both interpersonal and structural racism may affect the mental health of multitudes of adolescents.[29]

Studies have linked discrimination with stress, low self-esteem, and depressive symptoms in Black adolescents, and most Black youth have had at least one experience with discrimination. Using data from the National Survey of American Life Adolescent Supplement 2003, which is one of the largest national surveys of Black youth mental health, researchers at the University of Michigan examined the relationship between discrimination in Black adolescents and suicidal ideation. The sample included 1170 Black adolescents between the ages of 13 and 17 years. While 18 percent were interviewed on the telephone, the vast majority were interviewed in their homes. There were measures for sociodemographics, ethnicity, discrimination, and suicidal ideation. The researchers found an association between discrimination and suicidal ideation, regardless of gender, ethnicity, age, and socioeconomic status. This association was universal in nature; discrimination was related to suicidal ideation in Black adolescents.[30]

Researchers from Ohio, Pennsylvania, and New York studied suicides in Black youth ages 5 to 17 years. They used data from the web-based Injury Statistics Query and Reporting System and the National Violent Death Reporting System to understand trends and precipitating circumstances of Black youth suicide from 2003 to 2017. The precipitating circumstances in which the suicide occurred did not specifically address racism or discrimination, although there was a general category for interpersonal trauma and life stressors. As a result, racism as a cause of suicide did not appear in the data. Still, the researchers commented that Black youth suicide prevention programs need to be designed through a different lens; they must address the systematic racism and trauma regularly experienced by Black youth. Thus, as called for by the Congressional Black Caucus, there is a need for more research on Black youth and suicide. Screening for suicidal issues should consider risk factors pertinent to minority youth such as discrimination and racism and be culturally adapted to the target audience. Such screening could also involve religiosity and the Black church, which have been linked to reduced self-harm in Black youth.[31]

Suicidality has been increasing in children approaching adolescence as well as in early adolescent development. Is there an association between racial/ethnic discrimination and suicidality in Black and non-Black preadolescents? Researchers from Pennsylvania, the Netherlands, and Connecticut analyzed data from the Adolescent Brain Cognitive Development Study of 11,235 U.S. children, with a mean age of 10.9 years. They specifically sought to disentangle the association of racial/ethnic discrimination from other environmental adversities with childhood suicidality. In particular, they were able to assess the individuals over and above other forms of discrimination such as weight based, sexual orientation based, or non-U.S. born. The measures included exposures to discrimination, suicidality, and demographics such as race.

The results indicated that non-Black participants experienced far less racial/ethnic discrimination than Black participants. In fact, the Black participants reported over threefold more racial/ethnic discrimination compared to the non-Black participants. Regarding suicidality, Black participants reported more suicidal ideation and suicide attempts (9.7 percent) compared to non-Black participants (7.8 percent). However, once experienced, racial/ethnic discrimination was associated with suicidality in White, Black, and Hispanic youths. The messages from this study included that suicidality occurred in preadolescents and young adolescents, and the experiences of racial/ethnic discrimination were significant stressors for the racial groups studied. The association of racial/ethnic discrimination with suicidality is similar to that of other well-established risk factors such as sexual orientation or history of depression.[32]

Transgender/Gender Dysphoria

Because suicide is the third leading cause of death in adolescents between the ages of 12 and 24 years, there is increasing concern that youth with gender identity issues may be at even higher risk. Researchers from New York and Texas explored the prevalence of suicidal ideation among transgender youth in California. They also wanted to learn if there were established psychosocial factors that explained the higher suicide risk for transgender youth. Data were obtained from 910,885 high school students who participated in the California Healthy Kids Survey from 2013 to 2015. The measures included questions on sexual orientation and gender identity, suicidal ideation, demographics, and psychosocial mediators. Transgender identity was confirmed by 1.33 percent of the respondents. The researchers learned that 35 percent of the transgender youth reported suicidal ideation during the previous year, double the rate among the nontransgender sample and more than two times the national estimate among youth in grades 9 through 12. Depression and school-based victimization may partly explain the association between gender identity and suicidal ideation. The researchers implied that there is a need to screen for suicidal ideation in transgender students and develop interventions designed to meet their needs.[33]

More specifically, researchers from Arizona and Minnesota examined the prevalence of self-reported suicide behavior in six gender identity groups: male, female, transgender female, transgender male, transgender not exclusively male or female, and questioning adolescents. They reviewed data collected between 2012 and 2015 from the Profiles of Student Life: Attitudes and Behaviors Survey for 120,617 adolescents between the ages of 11 and 19 years. The measures included suicidality, gender identity, and several sociodemographic characteristics. With respect to all groups, 8.6 percent attempted suicide during the previous year, and 14.6 percent devised a plan or attempted suicide, also during the same time period. However, the researchers found disparities in suicidal behavior. Transgender male adolescents and nonbinary adolescents had the highest rates of suicidal behavior at 50.8 percent and 41.8 percent, respectively. In contrast, cisgender males had a rate of 9.8 percent. These data indicated that suicide prevention efforts should target transgender adolescents with particular emphasis on subgroups that have higher rates of suicidality.[34]

When compared to gay, lesbian, and bisexual individuals, transgender and gender diverse (TGD) adolescents have specific mental health risk factors. Researchers from several locations in New York City conducted a systematic review and meta-analysis to evaluate risky and protective factors for transgender adolescents. They located five studies that met their criteria. From these studies, the researchers learned that there was a relationship between symptoms of depression, gender-based victimization, and bullying and suicidal behaviors. One study determined that depression and school-based victimization mediated the association between gender identity and suicidal ideation. In addition, the researchers found four primary protective factors for TGD youth. The first included internal qualities that support resilience, healthy mental processing, and self-awareness. The other protective factors were external qualities including connections to family members, relationships with teachers and other non-familial adults, and feelings of community safety. These findings are aligned with the belief that there are multiple social groups that may foster protection to individuals with mental health issues.[35]

Violence

Teen dating violence has a significant negative impact on adolescent mental health. Physical dating violence may include shoving, slapping, punching, choking, and/or kicking a dating partner. It may cause negative mental health outcomes including anxiety, depression, substance abuse, and risky sexual practices that may lead to unintended teen pregnancy and sexually transmitted infection. Researchers in Texas and Ohio studied the prevalence of physical teen violence and suicidal ideation, suicidal plans, and suicidal attempts in adolescents ages 14 to 18 years, as well as the association between dating violence and suicidal behaviors. They used data from the 2015 Youth Risk Behavior Survey, with a sample of 9693 adolescents (50.4 percent male). The survey asked questions about suicidal behaviors during the previous 12 months and any history of physical teen dating violence also during the previous 12 months. Grade levels 9 to 12 were almost equally represented in the data. During the previous 12 months, 16.6 percent reported suicidal ideation, 13.7 percent had a suicide plan, and 7.6 percent attempted suicide. With respect to being a victim of bullying, 20.2 percent noted the affirmative, and 18.9 percent experienced cyberbullying victimization. The researchers learned that the adolescents who had a history of dating violence were more likely to have experienced all three suicidal behaviors. There were no associations between age, sex, and grade level with any of the three suicidal behaviors. Adolescents who self-identified as lesbian, gay, or bisexual were more likely to have engaged in suicidal behaviors including suicide attempts. Compared to Whites, Black, Hispanic, and Asian students had a higher risk of attempting suicide. The findings supported the need for suicide prevention efforts for adolescents with a history of dating violence, and these should be focused on certain groups such as LGBTQ and racial minorities.[36]

Treatment of Suicidality/Self-Harm

When an adolescent displays self-injurious behavior, a psychiatric evaluation is generally necessary. Warning signs of such injuries may include cuts, burns, or other injuries that are unexplained. There may be cuts in the same area of the body with different stages of healing. Or the adolescent may begin to show signs of psychological distress that could include a depressed mood, social withdrawal, changes in behavior, a lack of motivation, or a decline in academic performance. An emergency psychiatric evaluation may be indicated if the self-injurious behavior is out of control or escalating, there is potential for serious harm, there are threats of suicide, or there are dramatic changes in behavior. The plan of care will depend on the underlying psychiatric issues, as well as the driving forces for the behavior that could include social, academic, and family factors. Care may be as an outpatient, as an inpatient, or partial hospitalization. If a parent has concerns about suicidal behavior in their adolescent, then they should immediately take the adolescent to the nearest emergency department for evaluation.

According to the Substance Abuse and Mental Health Services Administration (SAMHSA), there is strong evidence that dialectical behavior therapy (DBT) is efficacious for the treatment of suicidal behaviors in adolescents. DBT emphasizes the development of four skills: mindfulness, interpersonal effectiveness, emotion regulation, and distress tolerance. DBT particularly combats emotional dysregulation or the inability to flexibly respond to and manage emotions. These aforementioned four skills are important tools in the prevention of suicidal behaviors. Individual or group therapy may help adolescents develop skills in these four areas in a systematic and gradual manner.

Studies have affirmed the efficacy of DBT for the treatment of suicidal behaviors in adolescents. Researchers from multiple locations in the United States compared the efficacy of DBT to individual and group supportive therapy (IGST) for reducing suicidal behaviors in adolescents at high risk for suicide. They designed a randomized clinical trial at four academic medical centers with 173 subjects (94.8 percent female) ages 12 to 18 years. Each of the subjects had a history of significant suicidal behavior and was placed in either a DBT treatment group or an IGST treatment group. Treatments occurred weekly for 6 months in individual and group settings with parent participation. Suicidal behaviors and ideation assessments were conducted at baseline and then at 3, 6, 9, and 12 months. From baseline until 6 months, 9.7 percent of the youth in the DBT group and 21.5 percent in the IGST group reported suicide attempts. From 6 months to 12 months, there were no significant differences between the groups. However, during the follow-up period, one adolescent in the IGST group died by suicide. The researchers concluded that their results supported DBT as the first well-established, empirically proven treatment for decreasing repeated suicide attempts and self-harm in youth.[37] In addition, in a preliminary study, DBT for adolescents was shown to be of benefit for LGBQ youth with a history of suicide attempts, NSSI, or self-destructive behaviors.[38]

Prevention of Suicidality/Self-Harm

Prevention of suicidal behaviors in adolescents may be approached in various ways and at different levels: it encompasses the adolescent, family, peers, school, medical facilities, community, and society in the form of social norms and policies. At all levels of interaction with adolescents, it is important to recognize the symptoms of suicidality. See Box 8.1 for the symptoms of suicidality in adolescents.

Some adolescents confide their suicidal thoughts to others, such as parents and/or peers. When that occurs, immediate action should be taken, whether it involves consulting a clinician or other authority or proceeding to the nearest emergency medical facility. Hotlines, such as the 988 Suicide & Crisis Lifeline and the Trevor Project (866-488-7386), are readily accessible, and the Trevor Project is especially useful for LGBTQ youth.

There are several best practice registries that list suicide prevention programs with evidence-based results. For example, the SAMHSA National Registry of Evidence-Based Practices may be accessed at the following website: https://www.samhsa.gov/nrepp.

Box 8.1 Symptoms of Suicidality in Adolescents (39)

Dramatic changes in personality or behavior
Changes in eating and sleeping habits (such as nightmares or difficulty falling asleep)
Worsening symptoms of depression or the appearance of psychotic symptoms
Neglect of hygiene or personal appearance
Increase in dangerous, self-destructive, or risk-taking behaviors
Withdrawal from family and friends
Giving away valued possessions
Talking about death and suicide
Preoccupation with thoughts about death or with the suicide of others
Restlessness, aggression, or insomnia
Expressions of guilt, worthlessness, or hopelessness
Decreased concentration or dramatic decline in academic performance
Suddenly appearing cheerful or relieved with no clear reason after a period of significant depression

From Hazen EP, Goldstein MA, Goldstein MC. *Mental Health Disorders in Adolescents: A Guide for Parents, Teachers, and Professionals.* Rutgers University Press; 2011.

The SAMHSA website describes a hospital-based suicide prevention program offered at the Children's Health System of Texas as a program that "shows promise." Named the Safe Alternative for Teens and Youth (SAFETY), SAFETY is an inpatient psychiatric unit and intensive care program for adolescents between the ages of 12 and 18 years. It offers individual, family, and group therapy as well as medication management. The program utilizes cognitive behavioral therapy family treatment as well as some elements of DBT and multisystemic therapy. Parents attend a weekly group to understand the skills that their adolescents are learning.

The Suicide Prevention Resource Center has an evidence-based prevention registry located at https://www.sprc.org. One of the resources highlighted by the center is the SOS Signs of Suicide Middle School and High Schools Prevention Programs. In one class period, students learn through video and discussion how to identify warning signs of suicide and depression. At the end of the session, students complete a seven-question screening for depression, and at-risk students are encouraged to seek help from adults. There is good evidence that this program is effective.

A team of researchers in Pennsylvania utilized the Patient Health Questionnaire-9 (PHQ-9) as a tool for in-school universal screening of adolescents for suicide risk. Students in 14 Pennsylvania high schools were randomized into the screening or the usual school practice of targeted referral for behaviors raising a concern for suicide risk. Adolescents in the universal screening arm had 7.1-fold greater odds of being identified as at risk for suicide compared to the control group. The team felt that the universal screening of adolescents for suicide risk would lead to increased identification and greater impact on treatment initiation.[40]

Pediatricians and other clinicians who provide services to youth have an important role in the prevention of adolescent suicidality. Screening for suicide risk should be a part of annual well adolescent visits as well as visits by youth to an emergency room. The screening should be not just for depression and substance use, but specifically for suicide risk. If the screen is positive, then arrangements must be made for the patient's safety as well as referrals for care as needed.[10] The Ask Suicide-Screening Questions (ASQ) is a four-question screening instrument that can be utilized to identify the risk for suicide in adolescents.[41]

On a federal level, the Suicide Training and Awareness Nationally Delivered for Universal Prevention Act of 2021 (STANDUP Act) became law in March 2022. This act provides for annual evidence-based suicide awareness and prevention training for students in grades 6 to 12 at certain state, local, and tribal levels. By federal action, 988 is now a nationwide phone number to connect directly to the 988 suicide and crisis lifeline.[42]

Conclusion

The third most common cause of death for adolescents is suicide. Biological, psychological, and social issues or a combination may drive suicidal behavior in adolescents. It is vitally important to recognize signs of suicidality in adolescents and promptly refer such youth to care.

References

1   Elflein J. Leading causes of death among teenagers aged 15–19 years in the United States 2020. Statista December 11, 2023.

2   Screening for suicide risk in primary care: a systematic evidence review for the U.S. Preventive Services Task Force. Agency for Healthcare Research and Quality (US). Rockville, MD; 2013.

3   Hooley JM, Fox KR, Boccagno C. Nonsuicidal self-injury: diagnostic challenges and current Perspectives. *Neuropsychiatr Dis Treat.* 2020;16:101–112.

4   Coon H, Darlington TM, DiBlasi E, et al. Genome-wide significant regions in 43 Utah high-risk families implicate multiple genes involved in risk for completed suicide. *Mol Psychiatry.* 2020;25:3077–3090.

5   Pandey GN. Biological basis of suicide and suicidal behavior. *Bipolar Disord.* 2013;15:524–541.

6   Carballo JJ, Llorente C, Kehrmann L, et al. Psychosocial risk factors for suicidality in children and adolescents. *Eur Child Adolesc Psychiatry.* 2020;29:759–776.

7   Benton TD, Muhrer E, Jones JD, Lewis J. Dysregulation and suicide in children and adolescents. *Child Adolesc Psychiatr Clin N Am.* 2021;30:389–399.

8   Yard E, Radhakrishnan L, Ballesteros MF, et al. Emergency department visits for suspected suicide attempts among persons aged 12–25 years before and during the COVID-19 pandemic—United States, January 2019–May 2021. *MMWR Morb Mortal Wkly Rep.* 2021;70:888–894

9   Cha CB, Franz PJ, Guzmán EM, Glenn CR, Kleiman EV, Nock MK. Annual research review: suicide among youth—epidemiology, (potential) etiology, and treatment. *J Child Psychol Psychiatry.* 2018;59:460–482.

10   Hua LL, Lee J, Rahmandar MH, Sigel EJ. Suicide and suicide risk in adolescents. *Pediatrics.* 2024 Jan 1;153(1):e2023064800.

11   Lindsey MA, Sheftall AH, Xiao Y, Joe S. Trends of suicidal behaviors among high school students in the United States: 1991–2017. *Pediatrics.* 2019;144:e20191187.

12   Shain BN. Increases in of suicide and suicide attempts among black adolescents. *Pediatrics.* 2019;144:e20191912.

13   Stone DM, Mack KA, Qualters J. Notes from the field: recent changes in suicide rates, by race and ethnicity and age group—United States, 2021. *MMWR Morb Mortal Wkly Rep.* 2023;72:160–162.

14   Fernandes SN, Zuckerman E, Miranda R, Baroni A. When night falls fast: sleep and suicidal behavior among adolescents and young adults. *Child Adolesc Psychiatr Clin N Am.* 2021;30:269–282.

15   Matamura M, Tochigi M, Usami S, et al. Associations between sleep habits and mental health status and suicidality in a longitudinal survey of monozygotic twin adolescents. *J Sleep Res.* 2014;23:290–294.

16   Weaver MD, Barger LS, Malone SK, Anderson LS, Klerman EB. Dose-dependent associations between sleep duration and unsafe behaviors among US high school students. *JAMA Pediatr.* 2018;172:1187–1189.

17   Liu X, Yang Y, Liu ZZ, Jia CX. Longitudinal associations of nightmare frequency and nightmare distress with suicidal behavior in adolescents: mediating role of depressive symptoms. *Sleep.* 2021;44:zsaa130.

18   Copeland M, Alqahtani RT, Moody J, et al. When friends bring you down: peer stress proliferation and suicidality. *Arch Suicide Res.* 2021;25:672–689.

19   Mackin DM, Perlman G, Davila J, Kotov R, Klein DN. Social support buffers the effect of interpersonal life stress on suicidal ideation and self-injury during adolescence. *Psychol Med.* 2017;47:1149–1161.

20 Galante J, Dufour G, Vainre M, et al. A mindfulness-based intervention to increase resilience to stress in university students (the mindful student study): a pragmatic randomised controlled trial. *Lancet Public Health.* 2018;3:e72–e81.

21 Twenge J, Joiner T, Rogers M, Martin GN. Increases in depressive symptoms, suicide-related outcomes, and suicide rates among U.S. adolescents after 2010 and links to increased new media screen time. *Clin Psychol Sci.* 2018;6:3–17.

22 Sumner SA, Ferguson B, Bason B, et al. Association of online risk factors with subsequent youth suicide-related behaviors in the US. *JAMA Netw Open.* 2021;4:e2125860.

23 Swedo EA, Beauregard JL, de Fijter S, et al. Associations between social media and suicidal behaviors during a youth suicide cluster in Ohio. *J Adolesc Health.* 2021;68:308–316.

24 Murthy VH. Protecting youth mental health: the U.S. surgeon general's advisory. Washington, DC; 2021.

25 Dupéré V, Leventhal T, Lacourse L. Neighborhood poverty and suicidal thoughts and attempts in late adolescence. *Psychol Med.* 2009;39:1295–1306.

26 Bernburg JG, Thorlindsson T, Sigfusdottir ID. The spreading of suicidal behavior: the contextual effect of community household poverty on adolescent suicidal behavior and the mediating role of suicide suggestion. *Soc Sci Med.* 2009;68:380–389.

27 Hoffmann JA, Farrell CA, Monuteaux MC, Fleegler EW, Lee LK. Association of pediatric suicide with county-level poverty in the United States 2007–2016. *JAMA Pediatr.* 2020;174:287–294.

28 Coleman BW. Ring the alarm: the crisis of black youth suicide in America. Washington, DC; 2019.

29 Bath E, Njoroge WFM. Coloring outside the lines: making black and brown lives matter in the prevention of youth suicide. *J Am Acad Child Adolesc Psychiatry.* 2021;60:17–21.

30 Assari SM, Lankarani M, Caldwell CH. Discrimination increases suicidal ideation in black adolescents regardless of ethnicity and gender. *Behav Sci.* 2017;7:75.

31 Sheftall AH, Vakil F, Ruch DA, et al. Black youth suicide: investigation of current trends and precipitating circumstances. *J Am Acad Child Adolesc Psychiatry.* 2022;61:662–675.

32 Argabright ST, Visoki E, Moore TM, et al. Association between discrimination stress and suicidality in preadolescent children. *J Am Acad Child Adolesc Psychiatry.* 2022;61:686–697.

33 Perez-Brumer A, Day JK, Russell ST, Hatzenbuehler ML. Prevalence and correlates of suicidal ideation among transgender youth in California: findings from a representative, population-based sample of high school students. *J Acad Child Adolesc Psychiatry.* 2017;56:739–746.

34 Toomey RB, Syvertsen AK, Shramko M. Transgender adolescent suicide behavior. *Pediatrics.* 2018;142:e20174218.

35 Bochicchio L, Reeder K, Aronson L, McTavish C, Stefancic A. Understanding factors associated with suicidality among transgender and gender-diverse identified youth. *LGBT Health.* 2021;8:245–253.

36 Baiden P, Mengo C, Small E. History of physical teen dating violence and its association with suicidal behaviors among adolescent high school students: results from the 2015 youth risk behavior survey. *J Interpers Violence.* 2021;36:NP9526–NP9547.

37 McCauley E, Berk MS, Asarnow JR, et al. Efficacy of dialectical behavior therapy for adolescents at high risk for suicide: a randomized clinical trial. *JAMA Psychiatry.* 2018;75:777–785.

38 Poo J, Galione JN, Grocott LR, Horowitz KJ, Kudinova AY, Kim K. Dialectical behavior therapy for adolescents (DBT-A): outcomes among sexual minorities at high risk for suicide. *Suicide Life Threat Behav.* 2022;52:383–391.

39 Hazen EP, Goldstein MA, Goldstein MC. *Mental Health Disorders in Adolescents: A Guide for Parents, Teachers, and Professionals.* Rutgers University Press; 2011.

40 Sekhar DL, Batra E, Schaefer EW, et al. Adolescent suicide risk screening: a secondary analysis of the SHIELD randomized clinical trial. *J Pediatr.* 2022;251:172–177.

41 Horowitz LM, Bridge JA, Teach SJ, et al. Ask suicide-screening questions (ASQ): a brief instrument for the pediatric emergency department. *Arch Pediatr Adolesc Med.* 2012;166:1170–1176.

42 Federal Communications Commission. 988 suicide and crisis lifeline. Washington, DC. November 30, 2022.

PART III
SOCIAL ISSUES

Social Media–Related Issues

9
Cyberbullying

Introduction

In contrast to adults, adolescents have a higher risk of being harmed by cyberbullying. While adults may encounter cyberbullying, especially if they are public figures, their reactions to such bullying are different from adolescents. Biologically, the brains and bodies of adolescents are still developing. Brain maturation and final growth end at about 25 years, when judgment and other cognitive abilities are fully matured. Though they may be the same age, different adolescents may be psychologically and emotionally at varying levels. While one teen may have the capacity to deal with difficult situations, another teen, at the same age, may feel totally threatened. Adolescents form cliques, discover and explore their sexuality, begin romantic relationships, and seek to fit in.

There is no standard definition for cyberbullying. Most are modeled on the definition of bullying, and there is overlap between the two. Cyberbullying often, but not always, involves in-school events, with students as both victims and perpetrators, and it incorporates electronic communications such as email, personal blogs, text messaging, and video content posted on streaming websites, such as YouTube, Instagram, Snapchat, and TikTok. The victims of cyberbullying may feel that they cannot escape from the bullying itself. Compared to traditional bullying, cyberbullying creates a larger audience, allows the perpetrator to be anonymous, reaches beyond school hours, and appears less likely to be reviewed by authority figures. Cyberbullying may cause its own psychological harm, and there is research suggesting that it is more likely to cause substance abuse and depression than more traditional bullying.[1]

The Department of Education of the Commonwealth of Massachusetts defines cyberbullying as

> the severe or repeated use by one or more students of a written, verbal, or electronic expression, or a physical act or gesture, or any combination thereof, directed at another student that has the effect of: (i) causing physical or emotional harm to the other student or damage to the other student's property; (ii) placing the other student in reasonable fear of harm to himself or of damage to his property; (iii) creating a hostile environment at school for the other student; (iv) infringing on the rights of the other student; or (v) materially and substantially disrupting the education process or the orderly operation of a school.[2]

There are several different subcategories of cyberbullying. Cyberbullying may include flaming, which is defined as online fighting using angry and/or vulgar language, repeatedly sending mean and insulting messages, and cyberstalking or continuous, intense provocation and denigration and threats that elicit fear. Other forms of cyberbullying include the online spreading of rumors and posting or sending gossip that damages a person's reputation or friendships. Another type of cyberbullying is outing or the sharing of someone's secrets or potentially embarrassing information or images. An individual may be deceived online into revealing a secret or information they would prefer to keep private. Impersonation occurs when one pretends to be someone else or communicates material that causes trouble or places a person in danger or damages someone's reputation or friendships. And finally, there is exclusion, or the intentional mean-spirited exclusion of someone from an online group.[3]

Symptoms and Signs of Cyberbullying

See Box 9.1 for symptoms and signs of cyberbullying.

In a study of 2218 students between the ages of 11 and 19 years and in four secondary schools in London, researchers from the United Kingdom observed posttraumatic stress symptomatology in cyberbullying victims and perpetrators. They designed a cross-sectional survey and self-report questionnaire. There were measures for cyber and traditional bullying as well as posttraumatic stress symptoms. The median age of the subjects was 15.0 years; the majority were female. Among participants, cyberbullying involvement was less common than the traditional form (25.46 percent vs. 33.48 percent). Those who were victims of cyberbullying or victim-perpetrators seemed to be associated with several types of posttraumatic stress symptoms. Female cyberbully victims seemed to be more symptomatic than their male counterparts. And there was a strong overlap between traditional bullying and cyberbullying, although perpetrators of cyberbullying were less likely to be involved in traditional bullying.[4]

Another study from the United Kingdom evaluated 2480 teenagers in East London participating in the Olympic Regeneration. (The Olympic Regeneration was a study of the impact of urban regeneration associated with the London 2012 Olympic Games on a prospective cohort of adolescents in East London.) About 14 percent of the adolescents reported that during the previous year they were victims of cyberbullying, 8 percent admitted to being cyberbullies, and 20 percent were both victims and

---

Box 9.1 Symptoms and Signs of Cyberbullying in Adolescents

Change in sleep patterns
Change in appetite
Restlessness
Decreased self-esteem
Increased school absenteeism
Increased anxiety
Increased self-harm behaviors such as cutting
Suicidal ideation
Suicide attempt

perpetrators of cyberbullying. When compared to noninvolved students, both victims and victims/cyberbullies were significantly more likely to report social anxiety or depressive symptoms. Because the victims may have internalized mental health symptomatology such as anxiety or depression, the researchers noted that cyberbullying might contribute to the public health burden.[5]

Researchers from Brazil conducted a literature search on cyberbullying that located 48 articles that met their criteria. They found that the prevalence of cyberbullying ranged from 6.5 percent to 35.4 percent. Whether victim or perpetrator, mental health symptoms for those involved in cyberbullying included depression, social anxiety, suicide attempts, low self-esteem, and substance use. Suicidal ideation was also seen among victims. The researchers maintained that the experiences of cyberbullying alone were unlikely to lead to youth suicide. Rather, cyberbullying may exacerbate an adolescent's instability and hopelessness at a time when they are already struggling with stressful life circumstances.[6]

Characteristics of Cyberbullying Perpetrators and Victims

In a study of adolescent males with attention-deficit/hyperactivity disorder (ADHD), researchers in Taiwan recruited 251 male subjects and asked about their cyberbullying experience. Thirty-six of the adolescents reported that they were perpetrators, and 48 said that they were victims. Aside from their ADHD, perpetrators had symptomatology consistent with depression, anxiety, and suicidality. Perpetrators likely had the hyperactivity types of ADHD, and victims would have a diagnosis consistent with the inattention form. There was no significant difference in victims who also had symptoms consistent with a mood disorder, anxiety, and depression. The researchers determined that cyberbullying perpetration was an extension of traditional bullying, and they suggested that approaching bullies with educational tools may prevent them from evolving into cyberbullies. Such transformations tend to occur at an older age when people have greater privacy and extensive connections to the internet. The researchers noted that cyberbullies had more significant problematic internet use (PIU) (as defined in Chapter 10) than nonperpetrators.[7]

Predictors of Cyberbullying

According to a researcher in Korea who studied South Korean adolescents, individual factors and social support are predictors of cyberbullying. Individual factors include gender, school satisfaction, self-esteem, self-control, and a history of being a cyberbully or a victim. Females are more likely to be victims than males, and males are more likely than females to be perpetrators. Students with low school satisfaction were more likely to receive or commit cyberbullying. In general, students with high self-esteem did not participate in cyberbullying activities. The higher the levels of self-control, the less likely it was that the student would encounter a cyberbullying experience. Students with high levels of self-control were able to avoid this type of behavior.[8]

Identifying Victims and Perpetrators of Cyberbullying

Victims of cyberbullying may demonstrate certain characteristics (see Box 9.2).

Perpetrators of cyberbullying may have certain behavioral characteristics such as becoming increasingly withdrawn or isolated from family, showing violent tendencies, laughing excessively while using device(s), and avoiding discussing what they are doing online. They may have increasing behavioral issues or disciplinary actions at school, hang out with the "wrong crowd," and use their devices at all hours of the day or night.[9,10]

Many victims of cyberbullying remain silent and are reluctant to seek help. As a result, it is important that social support networks, including family, teachers, health care providers, coaches, and clergy, recognize the symptoms of cyberbullying. While these symptoms may sometimes be difficult to observe, one of the most common and clearly evident symptoms is school avoidance, which may manifest itself in somatic complaints including stomachaches, headaches, and sleep issues such as nightmares. Victims may have depressive symptoms, outbursts, or self-injurious behaviors such as cutting. Adolescents may report cyberbullying in urgent and nonurgent settings. In a medical setting, such as a primary care or emergency room visit, screening questions could include the following: Have you ever been bullied? How often are you bullied or how often do you bully others? Where are you bullied or where do you bully others? How are you bullied or how do you bully others?[11]

Victims of cyberbullying may visit an emergency department or urgent care facility with mental health symptoms, including suicidal ideation or attempts at self-harm. Researchers from Canada performed a retrospective chart review of adolescents under the age of 18 years who presented with a mental health complaint and were seen by the psychiatry staff of two emergency departments. Of the 270 patients who were seen, 77 percent had a history of bullying. Of the 51 patients who said that they were victims of cyberbullying, 48 were suicidal. The adolescents who were cyberbullied were 11.5 times more likely to report suicidal ideation, and those with a history of verbal bullying were 8.4 times more likely to say they had suicidal ideation. Those patients with a history of any type of bullying were 19 times more likely to have documented suicidal ideation compared to those with no history of bullying.[12]

Box 9.2 Characteristics for Victims of Cyberbullying

Decreased self-esteem or feelings of helplessness
Increased symptoms of depression and/or anxiety
Sudden loss of friends, isolation from peers, or withdrawal at home
Increased truancy or school absences
Decline in academic performance or loss of interest in schoolwork
Changes in eating habits or appetite
Difficulty sleeping or frequent nightmares
Self-harm behaviors, such as cutting or suicidal ideation

Other researchers from Canada evaluated the prevalence of bullying victimization among adolescents referred for urgent psychiatric consultation. The study was conducted by a retrospective chart review of all adolescents who were referred to a hospital-based urgent consultation clinic during a 12-month period. Of the 375 patients who were assessed, 182 patients had a current or past history of being bullied. Teens who had a history of cybervictimization had more suicidal ideations than those who were verbally bullied. The researchers suggested that the students who were cyberbullied might seek help less often than those who were bullied by more traditional means. Because victims may fail to report cyberbullying, they may receive less support by networks including parents and schools, which increases their risk of suicidal ideation.[13]

Cyberbullies also carry certain predictive factors related to mental health. A group of researchers in California searched for articles on cyberbullying among tweens and teens on PubMed and George Scholar. They located 50 articles that met their criteria. The researchers learned that cyberbullies were more likely to be males with substandard academic performance, which seemed to affect their self-esteem. They had low peer support and attracted other students with similar issues, which effectively led to the moral approval of bullying and the normalization of violence. Moreover, cyberbullies tended to have low levels of empathy and were attracted to violent media and video games. They appeared to be unable to read nonverbal cues and express emotion. Their families may have had unclear rules and poorly defined boundaries, placing the adolescents at a higher risk for antisocial activities. It should be noted that other studies have found that a controlling parental style may be associated with a higher prevalence of adolescent involvement in cyberbullying, both as a victim and as a perpetrator.[14]

Epidemiology

Because there are varying definitions for cyberbullying, it is difficult to compare the findings of various studies. Nevertheless, there have been several studies that attempt to quantify the prevalence of cyberbullying and its associated risks in both the United States and worldwide. Researchers in Australia and the United Kingdom performed a systematic review of electronic databases and located 46 studies that met their cyberbullying criteria. The researchers learned that the children and adolescents in Australia had a lifetime prevalence of 25.13 percent for traditional bullying victimization and 7.02 percent for cyberbullying victimization. The percentages were lower for perpetration; the lifetime prevalence for perpetration was 11.61 percent for traditional bullying and 3.45 percent for cyberbullying.[15]

In the United States, researchers in Pennsylvania and Illinois examined the association of cyberbullying victimization with mental health conditions and violent behaviors among adolescents and potential differences by sex and race. Using data from the 2015 Youth Risk Behavior Survey from the Centers for Disease Control and Prevention, they created a cohort of 15,465 students from grades 9 through 12. The researchers learned that more than 15 percent reported that they were victims of cyberbullying; females were twice as likely as males to admit to victimization. In addition, the researchers found that negative mental health outcomes and violent behaviors were more pronounced in males, indicating a potential negative effect of being cyberbullied for that gender.[16]

This gendered dichotomy was supported by researchers in Canada who used data from the Ontario Student Drug Use and Health Survey to investigate the gender differences in the association between cyberbullying victimization and mental health, substance abuse–related outcomes, and suicide ideation in adolescents. The sample analyzed included 4940 students, 43.3 percent male, with a mean age of 15.1 years. The researchers learned that 13.3 percent of the female adolescents and 7.8 percent of the males admitted to two or more incidents of cyberbullying. Cyberbullying victims had increased odds of psychological distress, suicidal ideation, and delinquency, and the effects were more pronounced in females. While female victims had an increased risk of substance abuse, this finding was not seen in male victims.[17]

There is concern that adolescents with intellectual and developmental disabilities may be at increased risk for cyberbullying. Researchers from the Netherlands, Texas, California, and Italy examined the prevalence of cyberbullying among adolescents with these medical problems who studied in special education settings. The students in the cohort, which consisted of 114 students between the ages of 12 and 19 years, completed an electronic questionnaire with questions about bullying and victimization. The researchers determined that 4 to 9 percent of the students reported being a perpetrator or victim of cyberbullying at least one time per week. There was a significant association between cyberbullying and self-esteem as well as depressive feelings. Most online bullies admitted to also being online victims.[18]

Biopsychosocial Issues and Cyberbullying

Biological Issues and Cyberbullying

Sleep

Studies have found that compared to teens who are not victims of cyberbullying, victims of cyberbullying tend to have mental health issues. Using data from a longitudinal research study on physical and mental health, in two waves, researchers from China examined the association between cyberbullying perpetrations, sleep quality, and emotional distress in adolescents. The measures included cyberbullying perpetration and sleep quality as measured by the Chinese version of the Pittsburgh Sleep Quality Index and the Chinese version of the Depression Anxiety Stress Scales. The waves, T1 and T2, were 8 months apart. The researchers learned that the adolescents with higher levels of cyberbullying perpetration at T1 had poorer sleep quality at T2. And poorer sleep quality at T1 predicted cyberbullying at T2. The adolescents with more emotional distress at T1 were more likely to have higher levels of cyberbullying perpetration at T2.[19]

Researchers from Canada analyzed the link between cyberbullying victimization, perpetration, or both to sleep duration and screen time in adolescents. They used data from the Ontario Student Drug Use and Health Survey, which is a cross-sectional study of students in grades 7 to 12 in four public school systems. The 6834 students ranged in age from 11 to 20 years, with a mean age of 15.2 years; the majority were

White and male. There were questions on cyberbullying victimization and perpetration, sleep duration, and demographics. The researchers determined that all adolescents involved in cyberbullying, from victims to perpetrators, had greater odds of short sleep duration. The younger students who were not cyberbullied had a lower risk of short sleep duration. Gender and screen time did not moderate any of the associations between cyberbullying involvement and short sleep duration.[20]

Psychological Issues and Cyberbullying

Depression

To learn more about the health-related effects of cyberbullying on adolescents, researchers from Canada performed a scoping review of 36 studies; all of the studies involved social media sites. The adolescent subjects ranged in age from 12 to 18 years; the median reported prevalence of cyberbullying was 23.0 percent. The researchers noted that the most common forms of cyberbullying were name-calling or insults, spreading gossip and rumors, and circulating pictures. Ten of the studies attempted to determine if depressive symptoms or depression were associated with cyberbullying. In every study, the levels of depression increased significantly with exposure to cyberbullying. One longitudinal study found that over time, exposure to cyberbullying predicted increased depressive symptoms. This scoping review offers clear evidence of a consistent relationship between cyberbullying and depression in adolescents.[21]

More specifically, researchers from China and South Carolina examined the relationship between neuroticism, depression, and cyberbullying in young Chinese adolescents. Neurotic people tend to be emotionally labile, anxious, tense, and withdrawn. The cohort consisted of 3961 adolescents with a mean age of 10.85 years; the majority were males. They were studied at T1, T2, and T3; each evaluation was separated by 6 months. The researchers used the Abbreviated Junior Eysenck Personality Questionnaire to measure neuroticism and other tools to quantify cyberbullying perpetration and victimization. Using cascade models, or models that move information in a top-to-bottom manner, the researchers found concurrent correlations between neuroticism, depression, and both perpetrator and victimization cyberbullying at all three points. Neuroticism directly predicted subsequent cyberbullying victimization, and depression predicted both perpetrator and victimization cyberbullying. Yet either form of cyberbullying did not predict subsequent depression. The researchers concluded that adolescents with neurotic tendencies have an increased risk for perpetrator and victimization cyberbullying mediated by concurrent depression.[22]

PIU is associated with online risky activities, such as cyberbullying, that may cause physical, mental, and social harm, including the consumption of alcohol, tobacco use, depression, and low self-esteem. Researchers in Spain and England examined the correlation between cyberbullying victimization and PIU, depression, and substance use in adolescents. The cohort consisted of 845 adolescents, 59 percent female, ages 13 to 17 years, from 10 secondary schools in Spain. The teens completed a questionnaire for T1 and T2, the second of which did not include a defined time interval. There were measures for cyberbullying, depressive symptoms, substance use, and PIU. The researchers learned that cyberbullying victimization predicted an increase in PIU, but PIU did not predict cyberbullying. Cyberbullying victimization led to an increase in depressive symptoms, and depressive symptoms raised the probability of cyberbullying. The researchers advised intervention efforts for adolescents with PIU as well as those who were victims of cyberbullying.[23]

Substance Use
It is well known that victims of cyberbullying experience negative physical and mental health outcomes. Such outcomes may include increased risk to use substances. Researchers from Pennsylvania and Florida examined the relationship between bullying victimization (traditional, cyber, and both) and binge drinking and marijuana use among adolescents, as well as gender differences between bullying victimization and substance use. They used nationally representative data from the 2013 National High School Youth Risk Behavior Survey. There were two measures for substance use (a history of drinking five or more drinks of alcohol in a row in a few hours and any report of marijuana use) and a measure for bullying victimization. Interestingly, the researchers found no significant connection between traditional bullying victimization and binge drinking. However, the relationship between cyberbullying victimization and binge drinking and marijuana use was significant among females, and males and females who reported being victims of both traditional and cyberbullying were overall more likely to report binge drinking and marijuana use than those not involved in bullying of any form.[24]

To determine if different roles in cyberbullying were related to substance use, researchers from California and Colorado performed a longitudinal study. They studied roles that consisted of no involvement, witness and victim, witness and perpetrator, and witness, victim, and perpetrator. The cohort consisted of 2768 adolescents with a mean age of 15.5 years; the majority were female. The researchers surveyed the teens at baseline and 6 months later. Measures include cyberbullying and the past 6-month history of substance use. The researchers learned that even witnessing cyberbullying may increase the risk for future substance use. All types of roles/involvement with cyberbullying were related to the use of substances, including e-cigarettes, marijuana edibles, and prescription opioids. At the 6-month follow-up, the other three roles were much more likely to be using several substances than the witness-only role. This underscores the important need to prevent cyberbullying.[25]

Social Issues and Cyberbullying

Social Media
Social media sites are known settings for adolescent cyberbullying. Adolescent cyberbullying involves teenage perpetrators and victims, and it incorporates social media communication, including messages, photographs, and/or video. Social media sites, including Instagram, Snapchat, and TikTok, are often problematic for adolescents, who have a limited capacity for self-regulation and are susceptible to peer pressure. On these sites, they may easily and anonymously be drawn into cyberbullying. In the previously mentioned study from researchers in Italy and Singapore, the authors

noted that cyberbullying may spread quickly and the victim may feel a lack of control resulting in highly negative psychological consequences, including social anxiety, depression, and suicidality. This is particularly problematic when the bullying behavior continues over an extended period of time. The researchers did note that some social media sites have added features that enable people to report inappropriate content and comments.[26]

Researchers from Canada conducted a scoping review of social media studies on the prevalence and effect of cyberbullying on children and adolescents. Their definition of cyberbullying included three social media platforms: blogs (5.0 percent), social networking sites (4.0 to 20.0 percent), and message boards (26.0 percent). They found that the most hurtful or distressing types of social media cyberbullying included pictures or videos that teens were asked to send or coerced into sending or had been covertly filmed or photographed. The authors concluded that social media cyberbullying has emerged as a primary safety concern; there was evidence that exposure to cyberbullying was harmful.[27]

Researchers from the United Kingdom held six focus groups over 3 months with 54 adolescents between the ages of 11 and 18 years; the students were recruited from schools in Leicester and London to discuss social media. One of the topics addressed was whether social media placed people at increased risk for bullying and trolling. The teens in the focus groups blamed social media for fostering cyberbullying that they described as endemic to adolescence. Viewed positively, social media can be a useful way to share aspects of one's life with friends and family; in doing so, however, one can also become a victim of cyberbullying. Clearly, social media sites have created a platform for the bullying behaviors that extend beyond the boundaries and supervision of schools.[28]

Racism/Discrimination

Cyberbullying that is racially offensive or racist in nature is termed cyber racism. Researchers in North Carolina and California hypothesized that racial-ethnic minority adolescents experiencing offline victimization would also report online victimization as well as multiple types of victimization experiences including perceived racial discrimination. They drew a sample from the Teen Life Online and in Schools project, which was a longitudinal study of the risk and protective factors associated with online racial discrimination in diverse youth. The sample consisted of 735 adolescents, with a mean age of 14.5 years, majority female, endorsing non-White identities (Black, Hispanic, Latino, biracial, multiracial, Asian, Asian American, Native American, South Asian, and Middle Eastern). Three waves of data were collected in middle and high school; each wave was 10 to 12 months apart. The measures included offline bullying/harassment, online bullying/harassment, offline racial-ethnic discrimination, online racial-ethnic discrimination, time online, gender, age, parental education, and race/ethnicity.

The results showed that there was substantial co-occurrence of offline and online bullying/harassment and offline and online racial-ethnic discrimination. In addition, time spent online did not increase an adolescent's risk for later victimization experiences. The researchers suggested that an intervention targeting general bullying/harassment may protect racial-ethnic minority youth from future victimization experiences. Simply reducing time online did not appear to be an effective strategy for protecting adolescents from victimization in a digital age.[29]

LGBTQ

Hinduja and Patchin, cofounders and codirectors of the Cyberbullying Research Center, performed a survey of 4400 randomly selected students between the ages of 11 and 18 years, from one public school district. About 9 percent were nonheterosexual or questioning. Thirty-six percent of the nonheterosexual students indicated that they were victims of cyberbullying, in contrast to the 20 percent identified in the heterosexual group. Compared to 19 percent of the heterosexual group, 39 percent of the nonheterosexual group reported being a cyberbully perpetrator. Based on these results, sexual minority adolescents are at a higher risk for cyberbullying.[30]

Studies have shown that LGBTQ youth who are bullied have higher rates of depression, suicidal thoughts, and suicide attempts. In particular, one study determined that 48.7 percent of sexual minority youth had a history of being cyberbullied. In another study, researchers from Kentucky and Florida conducted a systematic literature review to clarify the effects of cyberbullying on LGBTQ youth. They found that the prevalence of cyberbullying varied from 10.5 percent to 71.3 percent depending on the paper. However, the authors felt that almost half of all sexual minority youth were victims of cyberbullying. The researchers noted that the negative effects of cyberbullying on LGBTQ youth included suicidality, lower self-esteem, body image issues, and impaired academic performance. The available programs recommended school-focused interventions for all youth. Furthermore, parents needed to be involved in the intervention efforts, including parental education on cyberbullying and parental involvement in their child's use of technology. It is likely that effective interventions for LGBTQ youth will differ from those designed for straight adolescents.[31]

Mortality

There are occasional reports of an adolescent's death by suicide related to cyberbullying. Are the two related? Researchers from the University of Hong Kong wanted to determine if the exposure to undesirable content on the internet was related to unnatural child death. The researchers used the EU Kids Online Survey, which provided data on internet-related behaviors of children and parents in 25 European countries. The data on 25,142 participants had been collected in a face-to face survey with adolescents aged 9 to 16 years. Four risks were studied: online information on self-harm or suicide, online and traditional bullying, experience of exclusively online bullying, and PIU. The researchers also used the European Detained Mortality Data, which had detailed information on deaths for each country stratified by year, cause of death, age, and death. The researchers found 1013 unnatural child deaths in children between the ages of 10 and 14 years. Suicide deaths accounted for 138 (13.6 percent); 48 (4.7 percent) were undetermined; 789 (77.9 percent) were accidental; and 38 (3.8 percent) were caused by assault. The researchers observed a statistically significant positive correlation between the prevalence of exclusively online bullying and unnatural death mortality, which was independent from offline bullying. The children's exposure to suicide content as well as PIU did not have a statistically significant association with unnatural child death.[32]

Researchers from the United Kingdom performed a systematic review on the relationship between cyberbullying as a victim or perpetrator and self-harm and suicidal behaviors in youth. They located 33 papers that met their criteria, with a total of 156,384 youth. Twenty-five articles reported either a positive association or negative influence of cyberbullying involvement—either victim or perpetrator—on self-harm and suicidal behaviors. When compared to nonvictims, victims of cyberbullying were at greater risk for both self-harm and suicidal behaviors. Although not as noteworthy, cyberbully perpetrators were at risk for suicidal ideation and suicidal behaviors.[33]

Washington State researchers examined the correlation between school connectedness and cyberbullying and suicide. Data were obtained from a middle school research program for youth and parents to help prevent health risk behaviors including suicidality. The program's intervention, which was administered in eighth grade, addressed stress and substance use. Measurements were taken at baseline and on multiple occasions up to and including 30 months after the interventions. The final evaluation, which had 93 subjects, one-third of whom were female, had questions on cyberbullying. Other measures included suicide risk, cybervictimization, and school connectedness. The findings suggested that victims of cyberbullying, but not perpetrators, had an increased risk of suicide. Students who were more connected to school were less likely to report suicidal behavior.[34]

Interventions

Not only should interventions target and mitigate cyberbullying, but also they should provide support for victims. In addition, perpetrators should undergo evaluations and treatments. There have been a number of interventions developed, and most of these have occurred in school settings. Still, whenever possible, families should be included in intervention efforts in addition to teachers and school staff. Researchers in Ohio conducted a systematic review of interventions for cyberbullying. Using Institute of Medicine guidelines, the researchers identified 17 programs that focused on children; they included lectures, discussion groups, role-playing, and group projects that lasted from 1 day to 1 year. The components included digital citizenship (defined as using technology in a responsible way or being a good citizen while online), acquiring coping skills (defined as the methods for youth to use to respond to cyberbullying), and education on cyberbullying. Only seven of the programs had educational content for parents. The researchers determined that the programs that significantly reduced cyberbullying and cyber victimization had sections on communication and social skills, empathy training, coping skills, and digital citizenship. While the 17 programs were all held in school settings, there is the possibility that certain elements, such as digital citizenship and cyberbullying education, could be used in a clinical setting, such as a medical provider's office. The researchers also commented that there was strong evidence of the value parental education may have on cyberbullying.[35]

Health care providers can play an important role in preventing cyberbullying. Studies have found that most adolescents would prefer disclosing their bullying experiences during an intake evaluation prior to seeing a health care provider. Other researchers suggest that health care providers ask their patients directly about bullying experiences. Once cyberbullying is acknowledged, interventions can be initiated. Of course, questions about cyberbullying may be asked during the annual well adolescent examination. This is particularly important if an adolescent has mental health symptoms. The annual exam is an opportunity for clinicians to raise questions that elucidate cyberbullying issues.[36]

At a clinical encounter, one can ask patients several questions if the provider is concerned about cyberbullying: How often do you get bullied (or bully others)? How long have you been bullied (or bullied others)? Where are you bullied (or bullied others)? How are you bullied (or how do you bully others)?[37]

Parents can have an important role in preventing cyberbullying. A researcher from Pennsylvania studied the cyberbullying of youth with autism spectrum disorder. The cohort consisted of 113 adolescents between the ages of 12 and 17 years who lived in the Midwest section of United States; 86 percent were male and had experienced cyberbullying. The researcher specifically focused on the association between parental mediation of technology use, defined as the use of prevention strategies to manage the child's relationship with digital media, and victim depression. Strategies included parental discussions of the appropriate use of digital media and time limits on the use of such media. Other strategies included guidelines on which sites they could view.

One year later, the researcher conducted a follow-up, and she learned that cyber-victimization was negatively associated with parental mediation of technology and perceived social support. At 1 year, lower levels of parental mediation and support were related to adolescent depression. Parental intervention via technology mediation and support may be a protective factor against cyberbullying and depression.[38]

Clinicians might advise parents whose adolescent is a victim of cyberbullying in a number of ways. First and foremost, make sure the adolescent is and remains safe. Ask the adolescent what they would like to happen, and collect evidence and keep detailed records of what has occurred. Parents should contact the school and inform the appropriate administrators of the situation. If there are physical threats, coercion, stalking, sexually explicit pictures, or videos of minors, the police should be contacted.

If the parents believe their adolescent is the perpetrator of cyberbullying, then they need to talk with them about the hurtful nature of cyberbullying. They should apply reasonable consequences to their actions and set firm limits. The parents might also consider installing tracking software, and they should closely monitor their child's use of technology.[39]

Prevention

Higher levels of resilience may help adolescents protect themselves from cyberbullying. In this context, resilience is the capacity to spring back, rebound, and successfully adapt in the face of adversity and develop social and academic competence despite exposure to severe stress—or simply the stress of today's world.[40] Hinduja and Patchin used data from a nationally representative sample of English-speaking 12- to 17-year-old students in the United States. The survey had measures for resilience, bullying, and cyberbullying. The sample size was 1204 students, with a mean age of

14.5 years, and 49.8 percent were female. In the sample, 15.7 percent reported they were cyberbullied. The results indicated that students with higher levels of resilience were less likely to report that they had been bullied at school or online. Of those who were bullied, resilience seemed to insulate them from significant disruption at school. These findings suggested that programs that improve youth resilience will be protective against cyberbullying.[41]

Researchers in Hungary questioned whether there were social-emotional skill differences between high school students who were cyberbullying victims and perpetrators. They examined empathy, intention to comfort, specific adaptive and maladaptive emotion regulation strategies, and moral disengagement. The cohort consisted of 524 students between the ages of 12 and 19 years; there were 214 males. The students answered questions on a self-reported questionnaire. The researchers determined that cyberbullying victims had empathy and regulated their emotions in adaptive and maladaptive ways. Meanwhile, cyberbullying perpetrators lacked empathy and were unable to appreciate the victims' perspective or feel vicarious emotions. There was an association between moral disengagement and cyberbullying perpetration. Cyberbullying victims used specific maladaptive emotional regulation strategies that included rumination and self-blame. The researchers commented that a prevention program should entail adolescents developing higher levels of empathy, adaptive emotional regulation, and intention to comfort others, as these could be protective against cyberbullying.[42]

Some school-based anti-cyberbullying programs have reported positive results. One of these is the Second Step Middle School Program, which aims to strengthen social connectedness through social belonging lessons at the start of middle school (grades 6 or 7) and again in grade 8, thus preparing students for the transition to high school. In a 3-year randomized clinical trial, researchers from Illinois, Arizona, Oregon, and Tennessee examined the direct and indirect impact of this program on cyberbullying. Thirty-six schools in Kansas and Illinois were assigned to either the Second Step program or a control activity. The students in the Second Step group participated in a total of 41 lessons. During the 3 years, 3651 sixth-grade students completed self-reported surveys four times. The researchers found that over the first 2 years, the students in the treatment group had decreases in self-reported delinquency that were significantly related to decreases in cyberbullying. Further, there were decreases in bullying and homophobic name-calling perpetration.[43]

The ViSC Social Competence Program, which was developed for middle school students, is one component of the Austrian national strategy to prevent violence in schools. Teachers are trained to recognize and deal with bullying cases and to implement preventive measures. The students are empowered to take responsibility for what happens in their classrooms. Using a longitudinal, randomized, controlled group study design, researchers in Austria investigated the usefulness and sustainability of the VISC program in preventing cyberbullying and cybervictimization. The study was conducted in 2009 to 2010, and 26 Vienna schools participated. The researchers learned that ViSC was effective in preventing cyberbullying and cybervictimization, and the positive outcome was still evident after 6 months.[44]

To be truly lasting, preventive efforts need to be offered from multiple fronts. Families, schools, health care workers, governments, and social media platforms should be initiating efforts. While adolescents and concerned adults should be wary of cyberbullying information websites endorsing the sale of products,[45] adolescent-friendly materials on various social media sites may be effective preventive tools.[46] Other resources include Kids Health and Connect Safely, a helpful site for adolescents who are being cyberbullied and their parents.[47] However, some content on popular sites like Facebook or the Centers for Disease Control and Prevention is either out of date or lacks interventions specifically for cyberbullying. The federal government thus has an extraordinary opportunity to lead and sponsor research, develop programming, and create and pass legislation on cyberbullying issues.[48]

Conclusion

Adolescents may be harmed by cyberbullying, and social media sites are known settings for this behavior. Youth may initially present to an emergency department with mental health symptoms, including suicidality. Families, health care providers, and schools have roles in recognizing and preventing cyberbullying among adolescents.

References

1 Englander E, Donnerstein E, Kowalski R, Lin CA, Parti K. Defining cyberbullying. *Pediatrics.* 2017;140(Suppl 2):S124–S151.
2 Massachusetts Anti-Bullying Law. MGL c71 §370.
3 Cantone E, Piras AP, Vellante M, et al. Interventions on bullying and cyberbullying in schools: a systematic review. *Clin Pract Epidemiol Ment Health.* 2015;11(Suppl 1 M4):58–76.
4 Mateu A, Pascual-Sánchez A, Martinez-Herves M, Hickey N, Nicholls D, Kramer T. Cyberbullying and post-traumatic stress symptoms in UK adolescents. *Arch Dis Child.* 2020;105:951–956.
5 Fahy AE, Stansfeld SA, Smuk M, et al. Longitudinal associations between cyberbullying involvement and adolescent mental health. *J Adolesc Health.* 2016;59:502–509.
6 Bottino SM, Bottino CM, Regina CG, Villa Lobo Correia A, Ribeiro WS. Cyberbullying and adolescent mental health: systematic review. *Cad Saude Publica.* 2015;31:463–475.
7 Yen CF, Chou WJ, Liu TL, et al. Cyberbullying among male adolescents with attention-deficit/hyperactivity disorder: prevalence, correlates, and association with poor mental health status. *Res Dev Disabil.* 2014;35:3543–3553.
8 Yoo C. What are the characteristics of cyberbullying victims and perpetrators among South Korean students and how do their experiences change? *Child Abuse Negl.* 2021;113:104923.
9 Hinduja S, Patchin JW. Cyberbullying identification, prevention, and response. Cyberbullying Research Center (cyberbullying.org); 2024.
10 Kumar VL, Goldstein MA. Cyberbullying and adolescents. *Curr Pediatr Rep.* 2020 Sep;8:86–92.
11 Lamb J, Pepler DJ, Craig W. Approach to bullying and victimization. *Can Fam Physician.* 2009;55:356–360.
12 Alavi N, Reshetukha T, Prost E, et al. Relationship between bullying and suicidal behaviour in youth presenting to the emergency department. *J Can Acad Child Adolesc Psychiatry.* 2017;26:70–77.

13 Alavi N, Roberts N, Sutton C, Axas N, Repetti L. Bullying victimization (being bullied) among adolescents referred for urgent psychiatric consultation: prevalence and association with suicidality. *Can J Psychiatry*. 2015;60:427–431.

14 Khan F, Limbana T, Zahid T, Eskander N, Jahan N. Traits, trends, and trajectory of tween and teen cyberbullies. *Cureus*. 2020;12:e9738.

15 Jadambaa A, Thomas HJ, Scott JG, Graves N, Brain D, Pacella R. Prevalence of traditional bullying and cyberbullying among children and adolescents in Australia: a systematic review and meta-analysis. *Aust N Z J Psychiatry*. 2019;53:878–888.

16 Alhajji M, Bass S, Dai T. Cyberbullying, mental health, and violence in adolescents and associations with sex, race: data from the 2015 youth risk behavior survey. *Glob Pediatr Health*. 2019;6:2333794x19868887.

17 Kim S, Kimber M, Boyle MH, Georglades K. Sex differences in the association between cyberbullying victimization and mental health, substance use, and suicidal ideation in adolescents. *Can J Psychiatry*. 2019;64:126–135.

18 Didden R, Scholte RH, Korzilius H, et al. Cyberbullying among students wit intellectual and developmental disability in special education settings. *Dev Neurorehabil*. 2009;12:146–151

19 Liu C, Liu Z, Yuan G. Associations between cyberbullying perpetration, sleep quality, and emotional distress among adolescents: a two-wave cross-lagged analysis. *J Nerv Ment Dis*. 2021;209:123–127.

20 Sampasa-Kanyinga H, Lien A, Hamilton HA, Chaput JP. Cyberbullying involvement and short sleep duration among adolescents. *Sleep Health*. 2022;8:183–190.

21 Hamm MP, Newton AS, Chisholm A, et al. Prevalence and effect of cyberbullying on children and young people: a scoping review of social media studies. *JAMA Pediatr*. 2015;169:770–777.

22 Zhang D, Huebner ES, Tian L. Longitudinal associations among neuroticism, depression, and cyberbullying in early adolescents. *Comput Hum Behav*. 2020;112:106475.

23 Gámez-Guadix M, Orue I, Smith PK, Calvete E. Longitudinal and reciprocal relations of cyberbullying with depression, substance use, and problematic internet use among adolescents. *J Adolesc Health*. 2013;53:446–452.

24 Priesman E, Newman R, Ford JA. Bullying victimization, binge drinking, and marijuana use among adolescents: results from the 2013 national youth risk behavior survey. *J Psychoactive Drugs*. 2018;50:133–142.

25 Yoon Y, Lee JO, Cho J, et al. Association of cyberbullying involvement with subsequent substance use among adolescents. *J Adolesc Health*. 2019;65:613–620.

26 Cataldo I, Lepri B, Neoh MJY, Esposito G. Social media usage and development of psychiatric disorders in childhood and adolescence: a review. *Front Psychiatry*. 2021;11:508595.

27 Hamm MP, Newton AS, Chisholm A, et al. Prevalence and effect of cyberbullying on children and young people: a scoping review of social media studies. *JAMA Pediatr*. 2015;169:770–777.

28 O'Reilly M, Dogra N, Whiteman N, Hughes J, Eruper S, Reilly P. Is social media bad for mental health and wellbeing? Exploring the perspectives of adolescents. *Clin Child Psychol Psychiatry*. 2018;23:601–613.

29 Weinstein M, Jensen MR, Tynes BM. Victimized in many ways: online and offline bullying/harassment and perceived racial discrimination in diverse racial-ethnic minority adolescents. *Cultur Divers Ethnic Minor Psychol*. 2021;27:397–407.

30 Hinduja S, Patchin J. Cyberbullying and sexual orientation. Cyberbullying Research Center. 2011.

31 Abreu RL, Kenny MC. Cyberbullying and LGBTQ youth: a systematic literature review and recommendations for prevention and intervention. *J Child Adolesc Trauma*. 2017;11:81–97.

32 Fu KW, Chan CH, Ip P. Exploring the relationship between cyberbullying and unnatural child death: an ecological study of twenty-four European countries. *BMC Pediatr.* 2014;14:195.

33 John A, Glendenning AC, Marchant A, et al. Self-harm, suicidal behaviours, and cyberbullying in children and young people: systematic review. *J Med Internet Res.* 2018;20:e129.

34 Kim J, Walsh E, Pike K, Thompson EA. Cyberbullying and victimization and youth suicide risk: the buffering effects of school connectedness. *J Sch Nurs.* 2020;36:251–257.

35 Hutson E, Kelly S, Militello LK. Systematic review of cyberbullying interventions for youth and parents with implications for evidence-based practice. *Worldviews Evid Based Nurs.* 2018;15:72–79.

36 Espelage D, Hong JS. Cyberbullying prevention and intervention efforts: current knowledge and future directions. *Can J Psychiatry.* 2017;62:374–380.

37 Moreno MA, Vaillancourt T. The role of health care providers in cyberbullying. *Can J Psychiatry.* 2017;62:364–367.

38 Wright MF. Victimization and depression among adolescents with autism spectrum disorder: the buffering effects of parental mediation and social support. *J Child Adolesc Trauma.* 2017;11:17–25.

39 Hinduja S, Patchin J. *Bullying Beyond the Schoolyard: Preventing and Responding to Cyberbullying.* 2nd ed. Corwin; 2015.

40 Henderson N, Milstein MM. *Resiliency in Schools: Making It Happen for Students and Educators.* Corwin Press; 2003.

41 Hinduja S, Patchin JW. Cultivating youth resilience to prevent bullying and cyberbullying victimization. *Child Abuse Negl.* 2017;73:51–62.

42 Arató J, Zsidó N, Lénárd K, Labadi B. Cybervictimization and cyberbullying: the role of socio-emotional skills. *Front Psychiatry.* 2020;11:248.

43 Espelage DL, Low S, Van Rzin MJ, Polanin JP. Clinical trial of second step middle school program: impact on bullying, cyberbullying, homophobic teasing, and sexual harassment perpetration. *School Psychol Rev.* 2015;44:464–479.

44 Gradinger P, Yanagida T, Strohmeier D, Spiel C. Effectiveness and sustainability of the ViSC social competence program to prevent cyberbullying and cyber-victimization: class and individual level moderators. *Aggress Behav.* 2016;42:181–193.

45 Espelage DL, Hong JS. Cyberbullying prevention and intervention efforts: current knowledge and future directions. *Can J Psychiatry.* 2017;62:374–380.

46 Healthychildren.org Social media & your child's mental health: what the research says. May 23, 2023.

47 Connect Safely. Family guide to parental controls. August 23, 2023.

48 Centers for Disease Control and Prevention. Fast facts: preventing bullying. Atlanta, GA. September 28, 2023.

10

Problematic Internet Use

Introduction

Also known as video game addiction, problematic internet gaming, problematic interactive media use, internet addiction, and problematic video gaming, problematic internet use (PIU) is a serious, widespread global social problem. Although definitions vary, PIU is essentially the inability to control one's use of the internet, leading to negative consequences in daily life such as avoiding academic work or social activities.[1] Some authorities also include use of noninternet games in the definition. It should be noted that PIU is not recognized as a disorder by the *Diagnostic and Statistical Manual of Mental Disorders*, fifth edition (DSM-5), or by the World Health Organization. The closest diagnosis in DSM-5 is internet gaming disorder (IGD), but that does not pertain to problems with the general use of the internet.[1]

Most adolescents spend more than 7 hours a day using media, but a subset of adolescents who suffer from PIU will spend more than that online. Adolescents with self-control and/or impulsivity issues appear to be at higher risk for PIU, and adolescents with PIU often show hostility and aggressiveness. The potential for worrying and nervousness (defined as neuroticism) has been identified as another risk, and family functioning may play an important role in PIU. Risk factors, according to Bickham, may include lower levels of family cohesion, increased family conflict and parental hostility, poorer family relationships, decreased time and affection with parents, and a lower-quality parenting style.[2]

Still, researchers have created ways to identify and categorize PIU despite its unrecognized status as a disorder. Investigators from Minnesota, Wisconsin, and Washington developed an 18-item scale to screen for PIU. Termed the Problematic and Risky Internet Use Screening Scale (PRIUSS), it uses a Likert scale (0–4) and has three subscales: social impairment, emotional impairment, and risky/impulsive internet use. A score of 25 or higher is a positive screen.[3] Researchers from Washington, California, and Michigan designed a shorter screening tool, the PRIUSS 3, to expedite the screening process (see Table 10.1). A score of 3 or more on the PRIUSS 3 should be followed by the PRIUSS test for a more thorough evaluation for possible PIU. The Chen Internet Addiction Scale is a 26-item self-report questionnaire that occasionally is utilized in research studies to determine PIU.

As shown in the table, the first question relates to social consequences, the second to emotional consequences, and the third to risk/impulsive internet use. This short screening tool makes it convenient to use in medical offices, schools, and other related venues where adolescents might be tested.

There may be a biological component to PIU. Based on models of brain functioning in gamblers and people addicted to substances, there is some evidence that adolescents with PIU may have some form of neurobiological dysfunction. Video games and

Table 10.1 PRIUSS

How Often Do You	Never 0	Rarely 1	Sometimes 2	Often 3	Very Often 4
Experience increased social anxiety due to your internet use					
Feel withdrawal when away from the internet					
Lose motivation to do other things that need to get done because of the internet					

Moreno MA, Arseniev-Koehler A, Selkie E. Development and testing of a 3-item screening tool for problematic internet use. *J Pediatr.* 2016 Sep;176:167–172.

other types of internet use may lead to the rapid release of dopamine, which in turn leads to immediate gratification, repetitive behaviors to maintain gratification, and increased tolerance to the release of dopamine. In patients with IGD, functional magnetic resonance imaging testing has demonstrated diminished impulse control and other behavioral patterns similar to those seen in people with gambling disorders.[5]

PIU may also have a genetic component. To test this hypothesis and further explain the genetic and environmental influences of adolescent PIU, researchers from China devised a twin study that consisted of 825 families with same-sex twin pairs who had a mean age of 15.47 years. There were 449 female pairs (328 monozygotic and 121 dizygotic) and 376 male pairs (279 monozygotic and 97 dizygotic). The measures include PIU and effortful control (the ability of an adolescent to regulate behavior, emotion, and cognition). Questions included "Is it easy for me to concentrate on homework?" or "When someone tells me to do something, is it easy for me to stop?" or "If I have a hard assignment, do I get started right away?" The researchers learned that PIU has a moderate to high heritability, and the remaining variance was explained by nonshared environmental influences. Heritability was slightly higher in males, and the magnitude of environmental effects was much lower in males than females. The most influential environmental factor was the accessibility to the internet.[6]

There appears to be an association with PIU and other psychological disorders. Researchers from Sweden, the United States, Italy, Germany, and Australia performed a systematic review on the associations between PIU and other psychological disorders. They located 20 papers that met their criteria for inclusion. Most of the studies were conducted in Asia and had a cross-sectional design. The researchers found that males had higher rates of PIU than females. Seventy-five percent of the studies showed a correlation between PIU and depression, and 100 percent of the studies showed this correlation with symptoms of attention-deficit/hyperactivity disorder (ADHD). As a result, adolescents with PIU should be screened for depression and ADHD.[7]

Researchers from New York, Brazil, Canada, and the National Institute of Mental Health also studied the relationship between PIU and psychiatric disorders in children and adolescents. Their cohort consisted of 564 participants between the ages of 7 and 15 years, with a mean age of 10.8 years. The subjects and/or parents had diagnostic interviews and completed questionnaires and Young's Internet Addiction Test (a measure of the severity of internet addiction).[8] The researchers learned that there was a positive association between PIU and autism spectrum disorder, depression, and ADHD.[9]

Epidemiology

Because PIU is not listed as a disease in the DSM-5 and because there is no standard PIU definition, it is difficult to compare the prevalence data from published studies. Nevertheless, in a cross-sectional study conducted from 2010 to 2011, researchers in Italy measured the prevalence of PIU in high school students. The cohort consisted of 2022 students, 48 percent male, with a mean age of 16.2 years. Data were collected over a 4-month period using a 43-item self-developed questionnaire that included demographic characteristics of the subjects and patterns of internet use (hours spent and types of activities pursued). The researchers learned that 99.4 percent of the students used the internet. The overall prevalence of PIU was 12.1 percent—14.2 percent in males and 10.1 percent in females. Gender was not associated with PIU in this study. Risk for PIU was related to the sensation of feeling lonely, the frequency of internet use, the number of hours of internet connection, and visiting pornographic websites.[10]

In India, researchers reviewed 38 studies on PIU from the Southeast Asian region that included students from precollege to postgraduate programs, with an age range of 11 to 26 years. Most of the studies used Young's Internet Addiction Test to quantify the level of internet use. The levels of "severe" PIU ranged from 0 to 47.4 percent depending on PIU definitions, study design, and the subjects studied. The highest levels were seen in a study of university students in Bangladesh who were 18 to 25 years old; 47.4 percent of the male students and 44.5 percent of the female students appeared to have PIU. Depression was noted among 44.7 percent of the males and 41.6 percent of the female adolescents.[11]

Given the difference in definitions, some researchers have focused instead on tracking the prevalence of IGD as the closest accepted disorder to PIU. It should be noted that IGD is not classified as a mental disorder in the DSM-5, even though it causes significant impairment or distress in several aspects of an individual's life. Additionally, in the World Health Organization *International Classification of Diseases*, it is classified as a disorder due to addictive behaviors. The official name is gaming disorder.[12]

To determine the overall and gender prevalence of IGD among adolescents, a researcher from Malaysia performed a meta-analysis of 16 studies investigating IGD primarily in Europe. The researcher found that the pooled prevalence for IGD was 5.6 percent. While the prevalence among female adolescents was 1.7 percent, the prevalence among male adolescents was 7.1 percent; male adolescents were four times more likely to engage in IGD.[13]

The prevalence of PIU appears to be higher in Asian countries, especially China, Taiwan, and South Korea. The reasons are unclear. Rates may be as high as 17.9 percent in Chinese high school students.[14]

Biopsychosocial Issues and PIU

Biological Issues and PIU

Stress

Some adolescents may develop PIU in response to increased stress from biopsychological changes that occur during adolescence as well as outside stressors from parents, peers, and schools. Researchers from China and New York wanted to further understand stress-induced PIU. Specifically, they wanted to evaluate how an adolescent's temperament and stressful life events predicted the development of PIU. The research team recruited 660 adolescents with a mean age of 14.1 years, 55 percent female, from southern China. The subjects completed a questionnaire that had measures for stressful life events such as serious family conflicts, parental divorce, fighting with friends, and academic issues. They also measured effortful control (ability to modulate behavior, thoughts, and emotions) and sensation seeking, maladaptive cognitions, and PIU. While the researchers found an association between stressful life events and PIU in adolescents, many female adolescents, but not all, were able to diminish or moderate this through effortful control. Those who were unable to lower their risk had higher incidences of PIU. Overall, male adolescents had a higher risk of developing PIU from stressful events than female adolescents.[15]

Personality traits may impact the prevalence of PIU. Researchers from China evaluated the correlation between stressful life events, adolescent personality traits, and PIU trajectories. The personality traits included neuroticism (neurotic individuals were defined as emotionally unstable, worried, and depressed), extraversion, agreeableness, conscientiousness, and openness to experience. The researchers used data from the Cumulative Risk and Adolescent PIU Project, which examined the trajectory of PIU in adolescents as well as other factors associated with PIU. The measures included PIU, stressful life events, and those five personality traits. Starting with a sample of 1365 adolescents between the ages of 11 and 18 years, data were collected in three waves over 3 years. The researchers determined that rates of PIU increased during the study, with males having higher levels of PIU than females. Adolescents who had more stressful life events had higher initial levels of PIU and experienced larger increases in PIU over time. Personality traits linked to high initial PIU included low agreeableness, low conscientiousness, high openness, and high neuroticism. The researchers determined that stressful life events and personality traits independently make unique contributions to the adolescents' PIU. So in developing programs to prevent PIU, researchers could consider an adolescent's stressful life events and certain personality traits including high neuroticism in targeting higher-risk adolescents.[16]

A researcher from Korea evaluated the relationships between physical activity, sleep satisfaction, perceived stress, and PIU in adolescents. Using data from the 2010 Korean Youth Risk Behavior Survey, the cohort consisted of 73,238 students, with a mean age of 15.1 years. Measures included physical activity, PIU, sleep satisfaction, and the level of perceived stress. The researcher found that physical activity was related to higher levels of sleep satisfaction, lower levels of perceived stress, and a low risk of PIU. The researcher concluded that high academic stress and low levels of physical activity and poor sleep may contribute to the high prevalence of PIU in Korean adolescents. These findings support the need for good-quality sleep and physical activity for overall biopsychological well-being in adolescents.[17]

Psychological Issues and PIU

Anxiety
There appears to be an association between PIU and anxiety in adolescents. To determine mental health comorbidities, researchers in Korea studied children and adolescents with internet addiction. Using data from Young's Internet Addiction Scale and the Beck Depression Inventory, the researchers assessed 836 adolescents with a mean age of 15.8 years. In the study group, 20.3 percent screened positive for internet addiction. Twelve randomly selected adolescents who screened positive had structured interviews to diagnose DMS-IV Axis 1 disorders (mental health diagnoses and substance use disorders). Three were diagnosed with major depression, one with schizophrenia, and one with obsessive-compulsive disorder (OCD). OCD is an anxiety disorder. The researchers commented that internet addiction is not a cause or a consequence of these disorders. Rather, there is an association between internet addiction and OCD.[18]

To identify students with potential internet addiction and its coexistence with other psychological problems, researchers from Lebanon and France studied health professional students. Students in medicine, dentistry, and pharmacy completed a cross-sectional questionnaire, and Young's Internet Addiction Test and the Depression Anxiety Stress Scale were used as measures. The cohort consisted of 600 subjects; 69.7 percent were female, and the mean age was 20.4 years. The researchers learned that the prevalence of internet addiction was 16.8 percent, with a significantly higher prevalence in males. There was a strong correlation between potential internet addiction and anxiety, stress, and depression. They recommended that students in this age group be screened for internet addiction, as it often coexists with other psychological problems.[19]

Depression
Depression may play a large role in PIU. Researchers from Korea hypothesized that internet addiction in adolescents was associated with psychiatric symptoms, and the more serious the level of addiction, the more severe the depressive symptoms. To test their hypothesis, the researchers enrolled 452 high school students, who had a mean age of 15.8 years; 42.7 were female. Young's Internet Addiction Test measured internet addiction, and depression was assessed by the Korean version of the Center for Epidemiologic Study for Depression. The 30-question Maudsley Obsessive Compulsive Inventory measured OCD. Of the 452 subjects, 29 percent had a mild degree of internet addiction and 1.8 percent had severe addiction; more males

(35.5 percent) than females (24.3 percent) were affected. The researchers noted that internet addiction is linked to depression in adolescents. Depressive symptoms had the most influence on the development of internet addiction. In addition, the association of OCD symptoms and internet addiction was noted. The researchers advised clinicians who treat adolescents with internet addiction to check for depression.[20]

These findings were supported by researchers in China who focused their research on a subset of adolescents highly prone to PIU based on previous data. Their study sought to understand the relationship between impulsivity, social support, and depression and internet addiction among male college freshmen. In 2019, the researchers administered a cross-sectional survey to 734 male college freshmen at one public college in China. The average age of the students was 19.7 years. There were measures for demographics, and scales for impulsiveness, social support, and depression and Young's Internet Addiction Test were used. The researchers believed that the severity of depression would be highest in the most profound internet-addicted group. The researchers determined that the levels of addiction among the students was either low (42.1 percent), medium (35.7 percent), or high (22.2 percent), and indeed, the levels of depression appeared to worsen internet addiction behavior in the male freshmen. The researchers speculated that the internet may provide a virtual space for coping with depression, thereby reinforcing each other. Likewise, impulsivity was positively correlated with internet addiction, and there was a significant inverse relationship between internet addiction and social support, which may help freshmen cope with stress and reduce their vulnerability to internet addiction.[21]

Eating Disorders
Studies have determined that PIU and eating disorders are independent health risk factors for adolescents. Researchers from Spain examined the relationship between PIU and eating disorders in college students. They performed a systematic review and meta-analysis of relevant studies; 12 papers were identified for the systematic review and 10 for the meta-analysis. The meta-analysis included 16,520 students, of whom 83.33 percent were in college. The researchers found a correlation between PIU and anorexia nervosa, bulimia, and binge eating disorder. The researchers noted that the interactions with social networks had a direct impact on the lives and behaviors of the subjects; the students appeared to be comparing themselves to other students. The meta-analysis confirmed that the students with PIU were more likely to develop eating disorders.[22]

Similarly, researchers in Turkey investigated the prevalence of disordered eating attitudes and internet addiction in Turkish high school students. The study group consisted of 584 adolescents, 34.8 percent male. Each student completed three questionnaires: the Eating Attitudes Test-26, the Internet Addiction Test, and a sociodemographic set of questions. The Eating Attitudes Test is a 26-item self-reported questionnaire that is useful for assessing eating disorder risk in high school– and college-age adolescents. The researchers found that 15.8 percent of the students had disordered eating attitudes, and 10.1 percent had scores consisted with internet addiction. There was a positive correlation ($p < .01$) between scores on the Internet Addiction Test and the Eating Attitudes Test-26.[23]

While PIU is seen in adolescents with eating disorders, there may be a way to screen for PIU before eating disorders manifest. Researchers in the Czech Republic and Slovakia wanted to determine if there are common factors or linkages between these types of behaviors. They assembled a cohort with 7083 adolescents in Slovakia with a mean age of 13.5 years, 50.3 percent female, and looked for linkages for internal symptoms (emotional) and external symptoms (behavioral, impulsivity) between PIU and eating disorder symptoms. The questionnaire contained measures for eating disorder symptoms, PIU, and internalizing and externalizing symptoms. After controlling for internalizing and externalizing symptoms, the researchers observed an association between PIU and eating disorder symptoms. Only externalizing symptoms were related to both PIU and eating disorder symptoms, and the findings were similar for both males and females. The researcher suggested that because externalizing symptoms such as poor self-control are shared factors for both PIU and eating disorder symptoms, such externalizing symptoms should be addressed in the intervention and prevention of both health risk behaviors.[24]

Suicidality/Self-Harm

PIU appears to have some relationship to suicidality. Suicide is the third leading cause of death in adolescents in the United States. To determine if internet addiction was related to suicidal behaviors, researchers from Taiwan, England, and Canada performed a systematic review and meta-analysis. They included 23 cross-sectional studies and two prospective studies with more than 271,000 subjects. Although most of the subjects were adolescents and young adults, the ages in some instances were not specified. When compared to the control subjects, the researchers found that the prevalence rates of suicidal ideation (odds ratio [OR] = 2.952), planning (OR = 3.172), and attempts (OR = 2.811) were all significantly elevated in adolescents with internet addiction. These findings were valid even after they adjusted for variables such as depression.[25]

Researchers in Taiwan and New York assessed the association of suicidal ideation and suicidal attempts with internet addiction in Taiwanese adolescents between the ages of 12 and 18 years. The cohort consisted of 9510 students (48.3 percent male) across junior high schools and senior high vocational schools in urban and rural districts. In the cross-sectional study, students were evaluated for suicidal ideation and attempts, internet addiction and activities, depression, self-esteem, and family support. The researchers discovered that 18.0 percent of the students had suicidal ideation and 5.7 percent had a history of suicide attempts in the preceding month. Internet addiction was documented as 18.7 percent. Online gaming was the most popular internet activity. After controlling for the effects of demographic characteristics, depression, family support, and self-esteem, the researchers observed that the adolescents who had internet addiction had a higher risk of suicidal ideation or attempts as compared to those without internet addiction. The researchers noted that spending more time anonymously online might result in more exposure to suicide information. Or there may be a common vulnerability in adolescents for internet addiction and suicide behavior. While prevention programs may be appropriate for those adolescents with internet addiction, the researchers suggested that certain webpages may need warning signs, or programs with detailed descriptions of suicide methods should

Table 10.2 Prevalence of Psychopathology and Self-Destructive Behaviors and PIU

Psychopathology	Adaptive Internet Users	Problematic Internet Users
Anxiety	5%	33.5%
Depression	5%	27.6%
Emotional issues	10.8%	32.0%
Self-injurious behaviors	4.5%	22.2%
Suicidal ideation	12.7%	42.3%
Suicidal attempts	0.3%	3.1%

Kaess M, Durkee T, Brunner R, et al. Pathological internet use among European adolescents: psycho-pathology and self-destructive behaviours. *Eur Child Adolesc Psychiatry.* 2014 Nov;23(11):1093–1102.

simply be disallowed on the internet. The federal government could take action on these issues.[26]

Additionally, location may influence incidences of suicidality among adolescents suffering from PIU. Researchers in 11 European countries wanted to learn more about the relationship between PIU, psychopathology, and self-destructive behaviors in adolescents and to consider the influence of gender and country. They designed a cross-sectional study that they administered to 11,356 adolescents (42.8 percent male) in Austria, Estonia, France, Germany, Ireland, Israel, Romania, Slovenia, and Spain. There were measurements for PIU, depression, anxiety, deliberate self-harm, emotional symptoms such as conduct issues, and suicidal behaviors. The overall prevalence of PIU was 4.2 percent: 4.7 percent in males and 3.9 percent in females. See Table 10.2 for further breakdown of the data.

The results demonstrated that the prevalence of self-injurious behavior, suicidal ideation, and suicide attempts was significantly correlated with PIU. Interestingly, nationality markedly influenced the relationship between PIU, psychopathology, and suicidal behaviors. The correlations between PIU, psychopathology, and self-destructive behaviors were strongest in Estonia and Ireland and weakest in France, Italy, and Hungary. According to the researchers, these findings corresponded with the prevalence of PIU and the national suicide rates in these countries. This underscores the role of the country in moderating these problems; it is noted that this moderation may be a result of gender and country, suggesting sociocultural influences such as cultural identity, family structure, and/or gender roles.[27]

Social Issues and PIU

Social Media

To learn more about the benefits and risks of social media, a researcher in Hong Kong designed a 1-year longitudinal panel survey that included 417 adolescents. Among the risks studied were adolescents being targeted for harassment, loss of privacy, and viewing pornographic and/or violent content. Forty-four percent of the adolescents were male, and the adolescents had a mean age of 14.46 years. They were studied at T1 (baseline) and T2, about a year later. Measures included internet addiction (or PIU), internet risk, social media use, and demographics. The researcher found that there was a consistent effect of social media instant messaging on overall internet addiction, especially the addictive symptoms of control loss and preoccupation. In addition, the adolescents who obtained the most gratification from social media at T1 were more likely to report internet addiction and symptoms at T2. When compared to online socializing, online gaming significantly predicted addictive symptoms.[28]

Researchers from the Netherlands hypothesized that the frequency and problematic use of social media by adolescents predicted delays in bedtimes and poorer perceived sleep quality. They also thought that these effects were mitigated when parents set strict rules regarding the use of smartphones and the internet before bedtimes. The researchers used data from the Digital Youth Project, a longitudinal research project on adolescent online behavior. There were two waves—one in 2017 and a second in 2018—and the cohort had a total of 2021 adolescents, with a mean age of 13.86 years in 2017. Measures included social media use, problematic social media use, perceived quality of sleep, bedtime, and two parental rules regarding the use of smartphones and the internet before bedtime. The researchers determined that the more frequent and more problematic use of social media in T1 predicted later bedtimes in T2. The strict use of parental rules on the bedtime use of smartphones and the internet was linked to earlier bedtimes and better quality of sleep for those adolescents who scored below average on social media use and/or problematic social media use. As a result, restricting the use of smartphones and the internet before bedtime may be helpful before adolescents become highly involved in social media use.[29]

Transgender/Gender Dysphoria

Youth who are transgender, nonbinary, or gender diverse (TNG) experience multiple barriers to psychological wellness. Discrimination, oppression, and a lack of parental and community support may lead to issues including stress, anxiety, depression, and suicidality. On the other hand, some TNG youth receive support from the web and social media sites. Researchers from Wisconsin investigated the relationship between psychosocial measures and digital technology use and its importance for cisgender and TNG youth. The study data were obtained from a cross-sectional 2019 survey performed on a nationally representative sample of 4575 adolescents, ages 13 to 18 years; 1.16 percent self-identified as TNG. The digital measures included the PRIUSS-3 and the Adolescent Digital Technology Interactions and Importance Scale. Psychosocial measures included overall well-being, parental relationships, body image, loneliness, and fear of missing out. The mean age of the cisgender and TNG teens was 14.6 years. Of the cisgender group, 52.9 percent identified as male; in the TNG group, 47.2 percent identified as male, 43.4 percent as nonbinary, and 9.4 percent as female. When TNG youth were compared to cisgender participants, they had statistically significant lower scores for well-being, parental relationship, and body image and higher scores for loneliness and fear of missing out consistent with barriers to psychosocial wellness in TNG youth. In contrast to the cisgender group, TNG adolescents who scored better on well-being and body image had higher PIU scores. Adolescents in the TNG group who had higher PIU scores tended to have low scores in parental relationship, loneliness, and fear of missing out. The associations between these psychosocial measures and PIU in TNG youth may reflect their use of the web and social media sites as a source of information and emotional support.[30]

Violence

Hoping to understand which adolescent internet activities could lead to aggressive behaviors, researchers from Taiwan evaluated the association between PIU and aggressive behaviors in teens. They used data from the Health of Adolescents in Southern Taiwan study, which included 9405 adolescents (51.8 percent female), with a mean age of 14.7 years, who completed the study questionnaire. The measures included demographics, aggressive behaviors, internet addiction (Chen Internet Addiction Scale), internet behaviors, frequency of exposure to violent television programs, family function, depression, and self-esteem. After controlling for factors such as watching violent television programs, the researchers learned that adolescents with PIU were more likely to have aggressive behaviors such as hitting, kicking, grabbing, shoving, or threatening someone during the previous year. This association was more often seen in younger adolescents and almost three times more likely in male adolescents. Internet activities such as online gaming and visiting adult sites were associated with aggressive behaviors, though that was not the case for online study and research. The researchers commented that clinicians treating adolescents for aggressive behaviors should consider PIU as a possible issue.[31]

Since addictive behaviors such as gambling have been linked to PIU, researchers in the Netherlands wanted to learn if pathological gaming, as a form of PIU, caused adolescents to exhibit increased levels of physical aggression. They developed a longitudinal study with four queries. Does pathological gaming in adolescents predict an increase in the frequency and duration of gaming sessions? Does pathological gaming result in an increase in physical aggression? Is the effect of pathological gaming on physical aggression a result of the violent content of the games? And are there any differences in adolescent females and males with respect to the possible effects of pathological gaming on physical aggression? The study had two waves, 6 months apart, with 540 game-playing adolescents (30 percent female). The mean age for the waves was 14.9 and 15.3 years. The measures included pathological gaming, time spent on games, violent game play, and physical aggression. The researchers determined that higher levels of pathological gaming at baseline were linked to a substantial increase in the frequency and duration of gaming sessions 6 months later. The researchers suggested that pathological gaming is a progressive process, and excessive gaming habits may worsen over time, displacing other activities. Higher levels of pathological gaming also correlated with an increase in self-reported physical aggression 6 months later. The effect was only seen in males, with both violent and nonviolent games. Time spent playing violent games seemed to cause an increase in aggressive behavior. Because the data demonstrated that pathological gaming is progressive, it is important to approach this issue as soon as possible and certainly prior to the point at which the adolescent leaves for college, technical training, or the workforce, when parental supervision wanes.[32]

Treatment

Unfortunately, since there is currently no agreement on the definition of PIU, there are no unified treatment protocols. Yet, PIU remains an ever-growing concern in the United States, and an even larger one in China, Taiwan, and South Korea. Possible treatments currently include parental-based interventions, cognitive behavioral therapy (CBT), applications of certain antidepressants or antipsychotics, or a combination of all of the above.

Researchers in China studied the effectiveness of multifamily group therapy to reduce internet addiction among adolescents. The intervention was designed to strengthen adolescent/parent communication and enhance relationships and replace the fulfillment provided by the internet. They recruited an intervention group of 17 males and 4 females with a mean age of 15 years; their parents were included in the study. The control group had 21 males and 4 females, with an average age of 15.7 years, and their parents. Assessments were conducted at baseline, after the intervention, and at a 3-month follow-up. The subjects in the intervention group met with therapists for six sessions; the subjects in the control group were on a waitlist. The measures included internet addiction, parent-adolescent relationships and communication, and adolescent psychological needs. The researchers observed a significant difference in the decline of the mean scores for internet addiction in the intervention group, and it was maintained for 3 months. The internet addiction rate dropped from 100 percent at baseline in the intervention group to 11.1 percent at the 3-month follow-up. The researchers commented that it is extremely important for parents to be involved in the treatment of adolescents with internet addiction.[33]

CBT is also being studied as a treatment for PIU. CBT attempts to change problematic thought patterns and works to have the adolescent deal with the thoughts in a healthy manner. One study performed in university students in China with PIU utilized CBT to modify maladaptive cognitions and coping and enhance self-regulation.[34] CBT seemed to have some usefulness, especially when combined with other therapeutic modalities.[35]

Motivational interviewing, which has been used for other addictions such as substance abuse, may help adolescents with PIU. The technique helps adolescents recover through four stages. The first is contemplation or "sitting on the fence" around change for PIU. The second is preparation or the adolescent is beginning to change. The third entails practicing new behaviors with respect to PIU. The fourth entails the adolescent being committed to maintaining the new behaviors.

Lastly, given the association between psychological issues including anxiety and depression with PIU, medications such as antidepressants and antipsychotics have been used with varying degrees of success as treatment. Bupropion has been studied extensively for the treatment of internet addiction, and it has shown some degree of success in adult patients.[36]

In particular, researchers from Korea and Utah devised a clinical trial that included 65 adolescents with major depression and video game addiction. Thirty-two adolescents were treated with bupropion and CBT, and 33 were treated only with bupropion. Measures included severity of internet use, depressive symptoms, anxiety symptoms, life satisfaction, and school adaptation. At 8 weeks, when the treatment was completed, the adolescents in the medication and CBT group experienced a significant decrease in the severity of their online game play. Life satisfaction and school adaptation were also improved. While both groups experienced improvements, the benefits in the combination group were more notable for video game addiction and life satisfaction. The researchers noted that the combination therapy may help adolescents with depression and online game addiction.[37]

Prevention

Prevention of PIU in adolescents involves more than simply trying to diminish risk and enhance protective factors for internet addiction, which may be why an effective prevention program has still not been developed. Yet, researchers are moving in that direction. Recently, researchers in the Czech Republic performed a systematic review on the prevention of internet addiction in adolescents. The following are some of their key findings:[38]

- Prevention of internet addiction should target children and adolescents.
- Prevention programs should be implemented in the school environment.
- Selective prevention programs may be aimed at children and adolescents who may be at higher risk for PIU because of medical problems such as attention-deficit disorder, depression, anxiety, social phobia, impulsivity, or hyperactivity as well as those teens who spend a large number of hours online.
- Children and adolescents at risk for PIU may benefit from developing skills in certain areas including internet use, coping with stress and emotions, and dealing with interpersonal situations.

Two key regulators of PIU are governments and schools. China has already regulated the distance between internet cafes and schools, and South Korea has a law requiring compulsory preventive education for internet addiction. Researchers have suggested that governments become proactive in educating parents about PIU.[39]

School-based prevention programs are more common; however, there has been no standard approach to program creation and implementation. Researchers in the United Kingdom conducted a systematic literature review of school-based programs to prevent internet addiction in adolescents in order to identify relevant prevention programs and their efficacy and highlight best practices for new initiatives. Some studies focused on internet addiction programs and others on multibehavior programs. The programs predominantly targeted internet use and gaming; multibehavioral programs targeted a variety of adolescent risk behaviors. Few programs involved parents. There were no studies on high-risk adolescents, such as those with impulse control issues. The studies had mixed outcomes and various design concerns such as the lack of a more precise definition of internet addiction and the need for increased and more robust assessment tools for measuring the effectiveness of programs.[40]

Dutch researchers created a secondary school-based program that simultaneously targeted a range of health behaviors, including internet use. Using an online questionnaire, the researchers collected preintervention health behavior information from 336 high school students, with an average age of 16 years, and then self-reported behavioral data collected on an annual basis for the 3-year intervention. The comparison groups therefore were at similar points in their secondary school careers, with one having received the intervention and the other without the integrated intervention. The researchers utilized a whole-school approach with health-promoting principles including making healthy choices easier, involving parents when possible, and focusing on personal skills development. In addition, the intervention program, which took place over a 3-year period, included the following modules: bullying, alcohol use, smoking, sedentary or screen time behaviors, drug use, nutrition, physical activity, and sexual behaviors. There was no control group. The researchers determined that for male adolescents, weekly computer and television screen time were significantly lower at the end of the intervention. For female adolescents, at the end of the intervention, the compulsive internet user score was significantly lower.[41]

Overall, there is no PIU prevention program that appears to have consistent positive results for adolescents. The prevention of PIU in adolescence is a joint responsibility of the family, schools, and government. The following are recommendations that parents should consider to help prevent PIU in their children:[42]

- Parents need to set boundaries with their children and adolescents on the amount of daily screen time, such as fewer than 2 hours per night.
- Screen time should be reserved primarily for educational matters.
- Consider designating screen-free time, such as during meals and within 1 hour of bedtime.
- At home, the computer used by an adolescent should be placed in a public area, not in the teen's bedroom.
- Work to prevent social isolation. Adolescents should be encouraged to get involved in other activities, such as sports or extracurricular pursuits, thus automatically reducing screen time.
- Parents should advise and monitor the areas adolescents are allowed to visit online, especially gaming and social media sites.
- Consider using an app to help limit the use of the internet through smartphones.
- Both parents should model appropriate use of the internet and smartphones.
- An excellent resource for parents and professionals on issues discussed in this chapter is "The Mediatrician's Guide: A Joyful Approach to Raising Healthy, Smart, Kind Kids in a Screen-Saturated World", written by Dr. Michael Rich of Boston Children's Hospital.

Conclusion

PIU is associated with certain mental health issues including anxiety, depression, self-injurious behaviors, and aggression, and it is a worldwide problem for adolescents. Treatment for PIU might include CBT, motivational interviewing, and medication. Schools and governments should take a leading role in the prevention of PIU; parents should set ground rules at home to control the adolescent's use of the internet.

References

1   Spada MM. An overview of problematic internet use. *Addict Behav.* 2014;39:3–6.

2   Bickham DS. Current research and viewpoints on internet addiction in adolescents. *Curr Pediatr Rep.* 2021;9:1–10.

3   Jelenchick LA, Eickhoff J, Christakis DA, et al. The problematic and risky internet use screening scale (PRIUSS) for adolescents and young adults: scale development and refinement. *Comput Human Behav.* 2014;35:10.1016/j.chb.2014.01.035.

4   Moreno MA, Arseniev-Koehler A, Selkie E. Development and testing of a 3-item screening tool for problematic internet use. *J Pediatr.* 2016;176:167–172.

5   Bickham DS. Current research and viewpoints on internet addiction in adolescents. *Curr Pediatr Rep.* 2021;9:1–10.

6   Li M, Chen J, Li N, Li X. A twin study of problematic internet use: its heritability and genetic association with effortful control. *Twin Res Hum Genet.* 2014;17:279–287.

7   Carli V, Durkee T, Wasserman D, et al. The association between pathological internet use and comorbid psychopathology: a systematic review. *Psychopathology.* 2013;46:1–13.

8   Kim SJ, Park DH, Ryu SH, Yu J, Ha JH. Usefulness of Young's internet addiction test for clinical populations. *Nord J Psychiatry.* 2013;67:393–399.

9   Restrepo A, Scheininger T, Clucas J, et al. Problematic internet use in children and adolescents: associations with psychiatric disorders and impairment. *BMC Psychiatry.* 2020;27:252.

10 Vigna-Taglianti F, Brambilla R, Priotto B, Angelino R, Cuomo G, Diecidue R. Problematic internet use among high school students: prevalence, associated factors and gender differences. *Psychiatry Res.* 2017;257:163–171.

11 Balhara YPS, Mahapatra A, Sharma P, Bhargava R. Problematic internet use among students in Southeast Asia: current state of evidence. *Indian J Public Health.* 2018;62:197–210.

12 Darvesh N, Radhakrishnan A, Lachance CC, Nincic V, Sharpe JP, Ghassemi M, et al. Exploring the prevalence of gaming disorder and Internet gaming disorder: a rapid scoping review. *Syst Rev.* 2020;9:68.

13 Fam JY. Prevalence of internet gaming disorder in adolescents: a meta-analysis across three decades. *Scand J Psychol.* 2018;59:524–531.

14 Jorgenson AG, Hsiao RC, Yen CF. Internet addiction and other behavioral addictions. *Child Adolesc Psychiatr Clin N Am.* 2016;25:509–520.

15 Li D, Zhang W, Xian, L, Zhen S, Wang Y. Stressful life events and problematic internet use by adolescent females and males: a mediated moderation model. *Comput Hum Behav.* 2010;26:1199–1207.

16 Xiao J, Li D, Jia J, Wang Y, Sun W, Li D. The role of stressful life events and the big five personality traits in adolescent trajectories of problematic internet use. *Psychol Addict Behav.* 2019;33:360–370.

17 Park S. Associations of physical activity with sleep satisfaction, perceived stress, and problematic internet use in Korean adolescents. *BMC Public Health.* 2014;14:1143.

18 Ha JH, Yoo HJ, Cho IH, Chin B, Shin D, Kim JH. Psychiatric comorbidity assessed in Korean children and adolescents who screen positive for internet addiction. *J Clin Psychiatry.* 2006;67:821–826.

19 Younes F, Halawi G, Jabbour H, et al. Internet addiction and relationships with insomnia, anxiety, depression, stress, and self-esteem in university students: a cross-sectional designed study. *PLoS One.* 2016;11:e0161126.

20 Ha JH, Kim SY, Bae S, et al. Depression and internet addiction in adolescents. *Psychopathology.* 2007;40:424–430.

21 Zhang Y, Liu Z, Zhao Y. Impulsivity, social support and depression are associated with latent profiles of internet addiction among male college freshmen. *Front Psychiatry.* 2021;12:642914.

22 Hinojo-Lucena FJ, Aznar-Diaz I, Cáceres-Reche MP, Trujillo-Torres JM, Romero-Rodriguez JM. Internet use as a predictor of eating disorders in students: a systematic review and meta-analysis study. *Nutrients.* 2019;11:2151.

23 Alpaslan AH, Koçak U, Avci K, Tas HU. The association between internet addiction and disordered eating attitudes among Turkish high school students. *Eat Weight Disord.* 2015;20:441–448.

24 Šablatúrová NJ, Gottfried L, Blinka L, Sevcikova A, Husarova D. Eating disorders symptoms and excessive internet use in adolescents: the role of internalising and externalising problems. *J Eat Disord.* 2021;9:152.

25 Cheng YS, Tseng PT, Lin PY, et al. Internet addiction and its relationship with suicidal behaviors: a meta-analysis of multinational observational studies. *J Clin Psychiatry.* 2018;79:17r11761.

26 Lin IH, Ko CH, Chang YP, et al. The association between suicidality and internet addiction and activities in Taiwanese adolescents. *Compr Psychiatry.* 2014;55:504–510.

27 Kaess M, Durkee T, Brunner R, et al. Pathological internet use among European adolescents: psychopathology and self-destructive behaviours. *Eur Child Adolesc Psychiatry.* 2014;23:1093–1102.

28 Leung L. Predicting internet risks: a longitudinal panel study of gratifications-sought, internet addiction symptoms, and social media use among children and adolescents. *Health Psychol Behav Med.* 2014;2:424–439.

29 van den Eijnden RJJM, Geurts SM, Ter Bogt TFM, van der Rijst VG, Koning IM. Social media use and adolescents' sleep: a longitudinal study on the protective role of parental rules regarding internet use before sleep. *Int J Environ Res Public Health.* 2012;18:1346.

30 Allen BJ, Streetman ZE, Kerr BR, Zhao Q, Moreno MA. Associations between psychosocial measures and digital media use among transgender youth: cross-sectional study. *JMIR Pediatr Parent.* 2021;4:e25801.

31 Ko CH, Yen JY, Liu SC, Huang CF, Yen CF. The association between aggressive behaviors and internet addiction and online activities in adolescents. *J Adolesc Health.* 2009;44:598–605.

32 Lemmens JS, Valkenburg PM, Peter J. The effects of pathological gaming on aggressive behavior. *J Youth Adolesc.* 2011;40:38–47.

33 Liu QX, Fang XY, Yan N, et al. Multi-family group therapy for adolescent internet addiction: exploring the underlying mechanisms. *Addict Behav.* 2015;42:1–8.

34 Anthony WL. Feasibility, acceptability, and preliminary outcome of a cognitive-behavioral group intervention for problematic internet use via smartphones in Chinese university students. *J Cogn Psychother.* 2022;1:112–128.

35 Bickham DS. Current research and viewpoints on internet addiction in adolescents. *Curr Pediatr Rep.* 2021;9:1–10.

36 Greenfield DN. Clinical considerations in internet and video game addiction treatment. *Child Adolesc Psychiatr Clin N Am.* 2022;31:99–119.

37 Kim SM, Han DH, Lee YS, Renshaw PF. Combined cognitive behavioral therapy and bupropion for the treatment of problematic on-line game play in adolescents with major depressive disorder. *Comput Hum Behav.* 2012;28:1954–1959.

38 Vondráčková P, Gabrhelík R. Prevention of internet addiction: a systematic review. *J Behav Addict.* 2016;5:568–579.

39 Zhan JD, Chan HC. Government regulation of online game addiction. *Commun Assoc Inf Syst.* 2012;30:13.

40 Throuvala MA, Griffiths MD, Rennoldson M, Kuss DJ. School-based prevention for adolescent internet addiction: prevention is the key: a systematic literature review. *Curr Neuropharmacol.* 2019;17:507–525.

41 Busch V, De Leeuw RJ, Schrijver AJ. Results of a multibehavioral health-promoting school pilot intervention in a Dutch secondary school. *J Adolesc Health.* 2013;52:400–406.

42 Jorgenson AG, Hsiao RC, Yen CF. Internet addiction and other behavioral addictions. *Child Adolesc Psychiatr Clin N Am.* 2016;25:509–520.

Discrimination-Related Issues

11

Racism and Discrimination

Introduction

Racism has profound effects on the biopsychosocial health of children, adolescents, and young adults. As a social determinant of health, racism may impact the development of adolescents, leading to issues into adulthood. As noted in previous chapters, studies of adolescents who are targets of racism have demonstrated associations with mental health issues, including anxiety and depression. Structural racism in the form of school segregation laws, which existed for many decades in parts of the United States, led to profound and permanent educational inequalities for Black children and adolescents. And racism may lead to numerous health inequalities including birth disparities and physical illnesses.

It is important to understand the following terminology to better understand the scope and impact of racism:

Racism

Racism is "a system of structuring opportunity and assigning value based on the social interpretation of how one looks."[1]

Systemic Racism

Systemic racism is the involvement of entire systems and often all systems such as political, economic, health care, legal, education, and criminal justice, as well as the structures that uphold the systems.[2]

The Aspen Institute offers the following definitions for additional terms used in this chapter:

Structural Racism

"A system in which public policies, institutional practices, cultural representatives, and other norms work in various, often reinforcing ways to perpetuate racial group inequity. It has been a feature of the social, economic and political systems in which we all exist."[5] This may be envisioned as the scaffolding for systemic racism.

It should be noted that systemic and structural racism may be terms that are used interchangeably in the literature. These constructs overlap to a considerable degree.

Institutional Racism

"Institutional racism refers to the policies and practices within and across institutions that, intentionally or not, produce outcomes that chronically favor, or put a racial group at a disadvantage."[5]

Individual Racism

Individual racism may "include face-to-face or covert actions toward a person that intentionally express prejudice, hate or bias based on race."[5]

Internalized Racism

The impacts from structural and personally mediated racism may result in internalized racism—that is, internalizing racial stereotypes about one's race.[3] This internalization may result in maladaptive cognitions and negative self-perceptions. And this may influence health and mental health outcomes.[4]

Ethnicity

Ethnicity "refers to the social characteristics that people may have in common, such as language, religion, regional background, culture, food etc."[5]

White Privilege

"White privilege refers to whites' historical and contemporary advantages in access to quality education, decent jobs and livable wages, homeownership, retirement benefits, wealth, and so on."[5]

Bias

Bias is a preconceived opinion for or against a person, thing, matter, or group that may be unfair. There are two overarching types of bias:

Implicit Bias
Implicit bias is a type of bias that is unconscious and the person is unaware of their evaluation. It can affect judgments, decisions, and behaviors.

Explicit Bias
Also known as conscious bias, the person is very aware that an evaluation is taking place.[6]

Redlining

Redlining is a discriminatory practice of categorizing neighborhoods on the basis of possible mortgage investment risk that led to racial residential segregation. This is turn has led to significant and persisting Black-White inequalities in health.[7] In addition, there are significant racial inequities linked to residential location. The majority of Black, Hispanic, and Native American children reside in very low and low opportunity neighborhoods compared to a minority of White and Asian children.[8]

Racism impacts the biopsychosocial health of adolescents in numerous ways, including reducing opportunities for education and shelter; directly affecting cognitive and emotional processes; diminishing opportunities for healthy food, exercise, and sleep; and exposing adolescents to violence. Violence may directly influence physical and mental health issues.

The impacts of racism on adolescents was studied by a group of Australian researchers who performed a systematic review of the relationship between racial discrimination and children and adolescents up to the age of 18 years. They included 88 articles that were primarily published in the United States since 2010. The studies tended to focus on exposure to racism self-reported by the subjects, and most of the studies collected data at two or three time points over intervals of 12 months or more. The researchers learned that there was a strong longitudinal association between racial discrimination exposure during childhood and adolescence and later health outcomes. The more common health outcomes were depression, emotional difficulties, self-esteem issues, anxiety, use of substances including alcohol and cigarettes, sleep difficulties, and asthma. The relationships between racial discrimination and mental health were stronger than with physical health issues. A few studies examined outcomes from racial discrimination during sensitive developmental periods, such as early and mid-adolescence. In those studies, depression and stress seemed to be linked to racial discrimination.[9]

Racism does affect physical health issues in adolescents. It is known that asthma is nearly three times more likely to cause death in non-Hispanic Black individuals compared to non-Hispanic White individuals. Researchers from California and New York wanted to understand the role of redlining on the incidence of asthma in those areas. The researchers obtained security maps for eight cities in California where the census tracts were categorized into mortgage risk. The worst risk levels were in cities that were historically redlined. The researchers also obtained emergency department visiting rates for children, adolescents, and adults, as well as air pollution and demographic data from a California State dataset for 2011 to 2013. The team determined that the median age-adjusted rates for emergency department asthma visits were 2.4 times higher in historically redlined census tracts than those not redlined in the 1930s. After adjusting for poverty, diesel particle emissions, and other issues, the asthma emergency visit rates remained elevated. This study implied that the redlining that occurred in the 1930s is likely contributing to present-day asthma health outcomes.[10]

A further study of asthma in children and adolescents and housing issues was performed by researchers from Ohio who sought to learn if the density of housing code violations, such as the presence of mold or cockroaches in a census tract, was associated with asthma morbidity. The study, which focused on the emergency department visits and hospitalizations of children for asthma, used data from January 1, 2009, through December 31, 2012, and included 4355 children between the ages of 1 and 16 years, with 8736 asthma-related emergency department visits and hospitalizations. Nearly 95 percent of the asthma-related hospitalizations in greater Cincinnati occurred at the Children's Medical Center. The researchers found a significant association between the density of housing code violations and the rates of children's asthma-related emergency department visits and hospitalizations that was independent of poverty. Children who were hospitalized for asthma had 1.84 greater odds of revisiting the emergency room or rehospitalization within 12 months.[11]

Another group of researchers from California and Illinois wanted to learn if recent school resegregation due to school districts being released from desegregation orders affected the health and health behaviors of Black children. They used data on child health and behaviors from the Panel Study of Income Dynamics, a nationally representative sample of families. The researchers restricted the analyses to 1248 Black children who were 5 to 17 years old in 1991 to 2014 and lived in districts under desegregation orders in 1991. The outcomes studied included asthma, obesity, mental/emotional issues, and behaviors such as physical activity and alcohol and tobacco use. To achieve even racial balance, about half of the Black and White students would have needed to move to another school in the same district. The children's mean age was 11 years at the interview (SD = 3.5 years). The findings were notable. The school resegregation that resulted from the school districts being released from desegregation orders was associated with behavioral problems among Black students and increased alcohol behaviors, especially among the female adolescents in the study group. The researchers suggested that the increased alcohol consumption might be due to an unhealthy coping mechanism to deal with the stress of school resegregation or peer influence. Clinicians should be aware from this study that school resegregation was associated with worse outcomes on several measures of well-being among Black children, which included behavioral problems and consumption of alcohol.[12]

Epidemiology

Whether it is implicit, explicit, institutional, or structural, racism is pervasive throughout the United States. Researchers in New York, California, and Rhode Island used a nationally representative dataset from the Pew Research Center 2016 Racial Attitudes in America, with 3631 respondents, to explore the prevalence of discrimination experiences among racial groups. The survey was administered by telephone to adults in all 50 states and the District of Columbia. The respondents were 57.67 percent White, 29.66 percent Black, 3.55 percent Asian, and 9.12 percent Hispanic. Overall, 37.24 percent of the respondents reported a discrimination experience from "time to time." Further breakdown of the data indicated the following reports of discrimination among these individuals: White (25.79 percent), Black (58.22 percent), Asian (45.74 percent), Hispanic (36.86 percent), Native American (38.78 percent), and Pacific Islander (57.14 percent). The researchers noted that the data supported continuing discrimination in the United States that could have significant outcomes in hiring, access to health care, health outcomes, housing, lending, education, prosecution, and sentencing.[13]

Narrowing down the focus to adolescents, researchers from California and Canada studied the experiences young adolescents had with racism and discrimination. They used cross-sectional data of adolescents ages 10 and 11 years from the Adolescent Brain Cognitive Development (ABCD) study, a large, diverse, population-based sample of 10,354 subjects during the period 2017 to 2019. The demographic breakdown for the adolescents was 19.2 percent Hispanic, 16.0 percent Black, and 5.5 percent Asian/Pacific Islander. Of the total population studied, 4.8 percent of the adolescents noted discrimination based on race/ethnicity. A further analysis showed that 10.0 percent of Black adolescents, 6.5 percent of Native American adolescents, 6.2 percent of Asian/Pacific Islander adolescents, 5.4 percent of Latino/Hispanic adolescents, and 2.8 percent of White adolescents reported this discrimination. These findings demonstrated that young adolescents encountered and observed discrimination based on race/ethnicity.[14]

A study from New York examined the prevalence of parent-reported ethnic discrimination and if children with special health care needs (CSHCN) were more likely to experience ethnic discrimination than children without these needs. Data were obtained from the National Survey of Children's Health 2011–2012, a telephone-based U.S. nationally representative survey with 95,677 subjects. The measures included two questions on ethnic discrimination: "Was [your child] ever treated or judged unfairly because of his/her race or ethnic group?" If so, "during the past year, how often was [your child] treated or judged unfairly?" Frequency was documented on a four-point Likert scale, and there was screening for CSHCN. The researchers determined that ethnic discrimination was much higher for Black (9.1 percent), other not Hispanic (9.9 percent), or Hispanic (4.7 percent) children than White children (1.4 percent). The researchers also learned that during the 12 months prior to the survey, CSHCN were two times more likely to experience frequent ethnic discrimination than comparable children in terms of age, sex, race, family income, parental education, and social capital. The researchers found that the parents had underestimated the prevalence of discrimination, and they may not have been aware of their child's experiences. This was most evident when the child was an adolescent. Likewise, the wording of the discrimination questions may not have addressed structural and systemic forms of ethnic/racial discrimination.[15]

Biopsychosocial Issues and Racism/Discrimination

Biological Issues and Racism/Discrimination

Obesity

Black and Hispanic adolescents have a disproportionate burden of obesity, and structural racism is a driver of this disparate health outcome.[16] Factors associated with these higher rates of obesity include less access to healthy foods, exercise, and health care and more limited housing options.

Researchers in New York wanted to understand if self-reported experiences of racial discrimination were associated with adiposity in children and adolescents. Using data from the ABCD study (2017–2019), the researchers administered the Perceived Discrimination Scale to quantify racial discrimination, and they had the weight, height, and waist circumference measured by research assistants. The mean age of the participants was 9.95 years. The study team determined that racial discrimination at baseline was associated with higher adiposity 1 year later. Personally mediated racial discrimination may be a risk factor for developing obesity in children and adolescents; therefore, interventions to reduce exposure to racial discrimination early in life may help reduce the risk of excessive weight gain throughout life.[17]

Some of the other causes for obesity in Black adolescents can be traced to redlining and housing segregation. Since Black individuals have historically had a reduced ability to secure a mortgage, it was far more difficult for them to build wealth. Accordingly, Black individuals often continued to live in food desert geographical areas where there were few grocery stores with healthier foods, including fruits and vegetables. Instead, they tended to rely on local convenience stores that carried highly processed foods with higher levels of fat and calories. The obesogenic (fostering obesity) environment had fewer recreational facilities and playgrounds and more fast-food restaurants.[18-20] The ability to exercise and participate in other recreational activities may depend on the perception that adolescents and their parents have about the safety of where they live. When there are obstacles to exercise, exercise is less likely to occur.[21,22]

Whatever their health insurance status, Black adolescents with obesity may have limited opportunities to obtain medical services for their obesity. This is especially true for Black adolescents who live in reduced socioeconomic circumstances.[23] Most likely, they will have more limited opportunities for local and convenient primary and specialized care. Specialized centers for the treatment of adolescent obesity are usually part of academic medical centers that may be located a significant distance away for the adolescent to travel. The costs for transportation and time off from work for the parent, as well as a lack of health insurance coverage, may be barriers for treatment of obesity.[24]

Researchers from Arkansas, Pennsylvania, and California designed a study to determine which neighborhood factors fostered an overweight or obese status of its residents. The researchers had multilevel data on 38,650 subjects in 18,381 households in 2104 U.S. counties that included information on individuals and households. For example, there were data on individual body mass index (BMI), diet features, household demographic characteristics—race and ethnicity, detailed food purchase information, and neighborhood variables—poverty rates, and the average number of food stores or restaurants per 10,000 county residents. The researchers found significant socioeconomic disparities in overweight and obesity status. In comparison with Whites and Asian children, adolescents, and adults, non-Hispanic Black individuals were more likely to be overweight or obese. A higher income and higher compliance with U.S. Department of Agriculture food guidelines were associated with a lower risk of obesity. And certain characteristics of the neighborhood food environment, including food desert status, were associated with obesity status, even after controlling for home food environment factors.[25]

Researchers from Michigan evaluated the ability of social environmental factors, such as racial discrimination, low household education, community violence, and cultural identity, to contribute to the risk for obesity. They recruited 198 Black adolescents, who were a subset of a larger sample, from Washtenaw County, Michigan, between the ages of 11 and 18 years; 60.6 percent were female. The measures included the Adolescent Discrimination Distress Index, a 15-item survey that is used to assess a subject's experience with discrimination. Household education was calculated with a seven-category item; community violence was gauged with the Survey of Children's Exposure to Community Violence; and acculturation was determined by the Acculturation, Habits, and Interests Multicultural Scale for Adolescents. The subjects' heights, weights, and BMI measurements were noted. The researchers learned that racial discrimination was positively related to BMI, while household education was inversely associated with BMI in female Black adolescents. Community violence and acculturation were not linked to BMI.[26]

Psychological Issues and Racism/Discrimination

Eating Disorders

As noted in Chapter 3, stress is ubiquitous and impacts all adolescents. Yet, as a result of their genetic makeup, development, and life experiences, adolescents respond in different ways to this stress. Chronic stress places a strain on the physiology of the body and leads to the "wear and tear" of many of the organs and systems, a concept described by McEwen and Stellar from Yale University as "allostatic load." For example, it is well known that increased stress may elevate heart rate and blood pressure, and chronic stress is associated with heart attacks, asthma, diabetes, and issues with the gastrointestinal system. While there appears to be no significant connection between racism/discrimination and the eating disorders anorexia nervosa, bulimia, and binge eating disorder, there may well be an association between racism/discrimination and disordered eating due to stress or emotional eating.[27]

During the process of acculturation, ethnic minorities and immigrants encounter stress that could result in disordered eating. Researchers from Baylor University studied the associations between acculturative stress (stress from being an immigrant or ethnic minority and going through the process of acculturation), emotional eating, and change in BMI scores in Latino adolescents over a 3-month period. They also compared Latino and non-Latino adolescents on measures of acculturative stress, emotional eating, and BMI. The sample was composed of 168 Latino and 278 non-Latino middle and high school students ranging in age from 12 to 17 years. The measures included the Emotional Eating Scale for children and adolescents; Social, Attitudinal, Familial, and Environmental Acculturative Stress Scale for children; BMI; and demographics. The study was cross-sectional except for the BMI, which was measured at two points 3 months apart. Compared to non-Latino adolescents, the results indicated that Latino adolescents endorsed significantly higher acculturative as well as higher total stress, general stress, process stress, and discrimination stress (p < .001). Acculturative stress was associated with higher levels of emotional eating in the Latino adolescents.[28]

Substance Use

Discrimination against certain groups of adolescents could result in youth using substances. It is well known that Native American individuals have been discriminated against for centuries. Most of the studies on this discrimination have been conducted on the adult population; however, researchers from Nebraska, Washington State, and Iowa examined the relationship between discrimination and substance abuse among Native American adolescents. The researchers hypothesized that discrimination toward Native American adolescents resulted in internalizing the symptoms that led to the early use of substances, or the stress from discrimination elicited an anger response that increased the likelihood of substance abuse. The cohort consisted of 195 Native American adolescents in grades 5 through 8 who were from three reservations; they had a mean age of 12.15 years. The measures used by the researchers included the age of the adolescents, household per capita income, perceived discrimination, substance abuse, internalizing symptoms (anxiety/depression, withdrawal, somatic complaints), anger, and delinquent behavior. Trained interviewers were tribal members or other trained individuals who were approved by the tribes. The researchers learned that 49 percent reported being insulted, 31 percent felt disrespected, and 24 percent thought peers excluded them because they were Native American adolescents. Perceived discrimination increased the likelihood that the subjects internalized symptoms. Yet, internalizing symptoms did not mediate the association between early onset substance abuse and discrimination, and internalizing symptoms were not related to the early onset of substance abuse. Rather, the perceived discrimination resulted in anger and delinquent behaviors among the adolescents, and then led to early substance abuse.[29]

While the results of the above study are not generalizable to other ethnic groups, a team of researchers from California examined the connection between perceived discrimination and substance use among Latino adolescents. They noted that Latino individuals born in the United States had significantly higher rates of alcohol, tobacco, and other drug use than Latino immigrants. The cohort consisted of 1332 Latino adolescents, with a mean age of 14.0 years; 49 percent were male. They were ninth-grade students who attended seven high schools in the Los Angeles area; most were second-generation immigrants. A questionnaire completed by the subjects included measures for substance use, demographic characteristics, acculturation, and perceived discrimination. Almost half of the subjects (47.6 percent) had a history of lifetime drinking, 26.4 percent had a history of smoking, and 19.3 percent had a history of marijuana use. The mean perceived discrimination score, determined by a 10-item scale with a range of one to four, was 1.71. The researchers concluded that perception of discrimination was significantly related to both recent and lifetime use of alcohol, cigarettes, and marijuana among young Latino adolescents. This was one of the first studies to demonstrate an association between the externalizing behavior of substance use and perceived discrimination in a population of Latino adolescents.[30]

Social Issues and Racism/Discrimination

Social Media

Online racial discrimination among adolescents, as a consequence of social media platforms, is a significant public health concern. Researchers in Illinois, California, and Massachusetts examined the associations between individual and vicarious racial discrimination via the internet and the psychological adjustment of adolescents. They designed an online cross-sectional survey, which they administered to 264 adolescents who ranged in age from 14 to 18 years. The study participants consisted of 51.1 percent White, 26.5 percent Black, 4.5 percent Asian, 2.3 percent Hispanic, and 9.8 percent multiracial adolescents with the remaining 5.7 percent of adolescents identifying their race as unknown or other. The researchers created measures for vicarious racial discrimination and online personal victimization across internet settings including social network sites, offline experiences with discrimination, and psychological adjustment. They learned that while vicarious racial discrimination occurred more often than discrimination directed against an individual, the adolescents experienced both individual and vicarious discrimination online. The findings also demonstrated that individual discrimination was directly related to an individual's symptoms of depression and anxiety. This study was one of the first to propose that online racial discrimination may negatively impact adolescents' psychological adjustment.[31]

Though offline civic engagement has been associated with positive psychosocial development in youths of color, online racial justice activities have been known to subject youths of color to individual racial discrimination directed to them personally or vicarious discrimination directed to people of the same race. Researchers at Fordham University proposed three hypotheses about online racial discrimination in youth. First, they maintained that more online media use results in more intergroup contacts and higher civic engagement, which in turn leads to increased exposure to individual and vicarious social media racial discrimination. Second, these uses of social media were related to increased risk for the symptoms of anxiety and depression as well as problems with alcohol and illicit drug use. And third, individual and vicarious racial discrimination mediates the association between these forms of social media use and mental health and substance use risk. The researchers formed a cohort of 407 teens between the ages of 15 and 18 years who were Black, Hispanic, East/Southeastern Asian, or Indigenous American; during the previous month, they had all used social media at least 5 days per week. The researchers crafted measures for demographics, hours of media use, social media intergroup contact, social media racial justice civic engagement and racial discrimination, symptoms of anxiety and depression, and alcohol and illicit drugs use screens.

The researchers learned that 94 percent of the adolescents experienced vicarious social media racial discrimination, and 79 percent had a history of individual social media racial discrimination, with the numbers significantly higher among the Black teens. In all racial groups, social media use was correlated with individual social media racial discrimination. The greater the number of hours on social media, the higher the number of symptoms of anxiety and depression, as well as substance use. The researchers believed that the coordination of online racial justice by subjects in the study caused an increase in their exposure to racism; those coordination efforts exposed these youth to unfriendly social media. In addition, the researchers felt that exposure to racism online might cause increases in depression, which then resulted in greater youth engagement in social media racial justice civic engagement as a coping mechanism. These findings highlighted the mental health vulnerabilities for adolescents of color when exposed to online vicarious and individual racial discrimination, especially while engaged in social justice activities on social media platforms.[32]

LGBTQ

Experiences that occur during adolescence help to shape a youth's identities and psychological well-being. For LGBTQ adolescents, a positive identity requires affirming relationships. Yet, in contrast, these adolescents often encounter isolation, bullying, and marginalization at school and, sometimes, within their own families. While many youths are forced to deal with outright discrimination and/or violence, these teens may also encounter covert and subtle types of discrimination such as microaggressions or humiliating actions that are brief, verbal, behavioral, or environmental. Microaggressions may be intentional or unintentional, and they communicate hostile, derogatory, or negative slights and insults. There are racial microaggressions as well as those against LGBTQ individuals, women, and people with disabilities.

Researchers from Ontario wanted to learn more about the type, nature, and impact of everyday microaggressions encountered by LGBTQ adolescents. They recruited 11 LGBTQ adolescents between the ages of 14 and 18 years who had a variety of sexual orientations including gay, queer, lesbian, pansexual, unsure, and biromantic/asexual. The teens participated in focus groups led by one of the researchers. The researchers determined that LGBTQ adolescents were faced with heterosexist expectations, and they were being denied the freedom to be themselves. At school, they encountered gender binary language such as "boys and girls" and erasure of trans identities. During focus groups, they described being surprised by friends who failed to use correct pronouns. They felt surrounded by "heteronormativity" and devalued by peers and family members, and they were continually reminded that they were different. Others described hearing that their gender identity was only a phase. While these actions are subtle forms of discrimination, they have the power to affect adolescents in a critical period of development.[33]

LGBTQ individuals of color experience racial discrimination. The Trevor Project surveyed LGBTQ youth ages 13 to 24 across the United States; 45 percent of the respondents were youth of color, and 38 percent were transgender or nonbinary. The results indicated that half of all LGBTQ youth of color reported discrimination in the past year based on their race or ethnicity; this included 67 percent of Black LGBTQ youth.[34] These results are not surprising. In a study from the Virginia Commonwealth University, 200 LGBTQ adult people of color were surveyed with measures for discrimination, mental health, and suicidal ideation. The researchers observed that racism exerted a direct effect on the mental health of individuals, although not apparently on suicidal ideation.[35]

Transgender/Gender Dysphoria

Transgender adolescents are also faced with discrimination. Youth assigned male at birth who later identify as transgender female are faced with a significant number of health disparities. They routinely cope with discrimination in various forms, including health care, education, and employment, and are at an increased risk of violence. In addition, racial discrimination in racial/ethnic minorities along with gender-based stigma for gender minority individuals may exert a profound effect on their mental health. One area of concern is the link between discrimination and mental health outcomes for transgender females. To determine the prevalence of discrimination and the relationship between discrimination and mental health, researchers in San Francisco studied transgender females between the ages of 16 and 24 years. They used data from a cross-sectional sample from SHINE, a study of HIV risk and resilience among transgender female youth in the San Francisco Bay area. The study, which was conducted from 2012 to 2013, had 300 subjects. Measures included sociodemographic factors, predictors (discrimination based on identity or race or both), psychological stress, depressive symptoms, and resilience-promoting factors. The researchers found that high transgender-based discrimination was significantly associated with greater odds of posttraumatic stress disorder, depression, and stress due to suicidal thinking. High racial discrimination was significantly associated with greater odds of psychological stress and stress related to suicidal thinking. According to the researchers, the data clearly showed the impact of discrimination on the mental health of the subjects in the study. Parental support was related to significantly lower odds for the mental health outcomes measured, and they suggested that interventions could include resources to build parent-child relationships.[36]

Mortality

Firearm injuries were the leading cause of death in children and adolescents ages 1 to 19 in 2020.[37] It has been repeatedly shown that structural racism is associated with disparities in rates of injury and death from firearms in urban youth. It has been well established that Black male youth are disproportionately affected by firearm injuries and death. Moreover, firearm injuries and hospitalizations are linked to economic disadvantage.[38] In all probability, racial segregation brought on by redlining and income inequalities are factors that increase the firearm homicide disparities between Black and White populations.[39]

As noted, structural racism led to the practice of redlining. In 2021, a researcher from Syracuse, New York, reported that from 2013 to 2014, the rates of firearm assaults and violent crimes in Philadelphia were highest in neighborhoods that were historically redlined. It appeared that structural racism was a key factor for the high rates of firearm violence experienced by urban youth, mediated by such factors as poverty, poor educational attainment, and preclusion from home ownership.[40,41]

Researchers from Texas, Georgia, Connecticut, and Iowa performed a longitudinal study of racial discrimination and death ideation (a part of the suicide spectrum) in Black adolescents. The researchers commented that although the literature on African American youth suicide was relatively sparse, racial discrimination is a particularly pernicious element in the lives of Black individuals, including preadolescents and adolescents, and comes out at a time when there may be direct and indirect consequences. Data were obtained from 722 Black adolescents, 54 percent female, with a mean age of 10.56 years during the first wave of the study; a second wave of data was obtained 2 years later. Measures included a 13-item schedule of racist events and a

47-item stressful life events inventory. Each subject had a structured psychiatric diagnostic interview appropriate for children and answered two questions on death ideation. The results were consistent with the belief that alienation and interpersonal rejection may serve as catalysts for suicide vulnerability. The researchers observed evidence of direct and indirect effects of racial discrimination on death ideation during the second wave. While depressive symptoms were not a robust predictor for death ideation in either gender, for females, the effects of racial discrimination were mediated by anxiety symptoms.[42]

A research group from Pennsylvania and Connecticut explored the contribution of racial/ethnic discrimination from other adversities associated with childhood suicidality. They analyzed data from the ABCD study of 11,235 subjects, 20.2 percent of whom were Black individuals, with a mean age of 10.9 years. The results indicated that Black individuals reported more discrimination and higher suicidality rates than non-Black subjects. The researchers concluded that racial/ethnic discrimination is disproportionately experienced by Black children and is associated with suicidality prior to adolescence over and above other adversities. They suggest addressing discrimination as part of suicide prevention strategies.[43]

Immigration

Approximately one out of every four adolescents in the United States is part of an immigrant family; Hispanic, Asian, and multiracial immigrant youth constitute about one-third of all children in this country.[44,45] It seems that there are rising mental health concerns in this population.[46] Researchers in Boston designed a study to examine three questions. First, is there a significant relationship between perceived discrimination (behavioral manifestation of a negative attitude, judgment, or unfair treatment toward members of a group) at school from peers and/or adults and depressive symptoms among immigrant adolescents? Second, does the association between this discrimination and depressive symptomology vary according to gender and nativity—foreign born or U.S. born? And third, does ethnic identity and social support play a protective role against the negative effects of perceived discrimination on depressive symptoms? The researchers assembled a cohort of 95 students who attended an urban high school with a high percentage of ethnic minority students; 53.7 percent were male, they had a mean age of 15.07 years, and 51.6 percent were born outside the United States. The subjects completed a survey that had measures for peer and adult discrimination, depressive symptoms, ethnic identity, social support, and demographics. Over 75 percent of the subjects had at least one incident of racial or ethnic discrimination by peers at school, and over half had an incident with adults at school. The correlation between perceived discrimination and depressive symptoms was significant for both males and females, but female adolescents reported higher levels of depressive symptoms. Although ethnic identity mitigated the negative effects of perceived adult discrimination for U.S.-born adolescents, social support did not moderate the relationship between peer and adult discrimination and depressive symptoms for the adolescents.[47]

Research findings on perceived discrimination show possible harm to an adolescent's well-being. A research team in Israel assessed the relationship between perceived discrimination and adolescent well-being at a baseline point (2002—2003) and a 2-year follow-up (2004—2005). They conducted face-to-face interviews with 1420 adolescents between the ages of 12 and 18 years who had immigrated to Israel from the former Soviet Union. Performed by Russian-speaking interviewers, the measures included self-efficacy, depressive mood, perceived discrimination, and social orientation. The researchers determined that perceived discrimination, espe-cially in school, perpetrated by peers and teachers increased depressive moods and reduced the adolescent's self-esteem and, most likely, school achievement. However, perceived discrimination did not increase their preference for in-group socialization. The researchers concluded that perceived discrimination seemed to be detrimental to psychological well-being, but it did not hinder social integration.[48]

Violence

Black youth who live in economically disadvantaged areas have a disproportional ex-posure to community violence.[49] This exposure is rooted in systemic racism. But there are other types of violence endured by Black youth. Anton Rose Jr. was a 17-year-old Black male who was a passenger in a car that was stopped by police in East Pittsburgh, Pennsylvania, in 2018. Suspected of being involved in a drive-by-shooting, he was shot and killed as he ran from the scene unarmed. This is only one example of the many adolescent and young adult Black males killed by the police in the past decade, supporting the growing body of research documenting the violence inflicted on this group. Racism underpins many of these violent acts. In addition, witnessing police vi-olence may have mental and physical consequences for adolescents including sleep is-sues, anxiety, chronic stress, and hypervigilance. In a study of Black adults conducted after a police killing of a Black individual, mental health effects were noted several months later in Black but not White individuals.[50] Living in neighborhoods with aggressive policing has been associated with hypertension, higher BMI, and overall poorer health. Additionally, police violence within the educational system may cause both physical harm to students and psychological humiliation and verbal abuse. In these types of situations, individual, institutional, and structural racism pertaining to law enforcement need to be addressed.[51]

Racism may motivate adolescent mass murderers. In May 2022, an 18-year-old teen armed with an assault rifle perpetrated anti-Black violence in a supermarket in Buffalo, New York, and murdered 10 innocent Black men and women. The motives were clearly racist, and there did not appear to be a direct link between mental ill-ness in the perpetrator and the mass murders. The act was well planned, not an im-pulsive act of adolescence. Adolescent perpetrators are likely to have low resilience, poor coping skills, and depressive symptoms. In one study, 70 percent of adolescent perpetrators of mass murders were loners. Days before a mass murder, the adoles-cent perpetrator may experience a precipitating event such as loss of a love interest, family argument, suspension from school, bullying, or physical injuries. Adolescent mass murderers are usually physically healthy, around age 16 years, attending public schools, but often have been raised in dysfunctional families and have problems with peer relationships. Exposure to previous mass murders through social media may reinforce their decision to be a copycat. The reasons for the mass murders included family dysfunction, bullying, voices heard commanding the event, war obsession, and White supremacy ideation.[52]

Prevention

With all its many facets, racism should also be considered as a public health problem that significantly impacts health, health disparities, and illness in people of color. Regrettably, racism has been embedded in the U.S. health care system since the earliest days of the country. Thus, although race is a social and not a biological construct, it has been included in some clinical practice guidelines (CPGs). In a systematic review of pediatric CPGs, 57.9 percent used race or ethnicity in a manner that could exacerbate health inequities, while 35.7 percent used race with potential for a positive effect.[53] Dismantling racism requires dramatic changes in systematic, institutional, and individual racism, as well as the concept of White privilege. Changes need to occur at all levels and sectors of society—individual, family, local, state, and federal—as well as in schools and sports. Acculturation to nonracist beliefs, values, attitudes, and thinking needs to begin at birth or even before conception.[54,55]

Some researchers have proposed the "weathering hypothesis." This suggests that the cumulative experiences of racism such as discrimination and segregation, especially those occurring in childhood and adolescence, are associated with a state of chronic inflammation. Proponents of this theory believe that chronic inflammation is associated with obesity as well as a number of other chronic illnesses. Preventive efforts here begin before the birth of the individual.[56,57]

In a prospective study, researchers in Georgia examined the relationship of perceived racial discrimination with allostatic load including a possible buffer of the association. They sampled 331 African American youth in the rural South and assessed perceived discrimination from ages 16 to 18. At age 18 their caregivers reported parental emotional support, and the adolescents were assessed for peer emotional support. The results indicated that perceived racial discrimination was positively associated with allostatic load. In addition, the association between perceived discrimination and allostatic load was ameliorated when adolescents received high levels of emotional support.[58]

Confronting Racism in Health Care

The Commonwealth Fund interviewed leaders of major medical institutions such as Mass General Brigham, University of California, Los Angeles, and the University of Chicago. They developed strategies for combatting racism in health care that begin during medical school training, and some are noted in Box 11.1.

Conclusion

Racism is pervasive in American society from individual to institutional, structural, and systemic levels, and this impacts adolescents in the biological, psychological, and social domains. Researchers have documented associations between racism and obesity as well as higher blood pressure, self-rated health, disordered eating, substance use, and inequalities to treatment for some medical conditions. Dismantling racism will require enormous systematic, institutional, and individual changes.

Box 11.1   Strategies for Combatting Racism in Health Care

- Examine institutional policies with an equity lens
- Audit medical school curricula for erroneous references to race
- Review clinical algorithms that erroneously rely on race
- Invest in scholarships for students of color who are interested in the health professions
- Train leadership and staff in diversity, equity, inclusion, and antiracism principles
- Listen to and learn from patients and health care professionals of color

Reproduced with the permission of the Commonwealth Fund. https://www.commonwealthfund.org/publications/2021/oct/confronting-racism-health-care. Accessed April 10, 2023.

References

1 Jones CP. Confronting institutionalized racism. *Phylon*. 2003;50:7–22.
2 Braveman PA, Arkin E, Proctor D, Kauh T, Holm N. Systematic and structural racism: definitions, examples, health damages, and approaches to dismantling. *Health Aff*. 2022;41:171–178.
3 Trent M, Dooley DG, Dougé J, Section on Adolescent Health; Council on Community Pediatrics; Committee on Adolescence. The impact of racism on child and adolescent health. *Pediatrics*. 2019;144(2):e20191765.
4 Bailey TM, Yeh CJ, Madu K. Exploring Black adolescent males' experiences with racism and internalized racial oppression. *J Couns Psychol*. 2022;69(4):375–388.
5 11 terms you should know to better understand structural racism. Aspen Institute. July 11, 2016.
6 Gopal DP, Chetty U, O'Donnell P, Gajria C, Blackadder-Weinstein J. Implict bias in healthcare: clinical practice, research and decision making. *Future Healthc J*. 2021;8:40–48.
7 Williams DR, Collins C. Racial residential segregation: a fundamental cause of racial disparities in health. *Public Health Rep*. 2001:116:404–416.
8 Acevedo-Garcia D, Noelke C, McArdle N, et al. Racial and ethnic inequities in children's neighborhoods: evidence from the new child opportunity index 2.0. *Health Aff (Millwood)*. 2020;39:1693–1701.
9 Cave L, Cooper MN, Zubrick SR, Shepherd CCJ. Racial discrimination and child and adolescent health in longitudinal studies: a systematic review. *Soc Sci Med*. 2020;250:112864.
10 Nardone A, Casey JA, Morello-Frosch R, Mujahid M, Balmes JR, Takur N. Associations between historical residential redlining and current age-adjusted rates of emergency department visits due to asthma across eight cities in California: an ecological study. *Lancet Planetary Health*. 2020;4:e24–e31.
11 Beck AF, Huang B, Chundur R, Kahn RS. Housing code violation density associated with emergency department and hospital use by children with asthma. *Health Aff*. 2014;33:1993–2002.
12 Wang G, Schwartz GL, Kim MM, et al. School racial segregation and the health of black children. *Pediatrics*. 2022;149:e2021055952.
13 Lee RT, Perez AD, Boykin CM, Mendoza-Denton R. On the prevalence of racial discrimination in the United States. *PLoS One*. 2019;14:e0210698.

178   SOCIAL ISSUES

14   Nagata JM, Ganson KT, Sajjad OM, Benabou SE, Bibbins-Domingo K. Prevalence of perceived racism and discrimination among US children aged 10 and 11 years: the adolescent brain cognitive development (ABCD) study. *JAMA Pediatr.* 2021;175:861–863.

15   Montes G. US children with special health care needs and ethnic discrimination: results from multivariate modeling. *World J Pediatr.* 2019;15:182–189.

16   Mackey ER, Burton ET, Cadieux A, Getzoff E, Santos M, Ward W, et al. Addressing structural racism is critical for ameliorating the childhood obesity epidemic in black youth. *Child Obes.*2022;18:75–83.

17   Cuevas AG, Krobath DM, Rhodes-Bratton B, et al. Association of racial discrimination with adiposity in children and adolescents. *JAMA Netw Open.* 2023;6:e2322839.

18   Booth SL, Sallis JF, Ritenbaugh C, et al. Environmental and societal factors affect food choice and physical activity: rationale, influences, and leverage points. *Nutr Rev.* 2001;59:S21–S39.

19   Boone-Heinonen J, Gordon-Larsen P, Kiefe CI, Shikany JM, Lewis CE, Popkin BM. Fast food restaurants and food stores: longitudinal associations with diet in young to middle-aged adults: the CARDIA study. *Arch Intern Med.* 2011;171:1162–1170.

20   Ohri-Vachaspati P, DeWeese RS, Acciai F, et al. Healthy food access in low-income high-minority communities: a longitudinal assessment—2009–2017. *Int J Environ Res Public Health.* 2019;16:2354.

21   Johnson KA, Showell NN, Flessa S, et al. Do neighborhoods matter? A systematic review of modifiable risk factors for obesity among low socio-economic status Black and Hispanic children. *Child Obes.* 2019;15:71–86.

22   Prins RG, Oenema A, van der Horst K, Brug J. Objective and perceived availability of physical activity opportunities: differences in associations with physical activity behavior among urban adolescents. *Int J Behav Nutr Phys Act.* 2009;6:70.

23   Byrd AS, Toth AT, Stanford FC. Racial disparities in obesity treatment. *Curr Obes Rep.* 2018;7:130–138.

24   Mackey ER, Burton ET, Cadieux A, et al. Addressing structural racism is critical for ameliorating the childhood obesity epidemic in black youth. *Child Obes.* 2022;18:75–83.

25   Chen D, Jaenicke EC, Volpe RJ. Food environments and obesity: household diet expenditures versus food deserts. *Am J Public Health.* 2016;106:881–888.

26   Nelson DS, Gerras JM, McGlumphy KC, et al. Racial discrimination and low household education predict higher body mass index in African American youth. *Child Obes.* 2018;14:114–121.

27   McEwen BS, Stellar E. Stress and the individual. Mechanisms leading to disease. *Arch Intern Med.* 1993;153:2093–2101.

28   Simmons S, Limbers CA. Acculturative stress and emotional eating in Latino adolescents. *Eat Weight Disord.* 2019;24:905–914.

29   Whitbeck LB, Hoyt DR, McMorris BJ, Chen X, Stubben JD. Perceived discrimination and early substance abuse among American Indian children. *J Health Soc Behav.* 2001;42:405–424.

30   Okamoto J, Ritt-Olson AD, Soto D, Baezconde-Garbanati L, Unger JB. Perceived discrimination and substance use among Latino adolescents. *Am J Health Behav.* 2009;33:718–727.

31   Tynes BM, Giang MT, Williams DR, Thompson GN. Online racial discrimination and psychological adjustment among adolescents. *J Adolesc Health.* 2008;43:565–569.

32   Tao X, Fisher CB. Exposure to social media racial discrimination and mental health among adolescents of color. *J Youth Adolesc.* 2022;51:30–44.

33   Munro LR, Travers R, Woodford MR. Overlooked and invisible: everyday experiences of microaggressions for LGBTQ adolescents. *J Homosex.* 2019;66:1439–1471.

34   National survey on LGBTQ Youth Mental Health 2021. The Trevor Project, West Hollywood, CA.

35 Sutter M, Perrin PB. Discrimination, mental health, and suicidal ideation among LGBTQ people of color. *J Couns Psychol.* 2016;63:98–105.
36 Wilson EC, Chen YH, Arayasirikul S, Raymond HF, McFarland W. The impact of discrimination on the mental health of trans* female youth and the protective effect of parental support. *AIDS Behav.* 2016;20:2203–2211.
37 Goldstick JE, Cunningham RM, Carter PM. Current causes of death in children and Adolescents in the United States. *N Engl J Med.* 2022;386(20):1955–1956.
38 Kalesan B, Vyliparambil MA, Bogue E, et al. Firearm Injury Research Group. Race and ethnicity, neighborhood poverty and pediatric firearm hospitalizations in the United States. *Ann Epidemiol.* 2016;26:1–6.
39 Beard JH, Morrison CN, Jacoby SF, et al. Quantifying disparities in urban firearm violence by race and place in Philadelphia, Pennsylvania: a cartographic study. *Am J Public Health.* 2017;107:371–373.
40 Formica MK. An eye on disparities, health equity, and racism—the case of firearm injuries in urban youth in the United States and globally. *Pediatr Clin North Am.* 2021;68:389–399.
41 Poulson M, Neufeld MY, Dechert T, Allee L, Kwnik KM. Historic redlining, structural racism, and firearm violence: a structural equation modeling approach. *Lancet Reg Health Am.* 2021;3:100052.
42 Walker R, Francis D, Brody G, Simons R, Cutrona C, Gibbons F. A longitudinal study of racial discrimination and risk for death ideation in African American youth. *Suicide Life Threat Behav.* 2017;47:86–102.
43 Argabright ST, Visoki E, Moore TM, et al. Association between discrimination stress and suicidality in preadolescent children. *J Am Acad Child Adolesc Psychiatry.* 2022;61:686–697.
44 Passel JS. Demography of immigrant youth: past, present, and future. *Future Child.* 2011;21:19–41.
45 Sirin SR, Ryce P, Gupta T, Rogers-Sirin L. The role of acculturative stress on mental health symptoms for immigrant adolescents: a longitudinal investigation. *Dev Psychol.* 2013;49:736–48.
46 Merikangas KR, He JP, Burstein M, et al. Service utilization for lifetime mental disorders in U.S. adolescents: results of the National Comorbidity Survey-Adolescent Supplement (NCS-A). *J Am Acad Child Adolesc Psychiatry.* 2011;50:32–45.
47 Tummala-Narra P, Claudius M. Perceived discrimination and depressive symptoms among immigrant-origin adolescents. *Cult Divers Ethn Minor Psychol.* 2013;19:257–269.
48 Mesch GV, Turjeman H, Fishman G. Perceived discrimination and the well-being of immigrant adolescents. *J Youth Adolesc.* 2008;37:592–604.
49 Roberts AL, Gilman SE, Breslau J, Koenen KC. Race/ethnic differences in exposure to traumatic events, development of post-traumatic stress disorder, and treatment-seeking for post-traumatic stress disorder in the United States. *Psychol Med.* 2011;41:71–83.
50 Bor J, Venkataramani AS, Williams DR, Tsai AC. Police killings and their spillover effects on the mental health of black Americans: a population-based, quasi-experimental study. *Lancet.* 2018;392:302–310.
51 Johnson TJ, Wright JL. Executions and police conflicts involving children, adolescents, and young adults. *Pediatr Clin North Am.* 2021;68:465–487.
52 Perasso G, Carraro E, De Marco J. Psychological predictors of mass-murdering in adolescents: exploring the psychological and criminological research. In Crews GA, Markey MA, Kerr SEM (Eds.), *Mitigating Mass Violence and Managing Threats in Contemporary Society.* IGI Global; 2021:18–34.
53 Gilliam CA, Lindo EG, Cannon S, Kennedy L, Jewell TE, Tieder JS. Use of race in pediatric clinical practice guidelines: a systematic review. *JAMA Pediatr.* 2022;176:804–810.

54 Wright JL, Davis WS, Joseph MM, Ellison AM, Heard-Garris NJ, Johnson TL. Eliminating race-based medicine. *Pediatrics.* 2022;150:e2022057998.

55 Hazelbaker T, Brown CS, Nenadal L, Mistry RS. Fostering anti-racism in white children and youth: Development within contexts. *Am Psychol.* 2022;77:497–509.

56 Mackey ER, Burton ET, Cadieux A, et al. Addressing structural racism Is critical for ameliorating the childhood obesity epidemic in black youth. *Child Obes.* 2022;18:75–83.

57 Simons RL, Lei MK, Beach SRH, et al. Discrimination, segregation, and chronic inflammation: testing the weathering explanation for the poor health of Black Americans. *Dev Psychol.* 2018;54:1993–2006.

58 Brody GH, Lei MK, Chae DH, Yu T, Kogan SM, Beach SRH. Perceived discrimination among African American adolescents and allostatic load: a longitudinal analysis with buffering effects. *Child Dev.* 2014;85(3):989–1002.

12
LGBTQ

Introduction

Adolescents who do not identify as straight or cisgender make up a very important and significant group. This chapter is devoted to those teens with a sexual identity other than heterosexual, and Chapter 13 addresses those with gender identities that are not cisgender. Obviously, there is some overlap, as researchers often study sexual and gender identities together. Since there is no universal acceptance of an abbreviation for these millions of teens, this book will use LGBTQ, which is further defined as follows:

Lesbian

A lesbian is a woman who is sexually and/or emotionally attracted to other women.

Gay

A gay man is sexually and/or emotionally attracted to other men, although the term "gay" may be used by anyone who is attracted to another person of the same sex or gender.

Bisexual

Bisexual individuals are attracted to men and women or to more than one gender identity.

Transgender

People who are transgender have an identity or expression that differs from the sex they were assigned at birth.

Queer

Queer is anyone who is not straight or cisgender. It may also be an individual who is questioning sexual orientation and/or gender identity and does not know how to identify themself.

Intersex

I stands for intersex or a person whose anatomy does not fit the definitions of male or female.

Asexual

A is used to denote asexual or a person who lacks sexual attraction or desire for other people.

+

The plus symbol is used to signify an individual who does not identify with any of the above categories.[1]

Pansexual

People who consider themselves to be pansexual are attracted to others regardless of their sexual or gender expression or gender identity.

Gender Fluid

People who are gender fluid do not identify as having a fixed gender.

Sexual orientation refers to the gender(s) for which an individual has romantic attraction or desire, while gender identity is the gender that is most aligned to the individual's inner self. Gender identity may or may not be the same as the biological or natal gender.

Although the exact causes for one's sexual orientation are not known, it is likely to be a combination of genetic and hormonal influences. There is no support that life experiences cause homosexuality or that an individual chooses their sexual orientation.[2] One's sexual orientation is biologically determined, and this most likely occurs at the molecular level. Compared to heterosexual men, gay men have a higher number of gay relatives, and there is evidence of familial clustering in families of gay men. In addition, the same sexual orientation in monozygotic twins is uniformly higher than the concordance rates in dizygotic twins or nontwin siblings. These findings suggest that sexual orientation is a highly inheritable trait.[3]

In addition, prenatal environmental exposures may play a part in female sexual orientation. Sexual hormones influence brain differentiation prenatally. Female fetuses that have a genetic disorder known as congenital adrenal hyperplasia (CAH) have an increased prenatal exposure to androgens in utero. After birth, these females receive treatment so that their testosterone levels normalize. The proportion of adult women with CAH who identify as lesbian is higher than in the general population. In animal models, there is compelling evidence that epigenetic mechanisms mediate the long-term effects of hormones and sexual differentiation in the brain. While it is unlikely that there are gay genes or straight genes, there may well be a network of genes that underlie sexual attraction, and this network may predispose a person's sexual orientation.[4,5] More than likely, nature is primarily involved in forging the sexual orientation of individuals.[6]

Health disparities in populations are an area of active research. LGBTQ individuals experience unique health disparities, and each of the LGBTQ populations has their own health concerns, which may be further impacted by race, ethnicity, socioeconomic status, age, and other factors. For adolescents and young adults, some of these disparities include an increased risk for depression and suicidal ideation. Among subgroups of LGBTQ youth, rates of smoking, alcohol consumption, and substance use may be higher than heterosexual youth; a disproportionate number of LGBTQ youth are unhoused. In comparison to heterosexual youth, LGBTQ youth are targets of increased levels of violence, victimization, and harassment.[7] Some health disparities between sexual minorities and heterosexual individuals persist into adulthood.[8]

LGBTQ adolescents can experience stigma from family, peers, and other social groups. Defined as the co-occurrence of labeling, stereotyping, separation, status loss, and discrimination in a setting in which power is exercised, stigma overlaps with racism and discrimination and is a fundamental cause of population health inequalities. Belonging to a sexual minority group increases the risk of stigmatization, which may negatively impact health through the disruption or alteration of systems including health care, social relationships, self-esteem, and coping mechanisms. Stress from stigmatization may create adverse health outcomes such as weight gain, anxiety, depression, and suicidality. Clearly, stigmatization may be considered as a social determinant of health.[9]

In addition, the health of LGBTQ adolescents is affected by stigmas that occur at multiple levels and from a vast number of sources. At the individual level, these youth must deal with internalized homophobia related to their sexual orientation or gender identity. Interpersonal stigma refers to discrimination that focuses on two forms: peer victimization and bullying. And there are structural forms of stigma, such as school settings, that could negatively influence opportunities, resources, and the well-being of the stigmatized.[10] For example, school settings could promote homophobia via lack of clubs for LGBTQ students, homophobic comments by teachers or administrators, or a lack of LGBTQ materials in the library.

In addition to issues due to stigmatization, LBGTQ youth report lower levels of parental closeness, increased rates of parental abuse, and homelessness.[11-13] They report a less secure maternal attachment. This occurs at a time when the adolescents are undergoing neurocognitive development as well as a maturation of coping skills. Since parents play an important role in these developmental tasks, the degree of attachment is especially important in helping youth meet developmental challenges in interpersonal, romantic, school, and work domains. Though parental rejection of LGBTQ youth may negatively affect their identity, coping mechanisms, and health, acceptance of these youth is critical to ensure that they develop a healthy sense of self.[14]

In the following sections, issues are reviewed that affect all adolescents including those who are LGBTQ. Every adolescent regardless of sexual orientation will have struggles with identity formation, career goals, family issues, and who they are in the context of their culture. LGBTQ youth face higher risks for certain issues such as anxiety and depression due to perceived nonacceptance by friends, family, the religious community, and society rather than due to a biological causation.

Epidemiology

To understand issues seen in LGBTQ adolescents, and to also plan services, it is important to understand the prevalence of sexual and gender identities among all youth. Researchers from Minnesota assessed the number of LGBTQ adolescents in their state to understand health disparities in respect to depressive symptoms and bias-based bullying. They obtained data from the Minnesota Student Survey, an anonymous survey of students in public or charter schools in grades 8, 9, and 11. In 2019, 81 percent of the school districts participated in this school-based survey. The students answered questions about sexual orientation and bullying on the basis of their sexual orientation and gender. They also complete a Patient Health Questionnaire-2 (PHQ-2) depressive symptom screen.

The researchers learned that 9.4 percent of the high school students identified as lesbian, gay, bisexual, queer, or pansexual. With respect to gender identity, 1.4 percent noted that they were transgender, gender queer, or gender fluid. The researchers observed that the students who identified as lesbian or gay had the highest predicted prevalence of sexual orientation–based bullying. The rates of depressive symptoms were highest among pansexual students, followed by queer, bisexual, gay, lesbian, and questioning individuals in descending order of prevalence. With respect to gender identities, depressive symptoms were highest among nonbinary and transmasculine youth. The researchers concluded that pansexual and queer youth as well as transmasculine and nonbinary youth whose sex is female carry a particularly high burden of bias and discrimination and should be screened for additional services and supports.[15]

Biopsychosocial Issues and LGBTQ

Biological Issues

Stress
LGBTQ teens may be forced to deal with the stresses associated with their minority status, such as discrimination, bias-related victimization, and family rejection. During adolescence, victimization by peers as well as family rejection may impact the psychosocial development of those in sexual minority groups. Peer victimization based on an adolescent's LGBTQ identity has been correlated with suicidal thought and attempts; family rejection may lead to stress related to becoming homeless. There appears to be a cumulative role for minority stress and suicide risk among LGBTQ adolescents. Researchers from the Trevor Project in California, a suicide prevention

and crisis intervention organization serving LGBTQ young people, studied the association of LGBTQ cumulative minority stress with suicide risk in adolescents and young adults in the United States. They obtained data from an online cross-sectional survey conducted between December 2019 and March 2020 of 39,126 LGBTQ youth ages 13 to 24 years in the United States. The measures include age, race/ethnicity, sexual orientation, gender identity, LGBTQ-based housing insecurity, perceived LGBTQ discrimination, physical harm or threats from LGBTQ status, LGBTQ identity change attempts from caregivers, and suicide attempts. Seventy percent of the sample reported one or more minority stress risk factors, with 20.4 percent of the adolescents ages 13 to 17 years reporting a suicide attempt. Compared to older youth, those under age 18 years had a greater risk (2.61) (p < .001) of a suicide attempt during the previous year. Exposure to a greater number of LGBTQ-related minority stressors resulted in a significantly greater odds of experiencing past-year suicide attempt. Marginalized members, including those with transgender and nonbinary identities and Native American and Alaskan Native youth, had a significantly greater chance of having more minority-related stress.[16] The results of the study underscored the need for suicide prevention programming and prioritizing those at highest risk.

A source of added stress for LGBTQ adolescents is microaggressions, which are brief, verbal, indirect, subtle or unintentional, behavioral, or environmental indignities that may be directed against a marginalized group. Examples of microaggressions against LGBTQ adolescents include endorsement of heteronormative or gender-normative culture or behaviors, use of heterosexist and transphobic language, and discomfort or disapproval of LGBTQ experiences. While microaggressions may not manifest in direct physical or verbal violence, they are clear signs of insensitivity and disrespect regarding LGBTQ sexual orientation and/or gender identity.

To further define these microaggressions, in a small study from Canada, researchers examined the impact of microaggressions on LGBTQ adolescents. They recruited 11 youth between the ages of 14 and 18 years to participate in two different focus groups. Three identified as female, two identified as male, three were trans male, one was gender queer/nonbinary, one was gender fluid, and a female was questioning. With respect to sexual orientation, two identified as gay, four were queer, one was lesbian, one was biromantic/asexual, two were pansexual, and one was unsure. The researchers learned that LGBTQ adolescents are consistently confronted with heterosexist expectations and are denied the freedom to be themselves. The adolescents expressed frustration at feeling overlooked and invisible from microaggressions. Although most of the microaggressions occurred at school, they also happened at home. And there were environmental microaggressions, such as gender markers on forms and achievement awards that marginalized transgender students. As a result of this study, the researchers suggested that schools create safe spaces for LGBTQ students, counseling services, and educational awareness.[17]

Psychological Issues

As previously discussed, LGBTQ teens have higher rates of anxiety, depression, suicide, posttraumatic stress disorder, and substance use during adolescence than their heterosexual peers. These disparities are believed to be the result of a minority stress model in which LGBTQ teens develop strain arising from their social positions as members of stigmatized, disadvantaged, and oppressed groups. Stressors expose LGBTQ adolescents to victimization and bullying; combined with the daily stressors all adolescents have, the stigma-related stressors may result in health disparities among teens who are LGBTQ.[18]

Anxiety

The Trevor Project in California conducted an online, cross-sectional survey that studied the prevalence of mental health symptoms among LGBTQ adolescents. The study sample, which was collected during the last quarter of 2021, included 44,828 LGBTQ individuals between the ages of 13 and 24 years, who were recruited by targeted ads on social media. Sixty-two percent of the respondents were between the ages of 13 and 17 years. The researchers learned that 73 percent of LGBTQ youth reported anxiety symptoms. As noted in Chapter 4, in a general national study, the lifetime prevalence of an anxiety disorder in adolescents was 32 percent. Although these two studies differ by methodology and participants, it can be stated that LGBTQ adolescents have a high prevalence of anxiety symptoms. With respect to sexual orientation, a majority of each group—lesbian, gay, bisexual, transgender, queer, and questioning—had anxiety symptoms, as did the majority of each gender group and the majority of each race/ethnicity. The researchers learned that there was widespread anxiety among LGBTQ youth, and 60 percent of these youth did not receive the mental health care they wanted.[19]

Depression

Prolonged exposure to stigmatization due to sexual minority status is likely to produce an increased prevalence of mental health symptoms. According to the 2015 Youth Risk Behavior Survey (YRBS), over 60 percent of lesbian, gay, and bisexual youth had prolonged feelings of hopelessness or sadness versus one-quarter of heterosexual youth who have those symptoms. In the Trevor Project survey, 58 percent of the LGBTQ youth had depressive symptoms, with gay males most at risk. Relatedly, data from the Trevor Project survey also indicated that 45 percent of LGBTQ youth seriously considered suicide in the past year, and 14 percent of these youth attempted suicide during this time period. However, the rates for suicidal ideation and suicide attempts were much higher in younger adolescents, suggesting that over time, suicidal thinking appears to diminish in these youth.[20]

Schools can serve as a crucial factor in mitigating depressive symptoms, suicidal ideation, anxiety, and other mental health issues among LGBTQ adolescents. Using data from the 2015 YRBS and the 2014 School Health Profiles, researchers in Pennsylvania wanted to learn if the proportion of schools teaching LGBTQ-inclusive sex education was associated with improved mental health outcomes. Further, they wanted to learn if associations were significantly different for sexual minority youth than their heterosexual peers. Data were obtained from 11 states. The measures included mental health symptoms (depression, suicidality), bullying victimization, LGBTQ-inclusive sex education, sexual identity, and demographic covariates. The researchers determined that LGBTQ-inclusive sex education was related to lower reports of adverse mental health among all youth as well as experiences of bullying among sexual minority youth. This sex education appeared to offer protection for depressive symptoms, suicidal thoughts, and the preparation of a suicide plan for all youth. For every 10 percent increase of schools teaching LGBTQ-inclusive sex education in a state, there was a 20 percent reduction in reported suicide plans. These data support research that inclusive school climates have positive implications for heterosexual youth as well as sexual minority youth.[21]

Eating Disorders

Both sexual majority and sexual minority adolescents are at risk for disordered eating and eating disorders. Disordered eating refers to an array of irregular eating behaviors such as significant weight loss, purging behaviors, or body image issues that may or may not meet the criteria for an eating disorder. Up to 80 percent of female adolescents have some degree of body dissatisfaction and feel a desire to change their weight or appearance. It is believed that female adolescents in the sexual minority—those with same-sex attraction or those who identify as lesbian, bisexual, or pansexual—have a higher prevalence of disordered eating.[22]

Parental and/or peer rejection and low support for their sexual identity may impact how sexual minority female adolescents feel about their bodies. Researchers based in Pennsylvania and Delaware hypothesized that sexual minority adolescents who have better-quality relationships with their parents and less victimization from their sexual orientation would have higher self-esteem and fewer symptoms of disordered eating, such as caloric restriction, purging, and binge eating. The researchers used ethnically diverse data from 528 sexual minority adolescent females recruited from a nationwide study on LGBTQ adolescent health. While their sexual orientations were primarily bisexual/pansexual, they also included lesbian/gay, queer/questioning, and other. The subjects completed an online survey with measures for demographics, parent-adolescent relationship quality, sexual orientation–based victimization, body esteem, and disordered eating behaviors. The researchers found evidence of a positive correlation between the quality of the parent-adolescent relationship and body esteem in these sexual minority female adolescents, and these females had lower levels of disordered eating. This relationship appeared to influence how the females felt about their appearance and weight. Their disordered eating was felt to be related to their sexual orientation victimization rather than body image issues. Disordered eating may be a coping mechanism for those sexual minority female adolescents who are victimized. These findings underscore the benefits of a positive parent-adolescent relationship and the need for educational efforts to help prevent sexual victimization.[23]

Regardless of sexual identity, all adolescents who are overweight or obese are subject to weight-based victimization. To further understand this victimization among LGBTQ adolescents, researchers from Connecticut studied sexual minority male and female adolescents. They used data from the 2017 LGBTQ National Teen Survey, an online instrument completed by 9838 sexual and gender minority adolescents with a mean age of 15.6 years and 159 straight adolescents. The measures included demographics, sexual orientation, gender identity, anthropometric data such as weight and height, and questions on weight-based victimization. The sexual identities included LGBTQ+ (98.4 percent) and straight (1.6 percent). The gender identities included cisgender female (44.0 percent), cisgender male (21.0 percent), transgender male (8.7 percent), transgender female (1.2 percent), assigned female at birth nonbinary (23.0 percent), and assigned male at birth nonbinary (2.2 percent). Compared to adolescents who identified as straight, respondents who identified as lesbian, gay, bisexual, queer, pansexual, asexual, or other had higher odds of weight-based victimization. Cisgender LGBTQ female adolescents had higher rates of teasing by family members and peers than cisgender male adolescents. The findings provided some evidence that weight-based teasing by family and/or peers is pervasive for both cisgender male adolescents and cisgender female adolescents who identify as LGBTQ, and this could occur for those who were underweight, healthy weight, overweight, or obese. The researchers further noted that previous research had determined that weight-based victimization in a primarily heterosexual adolescent population was disproportionally higher in those who were overweight or obese.[24]

A group of researchers from multiple countries studied 10,197 early adolescents from the United States in a cross-sectional analysis from the Adolescent Brain Cognitive Development Study. One of the study aims was to examine the association between sexual orientation and binge eating disorder and binge eating behaviors. Compared to their heterosexual peers, individuals who identified as gay or bisexual were found to have greater odds of binge eating disorder and binge eating behaviors. The researchers suggested that gay and bisexual adolescents face such stressors as stigma, bullying, discrimination, and internalized homophobia, which all compound to an increased risk of disordered eating.[25]

Substance Use

Many, if not most, adolescents participate in risky behaviors. Researchers at the Centers for Disease Control and Prevention studied these behaviors among sexual minority youth in grades 9 to 12 and compared their prevalence to that of sexual majority adolescents utilizing the Youth Risk Behavior Surveillance System (YRBSS). The YRBSS monitors the use of tobacco, alcohol, and other drugs. The researchers learned that of the 13 tobacco use–related risk behaviors, 11 were more often used by lesbian, gay, and bisexual students than by heterosexual students. With respect to 19 alcohol and other drug use behaviors, the use of 18 was higher among the lesbian, gay, and bisexual students than the students who were heterosexual. For example, while 32.0 percent of the lesbian, gay, and bisexual students used marijuana, 20.7 percent of the heterosexual students used this product. Compared to heterosexual students, the sexual minority students had a higher prevalence of many health risk behaviors. The researchers suggested that there should be an increased awareness of these disparities, and they recommended educational, health care, and evidence-based interventions for sexual minority youth.[26]

A researcher in Washington, DC noted some etiological factors to explain substance use disparities. Sexual minority students have normal adolescent stress, as well as stress from being a sexual minority. In addition to these external stressors, sexual minority youth often internalize stigma; they may internalize heterosexuality into their self-concept or how they view themselves. One way that these adolescents may cope with their internal and external stressors is by using substances. The researcher added that no empirically tested treatment interventions had been developed specifically for a sexually minority audience.[27]

However, these stressors can be mitigated by educational intervention. Researchers in Pennsylvania, Illinois, California, and New York wanted to determine if adolescents would drink alcohol less often if they lived in educational jurisdictions in which schools were more affirmative of LGBTQ youth. They used 2005 and 2007 data from the previously noted YRBSS for grades 9 to 12. There were three alcohol use measures, demographic questions including sexual orientation, and jurisdiction-level variables. From the jurisdiction-level questions, the researchers were able to create the LGBTQ school climate variable. The researchers found that during the previous month, the sexual minority students drank on significantly more days including days at school than their heterosexual counterparts. Living in jurisdictions with more versus less affirmative LGBTQ school climates was associated with fewer drinking days at school and fewer heavy episodic drinking days. The researchers recommended the following ways to help build a more affirmative LGBTQ school climate:

- Establish and enforce policies that protect adolescents from being bullied or harassed based on sexual orientation.
- Create safe spaces and clubs for LGBTQ adolescents.
- Train members of the school staff to be more knowledgeable about and support the LGBTQ adolescents.
- Develop and implement interventions that reduce anti-LGBTQ prejudice among both students and staff.
- Teach adolescents using LGBTQ-inclusive curricula especially in health and history.[28]

Suicidality

The earlier noted YRBSS survey also collected data on suicidality in adolescents. Table 12.1 compares rates of suicidal ideation, suicide plan, and suicide attempts in heterosexual, gay, lesbian, bisexual, or not sure adolescents. The data indicated higher rates of these behaviors in sexual minority adolescents.

Researchers in Minnesota, California, and Massachusetts wanted to learn if adolescents who attended schools and lived in communities with more supports for LGBTQ students and teen residents were at a lower risk for a past-year suicide attempt. Previous research had demonstrated that these benefits reduced suicidality in adults who had experienced school connectedness and engagement as teens. The researchers used data from multiple sources in Massachusetts, including students, schools, and communities. Students completed cross-sectional health surveys; school information was obtained from the School Environment Survey, and community data were obtained by structured internet keyword searches. The measures included student sexual orientation, sex/gender, suicide attempts, demographics, and school and community variables.

The mean age of the respondents was 16 years. Among the male adolescents, a past-year suicide attempt was reported in 15 percent of the gay, 20 percent of the bisexual, 10 percent of the questioning, and 4 percent of the heterosexual students. For female adolescents, a past-year suicide attempt was reported in 18 percent of the lesbian,

Table 12.1 Suicidal Behaviors Reported by Heterosexual, Gay, Lesbian, Bisexual, or Not Sure Adolescents

Type of Suicidality	Heterosexual	Gay, Lesbian, or Bisexual	Not Sure of Sexual Orientation
Ideation	14.8	42.8	31.9
Plan	11.9	38.2	27.9
Attempt	6.4	29.4	13.7

From Kann L, Olsen EO, McManus T, et al. Sexual identity, sex of sexual contacts, and health-related behaviors among students in grades 9-12—United States and Selected Sites, 2015. *MMWR Surveill Summ.* 2016 Aug 12;65(9):1–202.

24 percent of the bisexual, 11 percent of the questioning, and 4 percent of the heterosexual students. The availability of several school- and community-wide LGBTQ resources was related to a lower risk of suicide attempts among certain student subgroups. For example, compared to schools without these resources, a gender-neutral bathroom was linked to lower past suicide attempts in gay, bisexual, and questioning male adolescents. For questioning and heterosexual female adolescents, past-year suicide attempts were significantly lower if they lived in communities with more support. The researchers commented that this type of encouragement and assistance in schools and communities may be beneficial for all adolescents regardless of their sexual orientation.[29]

Social Issues and LGBTQ

Social Media

Many LGBTQ adolescents use social media as a primary means to interact with other LGBTQ adolescents. They search online for information on sexuality, and the internet plays a role in their identity formation. Researchers in Australia and New York City studied the ways LGBTQ adolescents used social media to explore their identity and seek support from LGBTQ peers. They interviewed 30 LGBTQ individuals with a mean age of 16.17 years; 23 were cisgender, 4 were nonbinary, and 3 were transgender male adolescents. The team concluded that LGBTQ adolescents used social media for identity, relationship, and well-being support. In addition, they obtained and provided information on sex, relationships, and sexual health through social media. However, the researchers found that social media groups could be a source of discrimination and stigma for LGBTQ adolescents. The investigators concluded that social media networks were perceived as an effective method for LGBTQ adolescents to secure social support, and they viewed social media as protective against some mental health issues. However, these adolescents reported experiences of homophobia, transphobia, discrimination, and racism through social media. LGBTQ adolescents used social media in ways that provided positive influences on their well-being.[30]

As noted, LGBTQ youth also face online harassment because of their sexuality and/ or gender identity. Researchers from Canada and Ohio were looking to understand the total impact of social media use among LGBTQ teens. They sought to answer three questions: How often do LGBTQ youth use social media sites? Why do these youth use social media sites? How do the benefits obtained from using these sites enhance the well-being of these youth? The 6178 subjects self-identified as LGBTQ youth and were between the ages of 14 and 29 years, with a mean age of 18.21 years; they all lived in the United States or Canada. The clear majority (65.4 percent) was between the ages of 14 and 18 years. The study measured social media benefits, five favorite social media sites, and the reasons the subjects used the sites.

The researchers learned that social media helped stigmatized youth, in this instance LGBTQ youth. This study also confirmed that social media assisted these youth in accessing emotional support, developing their identities, obtaining important information, and finding entertainment. These positive findings stand in sharp contrast to the potential negative effects of social media, such as increasing anxiety and depression as well as lowering self-esteem and other aspects of mental health in youth.[31]

However, use of social media may be harmful as these sites could increase sexual victimization of LGBTQ adolescents and young adults. Researchers in New York City studied 175 gay, bisexual, and other men who had sex with men who were recruited by broadcast advertisements on Grindr. The demographics indicated that 38 percent of the participants were ages 18 to 25 years and 85 percent identified as gay. The researchers found that 38 percent of the participants reported a history of intimate partner violence.[32] Many LGBTQ young adults use apps such as Grindr or Tinder to meet other gay and lesbian youth and can be at risk of being lured into unwanted sexual situations. Primary care clinicians should provide some preventive counseling on these issues to this population.

Discrimination

Studies have found that social stigma and negative societal responses are harmful to the physical, emotional, and social health of sexual minority adolescents. Researchers in California and Utah examined the association between family rejection and negative health outcomes in LGBTQ young adults. The researchers recruited 224 subjects between the ages of 21 and 25 years who were lesbian, gay, or bisexual. Their survey had measures for family rejection, subjects' mental health (current depression, suicidal ideation in the last 6 months, and lifetime suicide attempts), substance use and abuse, and sexual risk behavior. The researchers found a correlation between negative family reactions to an adolescent's sexual orientation and health problems in lesbian, gay, or bisexual young adults. Those subjects who reported higher levels of family rejection during adolescence were 8.4 times more likely to have attempted suicide, 5.9 times more likely to have high levels of depression, 3.4 times more likely to use illegal drugs, and 3.4 times more likely to have engaged in unprotected sex compared to those in the study group who had no or low levels of family rejection. This study provided solid evidence that family support for lesbian, gay, or bisexual adolescents may make a critical difference in helping to decrease their risk for negative health outcomes as young adults. Clinicians who serve this population should help to educate families on the potential impact of rejecting behaviors.[33]

Given the strong influence that family has on LGBTQ stigmatization and discrimination and the serious negative health concerns that may follow, researchers in New York City conducted a scoping study to find existing intervention programs and policies that may help promote more supportive family environments for LGBTQ youth. The researchers found only nine peer-reviewed publications between 2010 and 2017 that described interventions. Surprisingly, only 1 of the 18 programs the researchers located had outcomes data. That program was an intervention for gender variant children rather than LGBTQ individuals. The researchers concluded that there was little published research, evidence-based interventions, or policies that addressed family-based stigma and discrimination against LGBTQ youth. Much of the work was ongoing to improve family environments for LGBTQ youth, and governments or nongovernmental organizations conducted it. Tackling family-based stigma and discrimination requires community and structural level programs and policies that impact an audience beyond those who participate in the intervention. Such programs could include pro-acceptance campaigns, and policies could include anti–conversion therapy laws. Structural policies to reduce sexual minority discrimination in schools or health care settings could also be a strategy that might improve the family environment for LGBTQ youth.[34]

Violence

Youth violence, such as peer victimization, bullying, and dating violence, are relatively common during the adolescent years. According to the minority stress model, LGBTQ individuals undergoing such violence may demonstrate health disparities compared to their heterosexual peers. Researchers in Illinois compared peer victimization, perceptions of school violence and crime, and teen dating violence and victimization among LGBTQ and non-LGBTQ students and whether they were linked to anxiety and suicidality. They sampled 11,794 high school students from Dane County, Wisconsin, with a mean age of 16 years; 51 percent were female. Regarding sexual orientation, 93 percent were heterosexual, 1.1 percent were gay/lesbian, 3.2 percent were bisexual, and 2.2 percent were questioning. The subjects completed questions via SurveyMonkey; measures included anxiety, suicidality, peer victimization, and teen dating violence/victimization. The results supported the minority stress model. The researchers learned that LGBTQ adolescents with lower rates of victimization had significantly lower rates of suicidality compared to LGBTQ individuals with higher rates of victimization. In addition, the LGBTQ adolescents in schools with greater student perceptions of school violence and crime had higher suicidality than non-LGBTQ counterparts. Peer victimization appeared to moderate the associations between sexual orientation mental health outcomes, and LGBTQ youth reported greater teen dating victimization and violence. The researchers recommended that prevention programs address multiple forms of victimization including those from peers and dating, paying particular attention to the experiences of LGBTQ youth.[35]

Taking this issue a step further, researchers from New Hampshire and Illinois questioned if LGBTQ college students had a higher risk for violence than heterosexual students during the previous 6 months. From September 2011 to February 2012, they studied 6030 students from eight New England universities who were between the ages of 18 and 24 years. The majority were female and had exclusively heterosexual experiences. The questionnaire used included measures of sexual minority status, victimization by physical dating violence, sexual assault, and unwanted pursuit. The findings demonstrated that sexual minority students noted a significantly higher 6-month incidence of physical dating violence (30.3 versus 18.5 percent), sexual assault (24.3 versus 11.0 percent), and unwanted pursuit victimization (53.1 versus 36.0 percent). Female sexual minority students had significantly higher rates of physical dating violence than heterosexual female students. The research supported the significant prevalence of victimization on university campuses and the need to develop intervention and prevention programming that are appropriate for both LGBTQ and heterosexual students.[36]

Researchers in Wisconsin, North Carolina, New Hampshire, and Florida interviewed college campus practitioners who identified as LGBTQ and who were working on sexual and relationship violence (SRV) and LGBTQ issues. The aim of the study was to determine which strategies could better affirm LGBTQ students in campus SRV prevention. The strategies were grouped into those at the individual, relationship, community, and societal levels. At the individual level, some strategies included programming for bystander interventions and SRV training for LGBTQ students, staff, and faculty. At the relationship level, among the recommendations was hiring LGBTQ individuals for SRV-related roles and senior leadership positions. Strategies at the community level included providing LGBTQ-specific health and advocacy services. At the societal level, two of the recommendations were comprehensive sexual education in K–12 schools and establishing LGBTQ-affirming federal anti-harassment and nondiscrimination guidance.[37]

Prevention

Researchers in San Francisco studied whether family acceptance would be a protective factor for LGBTQ adolescents and young adults. They recruited a sample of 245 LGBTQ young adults in the San Francisco area and developed measures for family acceptance, demographics, and young adult adjustment and health. The results indicated that family acceptance did not vary based on the gender or sexual identity or transgender identity of the study participants. In addition, family acceptance in adolescence was associated with young adult positive health outcomes. These outcomes included self-esteem, social support, and general health. Furthermore, family acceptance was a protective factor for such negative health outcomes as depression, substance abuse, suicidal ideation, and suicide attempts. Thus, intervention at the family level through acceptance is associated with positive LGBTQ young adult mental and physical health.[38]

Since middle and high school settings may be domains where homophobia exists alongside anti-gay harassment and bullying, these institutions may place LGBTQ students at risk for safety, mental health, and academic problems. Fortunately, there are strategies that have been shown to promote the safety and well-being of LGBTQ youths in the school setting. They have been previously outlined and are further elaborated in Box 12.1.[39]

In addition, researchers from New York, Illinois, Massachusetts, and California studied whether sexual minority youths living in states with more protective school climates were at lower risk of suicidality. Using data from the YRBSS, they determined that lesbian, gay, and bisexual students living in states and cities with more protective school climates reported fewer past-year suicidal thoughts than those living in states and cities with less protective climates.[40]

Homophobia prevention efforts do not start or stop at schools. Community activities have been shown to promote psychosocial health for LGBTQ youth. In a recent study of LGBTQ youth of color, there was an association of community social activities and involvement with the psychosocial health of Black and Latinx youth. This was especially noted through social activities tailored to LGBTQ individuals.[41]

Conclusion

Based on their sexual and gender identities, LGBTQ adolescents experience distinctive health disparities. These include the increased prevalence of mood disorders and suicidal thinking. Due to a loss of social supports during the COVID-19 pandemic, these problems may well have worsened. And it is not uncommon for LGBTQ adolescents to be subjected to discrimination and stigmatization from peers, family members, schools, and other structural organizations.

That said, many adolescents who identify as LGBTQ do not experience mood disorders, victimization, stigmatization, and the other issues noted previously. These individuals are very successful in meeting the goals of adolescence and young adulthood.

For teens who are in the sexual minority, a positive parental relationship may help prevent mental health symptomatology. Effective interventions and prevention programs need to be created to educate groups including families, schools, governments, and other institutions to promote acceptance of LGBTQ adolescents. These efforts should begin at the family level and flow through peers, schools, communities, and local, state, and federal governments.

References

1 The Lesbian, Gay, Bisexual & Transgender Community Center. What is LGBTQIA? New York, NY; 2024.
2 O'Hanlan KA, Gordon JC, Sullivan MW. Biological origins of sexual orientation and gender identity: impact on health. *Gynecol Oncol.* 2018;149:33–42.
3 O'Hanlan KA, Gordon JC, Sullivan MW. Biological origins of sexual orientation and gender identity: impact on health. *Gynecol Oncol.* 2018;149:33–42.
4 Ngun TC, Vilain E. The biological basis of human sexual orientation: is there a role for epigenetics? *Adv Genet.* 2014;86:167–184.
5 Gondim R, Teles F, Barroso U Jr. Sexual orientation of 46,XX patients with congenital adrenal hyperplasia: a descriptive review. *J Pediatr Urol.* 2018 Dec;14(6):486–493.
6 Balthazart J. Fraternal birth order effect on sexual orientation explained. *Proc Natl Acad Sci U S A.* 2018;115:234–236.

7   Institute of Medicine (US) Committee on Lesbian, Gay, Bisexual, and Transgender Health Issues and Research Gaps and Opportunities. *The Health of Lesbian, Gay, Bisexual, and Transgender People: Building a Foundation for Better Understanding.* National Academic Press; 2011.

8   Liu M, Sandhu S, Reisner SL, Gonzales G, Keuroghlian A. Health status and health care access among lesbian, gay, and bisexual adults in the US, 2013 to 2018. *JAMA Intern Med.* 2023;183:380–383.

9   Hatzenbuehler ML, Phelan JC, Link BG. Stigma as a fundamental cause of population health inequalities. *Am J Public Health.* 2013;103:813–821.

10 Hatzenbuehler M, Pachankis JE. Stigma and minority stress as social determinants of health among lesbian, gay, bisexual, and transgender youth: research evidence and clinical implications. *Pediatr Clin North Am.* 2016;63:985–997.

11 Pearson J, Wilkinson L. Family relationships and adolescent well-being: are families equally protective for same-sex attracted youth? *J Youth Adolesc.* 2013;42:376–393.

12 Corliss HL, Cochran SD, Mays VM. Reports of parental maltreatment during childhood in a United States population-based survey of homosexual, bisexual, and heterosexual adults. *Child Abuse Negl.* 2002;26:1165–1178.

13 Corliss HL, Goodenow CS, Nichols L, Austin SB. High burden of homelessness among sexual-minority adolescents: findings from a representative Massachusetts high school sample. *Am J Public Health.* 2011;101:1683–1689.

14 Katz-Wise SL, Rosario M, Tsappis M. Lesbian, gay, bisexual, and transgender youth and family acceptance. *Pediatr Clin North Am.* 2016;63:1011–1025.

15 Gower AL, Rider GN, Brown C, Eisenberg ME. Diverse sexual and gender identity, bullying, and depression among adolescents. *Pediatrics.* 2022;149:e2021053000.

16 Green AE, Price MN, Dorison SH. Cumulative minority stress and suicide risk among LGBTQ youth. *Am J Community Psychol.* 2022;69:157–168.

17 Munro L, Travers R, Woodford MR. Overlooked and invisible: everyday experiences of microaggressions for LGBTQ adolescents. *J Homosex.* 2019;66:1439–1471.

18 Espelage DI, Herrin GJ, Hatchel T. Peer victimization and dating violence among LGBTQ youth: the impact of. school violence and crime on mental health outcomes. *Youth Violence Juv Justice.* 2018;16:156–173.

19 The Trevor Project. 2022 national survey on LGBTQ youth mental health. West Hollywood, CA; 2022.

20 Ibid.

21 Proulx CN, Coulter RWS, Egan JE, Matthews DD, Mair C. Associations of lesbian, gay, bisexual, transgender, and questioning-inclusive sex education with mental health outcomes and school-based victimization in U.S. high school students. *J Adolesc Health.* 2019;54:608–614.

22 Parker LL, Harriger JA. Eating disorders and disordered eating behaviors in the LGBT population: a review of the literature. *J Eat Disord.* 2020;8:51.

23 Rezeppa TL, Roberts SR, Maheux AJ, Choukas-Bradley S, Salk R, Thom BC. Psychosocial correlates of body esteem and disordered eating among sexual minority adolescent girls. *Body Image.* 2021;39:184–193.

24 Puhl RM, Himmelstein MS, Watson RJ. Weight-based victimization among sexual and gender minority adolescents: feelings from a diverse national sample. *Pediatr Obes.* 2019;14:e12514.

25 Nagata JM, Smith-Russack Z, Paul A, et al. The social epidemiology of binge-eating disorder and behaviors in early adolescents. *J Eat Disord.* 2023;11(1):182.

26 Kann L, O'Malley Olsen E, McManus T, et al. Sexual identity, sex of sexual contacts, and health-related behaviors among students in grades 9–12—United States and selected sites, 2015. *MMWR Surveill Summ.* 2016;65:1–202.

27 Mereish EH. Substance use and misuse among sexual and gender minority youth. *Curr Opin Psychol.* 2019;30:123–127.

28 Coulter RW, Birkett M, Corliss HL, Hatzenbuehler ML, Mustanski B, Stall RD. Associations between LGBTQ-affirmative school climate and adolescent drinking behaviors. *Drug Alcohol Depend.* 2016;161:340–347.

29 Eisenberg ME, Wood BA, Erickson DJ, Gower AL, Schneider SK, Corliss HL. Associations between LGBTQ+-supportive school and community resources and suicide attempts among adolescents in Massachusetts. *Am J Orthopsychiatry.* 2021;91:800–811.

30 Berger MN, Taba M, Marino JL, et al. Social media's role in support networks among LGBTQ adolescents: a qualitative study. *Sex Health.* 2021;18:421–431.

31 Craig S, Eaton AD, McInroy LB. Can social media participation enhance LGBTQ+ youth well-being? Development of the social media benefits scale. *Soc Media Soc.* 2021;7:1–13.

32 Duncan DT, Goedel WC, Stults CB, et al. A study of intimate partner violence, substance abuse, and sexual risk behaviors among gay, bisexual, and other men who have sex with men in a sample of geosocial-networking smartphone application users. *Am J Mens Health.* 2018;12:292–2301.

33 Ryan C, Huebner D, Diaz RM, Sanchez J. Family rejection as a predictor of negative health outcomes in white and Latino lesbian, gay and bisexual young adults. *Pediatrics.* 2009;123:346–352.

34 Parker CM, Hirsch JS, Philbin MM, Parker RG. The urgent need for research and interventions to address family-based stigma and discrimination against Lesbian, Gay, Bisexual, Transgender and Queer youth. *J Adolesc Health.* 2018;63:383–393.

35 Espelage DI, Harrin GJ, Hatchel T. Peer victimization and dating violence among LGBTQ youth: the impact of school violence and crime on mental health outcomes. *Youth Violence Juv Justice.* 2018;16:156–173.

36 Edwards KM, Sylaska KM, Barry JE, et al. Physical dating violence, sexual violence, and unwanted pursuit victimization: a comparison of incidence rates among sexual-minority and heterosexual college students. *J Interpers Violence.* 2015;30:580–600.

37 Klein LB, Doyle LJ, Hall WJ, et al. LGBTQ+-affirming campus sexual and relationship violence prevention: a qualitative study. *J Interpers Violence.* 2023;38:4061–4087.

38 Ryan C, Russell ST, Huebner D, Diaz R, Sanchez J. Family acceptance in adolescence and the health of LGBT young adults. *J Child Adolesc Psychiatr Nurs.* 2010;23:205–213.

39 Russell S. Challenging homophobia in schools: policies and programs for safe school climates. *Educ Rev.* 2011;39:123–138.

40 Hatzenbuehler ML, Birkett M, Van Wagenen A, Meyer IH. Protective school climates and reduced risk for suicide ideation in sexual minority youths. *Am J Public Health.* 2014;104:279–286.

41 Heath RD, Keene L. The role of school and community involvement in the psychosocial health outcomes of Black and Latinx LGBTQ youth. *J Adolesc Health.* 2023;72(5):650–657.

13
Transgender Adolescents and Gender-Incongruence

Introduction

In the previous chapter on LGBTQ adolescents, there were references in some sections that applied to transgender adolescents. However, transgender adolescents have unique issues apart from those of LGBQ adolescents. In addition, medical treatments for transgender individuals may include puberty blockers, gender-affirming hormones, and surgical procedures. Research on transgender issues is also limited in some areas, and at this time, there is significant political activity around transgender matters.

Gender incongruence is not a new condition; treatment guidelines were published more than 40 years ago. Around 1987, Patient Zero was referred to Henriette A. Delemarre-can de Waal, a pediatric endocrinologist who founded the first gender clinic in Amsterdam with child psychologist Peggy Cohen-Kettenis. In despair about being forced to live through female puberty, Patient Zero was placed on puberty suppressants, which paused further sexual development.[1] Dr. Norman Spack, a pediatric endocrinologist and specialist in adolescent medicine at Boston Children's Hospital, began to treat transgender adults in the 1980s. Subsequently, he founded the first pediatric transgender program in the United States in 2007, also at Boston Children's Hospital.[2] There is greater awareness today with over 100 clinics in the United States offering care to gender diverse children and adolescents.

When discussing transgender issues, it is useful to know the definitions of a few frequently used terms.[3]

Gender dysphoria: psychological distress from an incongruence between one's sex assigned at birth and one's gender identity.

Gender expression: the way an individual expresses their gender such as through dress, actions, and social roles.

Gender attribution: how strangers perceive an individual's gender.

Gender identity: an individual's sense of being male, female, both, neither, or another combination.

Gender incongruence: characterized by a marked incompatibility between an individual's experienced/expressed gender and the assigned sex. The individual may not necessarily have psychological distress due to the incongruence.

Nonbinary: a term used for people who do not identify as either 100 percent male or 100 percent female. The term is used interchangeably with the terms "gender nonconforming," "gender expansive," and "gender fluid."

Transgender male: an individual whose gender identity is male, which differs from the gender assigned at birth.

Transgender female: an individual whose gender identity is female, which differs from the gender assigned at birth.

Cisgender male: an individual whose gender identity is male, which aligns with the gender assigned at birth.

Cisgender female: an individual whose gender identity is female, which aligns with the gender assigned at birth.

Gender identity is not the choice of an individual.[4] There is no evidence that social media, peer pressure, mental health issues, or trauma causes gender incongruence. The cause of gender incongruence may be a combination of different biopsychosocial factors, according to clinicians at Cincinnati Children's Hospital Medical Center. Investigators in the Netherlands conducted brain neuroimaging research that suggests adolescents with gender incongruence have structural characteristics resembling peers of their gender identity. Other authorities maintain that genetic factors contribute to gender development. Some believe that hormonal influences that occur prenatally may influence gender development. Environmental factors, such as cultural norms and social relationships, may also play a part in gender development and expression.[5]

While researchers still have much to learn about the origins of transgender development, it is clear that gender identity begins as early as 3 to 4 years. The majority of respondents to the United States Transgender Survey indicated that by the age of 10 years, they began to feel that their gender was different from the one on their birth certificate. By the age of 15, most knew that they were transgender, and by the age of 25, they started to share their transgender status with others.[6,7]

Children and adolescents who are transgender appear to have a higher prevalence of mental health issues including anxiety, depression, eating disorders, and suicidality. This is due to their nonacceptance or fear of nonacceptance of their gender identity as well as not being able to live in their gender identity. Some researchers believe there is no overrepresentation of gender diversity with neurodiversity (such as autism spectrum disorder) or the converse.[8] Yet others believe or have shown that transgender and gender diverse (TGD) individuals score higher on self-report measures of autistic traits.[9] Thus, the linkages, if any, between neurodiversity and gender diversity are not conclusive.

Researchers from multiple institutions developed the Study of Transition, Outcomes, and Gender (STRONG) to assess morbidity among transgender and/ or gender nonconforming (TGNC) adolescents between the ages of 3 and 17 years. STRONG was an electronic medical record–based prospective and retrospective cohort study of the members of several Kaiser Permanente sites. On the basis of the diagnosis in the electronic records, it identified persons who were showing evidence of TGNC status between January 1, 2006, and December 31, 2014. For each validated TGNC subject, 10 cisgender male and 10 cisgender female Kaiser enrollees were matched based on birth year, race/ethnicity, and site. There were 588 subjects in the trans female cohort and 745 in the trans male cohort. The results for all diagnostic categories or the prevalence of mental health diagnoses were severalfold higher among the TGNC group than in the matched cisgender group. For example, in the trans fe-male group, 40.3 percent of the subjects had depression, compared to 22.8 percent in the cisgender male group and 13.3 percent in the cisgender female group. For the trans male subjects, the prevalence of depression was 49.8 percent. The results sug-gested that TGNC youth require immediate evaluation and implementation of mul-tispecialty gender-affirming health care including a mental health specialist familiar with issues of gender in youth.[10]

Initial evaluations for children and adolescents with gender incongruence are usu-ally provided at multispecialty clinics located in academic medical centers. This care embodies the principles that transgender identities and diverse gender expression are not mental or psychiatric disorders. Instead, these variations are normal aspects of human diversity. Clinic staff understand that gender identity evolves as an inter-play of biology, development, socialization, and culture. And if a mental health issue is present in the patient, it most often stems from stigma and negative experiences, rather than being intrinsic to the child. An underlying principle is that adolescents who identify as transgender or gender diverse should have access to comprehensive gender-affirming and medically appropriate health care that is provided in a safe and inclusive clinical space. Treatment for children and adolescents with gender incon-gruence may be provided in academic medical centers as well as in the offices of pedi-atricians, family medicine providers, and adolescent medicine specialists.

Does gender-affirming care significantly improve the mental health symptoms of TGNC individuals? Researchers in Illinois, California, and Massachusetts studied the longitudinal course of psychosocial functioning in a cohort of transgender and non-binary youth for 2 years after initiation of gender-affirming hormone care. The group consisted of 315 adolescents ages 12 to 20 years with a mean age of 16 (SD 1.9 years), 60.3 percent transmasculine, in four different sites. They were studied at baseline and at 6, 12, 18, and 24 months after gender-affirming hormone initiation. At the visits, they completed scales for depression, anxiety, life satisfaction, and emotion battery. The results showed significant reductions in depression and anxiety and increases in overall well-being in those youth designated female at birth but not among those des-ignated male at birth. The investigators speculated that key estrogen-mediated body changes can take between 2 and 5 years to reach their maximum effect and a longer follow-up period would be needed to demonstrate improvements in anxiety, depres-sion, and life satisfaction in those subjects. Suicidal ideation in 11 individuals and death by suicide in 2 were the most common adverse events during the study.[11] In a study from Massachusetts, researchers performed a cross-sectional survey of 20,619 transgender adults who reported a history of pubertal suppression during adoles-cence. The researchers examined associations between access to pubertal suppression and adult suicidality. They determined an inverse association between pubertal sup-pression treatment during adolescence and lifetime suicidal ideation in transgender adults. These results suggested that pubertal suppression is associated with favorable mental health outcomes during adulthood.[12]

Does gender incongruence improve after treatment? Researchers from the Netherlands and Washington State evaluated 55 transgender young adult males and 22 transgender young adult females who had undergone puberty suppression during adolescence. They were assessed before the start of puberty suppression (mean age of

13.6 years), when hormones were introduced (mean age of 16.7 years), and 1 year or more after gender-affirming surgery (mean age of 20.7 years). The measures included gender incongruence, psychological functioning, and objective and subjective well-being. The findings were important and consequential for the transgender community and their medical providers since by the end of treatment, gender incongruence had resolved, and the well-being of the subjects was comparable or even better than peers from the general population. The researchers determined that improvements in psychological functioning were positively correlated with postsurgical subjective well-being. The treatment offered adolescents and young adults with gender incongruence who sought gender assignment from early puberty the opportunity to develop into well-functioning young adults.[13]

A decision to offer gender-affirming hormone therapy should follow an evaluation performed ideally by a multidisciplinary team consisting of medical and mental health clinicians, although recent standard of care guidelines from the World Professional Association for Transgender Health (2022) allow a medical provider to initiate the biopsychosocial evaluation.[14] There are many medical interventions that may be offered to adolescents who identify as TGD. Some do not need any medical or surgical treatments and will do well with support groups for themselves and their families. Management of a transgender adolescent may include the suppression of puberty at its onset. Blocking of gonadotropin-releasing hormones prevents the development of secondary sex characteristics, such as breasts, beards, and menses, and allows time for the teen and family to explore gender identity and define treatment goals. Pubertal suppression may relieve some mental health symptoms including anxiety, and pharmacologic affirmation may follow, which can start as early as age 13 years. That involves the administration of hormones that allow for the puberty that matches the individual's gender identity. The adolescent will then develop the secondary sexual characteristics of their gender identity. Generally, surgeons wait until adolescents are 18 years old to conduct affirmation surgery, which includes procedures to match their physical appearance with their gender identity. This may be top surgery to remove the breasts, augmentation surgery to enlarge the breasts, or bottom surgery to alter the genitalia or even the removal of internal organs, such as the ovaries and/or uterus.[15]

Epidemiology

The Williams Institute at the UCLA School of Law used data from the Centers for Disease Control and Prevention Behavior Risk Factor Surveillance System and the Youth Risk Behavior Survey beginning in 2017 to estimate the number of adolescents ages 13 to 17 years who identified as transgender. In the United States, 1.4 percent of this group of adolescents identified as transgender. In the West, 1.62 percent of adolescents identified as transgender; in the Midwest, 1.24 percent; in the South, 1.25 percent; and in the Northeast, 1.82 percent. New York had the highest percentage of transgender adolescents at 3.0 percent; it was followed by 2.62 percent in New Mexico. New Jersey had the least reported adolescents who identified as transgender at 0.67 percent, followed by Kentucky and West Virginia at 0.68 percent.[16]

More granular transgender data may be difficult to determine. While it is thought that there are more transgender males than transgender females, there are no data on those who either identify no specific gender or identify as having both genders.

Biopsychosocial Issues, Transgender Adolescents, and Gender Incongruence

Biological Issues

Sleep

In cisgender adolescents, poor sleep is associated with worsening mood and anxiety. After a week of experimentally restricted sleep of 6.5 hours in bed per night instead of 10 hours in bed per night, cisgender adolescents had higher levels of irritability, emotional problems, and anxiety symptoms. Researchers in Colorado studied transgender male adolescents to determine if they had poorer measured sleep and higher levels of symptoms of insomnia associated with more depression and anxiety and poorer health-related quality of life (HRQOL). The researchers recruited 10 transgender adolescent males between the ages of 13 and 16 years, with a mean age of 15.4 years; the teens had not yet begun taking testosterone therapy. Measures included actigraphy to quantify sleep, chronotype or the preferred times for sleeping (morning type, evening type, or intermediate type), insomnia symptoms, mood symptoms, and HRQOL. The researchers learned that the morning-type chronotype (early to bed, early to rise) was linked to a better HRQOL; the adolescents who were evening types had poorer HRQOL. Moreover, self-reported insomnia symptoms were correlated with more anxiety and depression and poorer HRQOL. The researchers commented that their findings were consistent with those of cisgender adolescents and transgender adults. It would be interesting if future research determined if hormonal treatment improved sleep quality and HRQOL and lessened the symptoms of anxiety and depression.[17]

Stress

While adolescents experience stress from factors such as academics, college applications, future training, and employment concerns, transgender adolescents are faced with a unique set of additional stressors. They must deal with the overt stress associated with harassment or victimization, as well as subtle forms of discrimination and prejudice, which may impact health outcomes. In addition, internalized transphobia is felt to be another stressor. Not every trans youth has gender dysphoria, especially if family and community affirm them. However, according to Russell Tommey of the University of Arizona, transgender adolescents face three additional stressors: interpersonal gender dysphoria, intrapersonal gender dysphoria, and limited affirmative health care services. Interpersonal gender dysphoria may occur when others refuse to let the transgender teen use their chosen name or pronouns or permit access to bathrooms that respond to their gender identity. Intrapersonal gender dysphoria is the emotional distress caused by the incongruence between a transgender adolescent's gender identity and their physical anatomy. Transgender teens often have a limited availability of affirmative health care services. When they are able to use such affirmative health care services, health disparities such as mental health outcomes and suicidality are diminished.[18]

Psychological Issues, Transgender Adolescents, and Gender Incongruence

Researchers at the University of Minnesota identified health disparities in transgender adolescents by examining school-based 2016 survey data provided by 9th and 11th grade students. The survey instrument identified numerous demographic and personal characteristics of the students, including risk behaviors and experiences and protective factors for such risk behaviors, in 2168 transgender and 78,761 cisgender adolescents. When compared to the cisgender adolescents, the transgender teens had high-risk behaviors ($p < .001$) in four domains: substance use, sexual behaviors, emotional distress (depression and suicidality), and bullying victimization. Protective factors were lower for transgender adolescents than their cisgender peers ($p < .001$) for internal assets (resilience), family connectedness, student-teacher relationships, and feeling safe in the community. This study provided the first large-scale population-based evidence of substantial health disparities for transgender youth.[19]

Since there are mental health disparities for transgender youth, would affirming care help to reduce these disparities? The military has records of all inpatient and outpatient care and outpatient prescriptions provided to military dependents domestically and abroad. Using electronic medical records, researchers from multiple military locations in the United States performed a retrospective cohort study on the use of mental health services among TGD military dependents between October 2010 and September 2018. They compared the use of psychotropic medications in these youth and their cisgender siblings. They theorized that the TGD youth would have greater mental health needs, and pharmaceutical interventions would be correlated with decreased treatment requirements. At the time of first contact, all of the TGB youth were under the age of 18 years. There were 3754 TGD youth and 6603 cisgender siblings; they were tracked for 8.5 years. The researchers learned that each year the median number of visits of the TGD youth was 18.7; that was in contrast to the 9.5 median number of visits of the cisgender siblings ($p < .001$). During the study period, puberty suppression or gender-affirming hormones were administered to 5.6 percent of the TGD youth, and the majority of this treatment group also received a psychotropic medication. Over 89 percent of the TGD youth had a mental health diagnosis, compared to 50 percent of the cisgender siblings with disparities in diagnoses. For example, 18 percent of the TGD youth had a suicidality diagnosis, compared to 2.5 percent of the cisgender siblings. And TGD youth had a considerably greater use of psychotropic medications. This study supports the need for continued mental health services for TGD youth undergoing affirming treatment. This is an especially important finding as some states may limit gender-affirming care for adolescents. In addition, these results demonstrated that mental health care should be readily available to the cisgender siblings who also significantly utilized these services.[20]

Another study found fewer psychiatric comorbidities in adolescents with gender dysphoria. To determine *Diagnostic and Statistical Manual of Mental Disorders,* fourth edition psychiatric comorbidities, researchers in the Netherlands studied adolescents with gender dysphoria. The cohort consisted of 105 adolescents between the ages of 12 and 17 with gender dysphoria who were patients at the Amsterdam Gender Identity Clinic. The parents of the teens were administered the Diagnostic Interview Schedule for Children. Measures included intelligence (Wechsler Intelligence Scale for Children or the Wechsler Adults Intelligence Scale), behavioral problems, living arrangements, and education level of parents; gender dysphoria diagnosis; and psychiatric comorbidities. The researchers found that 67.6 percent of the adolescents with gender dysphoria had no current psychiatric disorder. Anxiety disorders occurred in 21 percent, mood disorders in 12.4 percent, and disruptive disorders in 11.4 percent. Gender dysphoric youth born as natal males more often had two or more comorbid diagnoses than those born as natal females. These results differed from the military study with respect to concurrent psychiatric comorbidities in gender dysphoric youth. However, this cohort was considerably smaller, and the study was cross-sectional in design, not longitudinal.[21]

There also appears to be heightened rates of disordered eating and eating disorders in TGD adolescents. This may be due to the minority stress hypothesis resulting from transgender adolescents being part of a marginalized community, higher rates of discrimination, and harassment. Gender-affirming care is critically important to support those adolescents with an eating disorder. This care should also be trauma informed.[22]

Social Issues and Transgender/Gender Incongruence

Social Media

For most people, adolescence is a time for development of identity, self-concept, and personality, but for many in the transgender community, this development may come later. As part of his graduate thesis, a researcher conducted five interviews with adult trans individuals, using social media to explore their identity development. The subjects explained that social support was a key element in this development, and social media had provided them access to social support. However, social media use also had negative effects on identity formation and self-image.[23]

Noting that social stigma, shame, and family pressure may delay the coming-out process for transgender teens, researchers from North Carolina and California examined how media influenced the development of the transgendered individual's identity. Using a semistructured format, the lead researcher interviewed 41 people who were transgender. From these interviews, the researchers learned that people who were transgender obtained information about gender and sexuality from traditional media and emerging media technologies. This included posting photos in online forums and reviewing the comments, using the internet to understand transgender sexuality, and creating a sense of community in online transgender sites. The internet facilitated identity-related conversations with relational partners. The researchers concluded that the internet was the primary medium cited by the study participants for understanding sex and transition options.[24]

While transgender adolescents are at a higher risk for mental health disparities including anxiety, depression, and suicidality than their cisgender peers, social media can be especially helpful to support them. Researchers from the University of Michigan, Oberlin College, and Oakland University investigated how transgender youth use social media for social support. During semistructured interviews with 25 subjects between the ages of 15 and 18 years who attended a pediatric gender services clinic, the researchers learned that 11 identified as transgender female, 13 as transgender male, and 1 as nonbinary. The researchers determined that social media was a place where transgender teens could interact with other transgendered individuals, and social media was useful for dealing with offline concerns. They felt validated by transgender-related content and informational support. To these adolescents, the experience was generally positive with notable negative experiences, such as harassment expressed openly through transphobia and hurtful comments. The researchers noted that transgender youth should be counseled to be cautious in their use of social media while exploring online support.[25]

Cyberbullying/Bullying

As noted in Chapter 9, sexual minority adolescents are bullied 1.5 to 2 times more than those in the sexual majority. There also appear to be differences between gender minority and cisgender youth. Researchers in Finland evaluated bullying among gender minority and cisgender adolescents in middle and high school. The researchers were interested in the prevalence of both perpetrator and victim bullying among transgender adolescents. They used data from the School Health Promotion study, a school-based cross-sectional anonymous survey completed by students throughout Finland. The measures included sexual and gender identity, questions on bullying, and internalizing and externalizing symptoms. The study included 139,829 adolescents in middle and high school, 51.3 percent female; the mean age for the middle school students was 14.8 years and for the high school students was 17.9 years. In middle school, 0.7 percent reported that they were transgender, and 3.6 percent said they were nonbinary. For high school students, the results for these identities were 0.5 percent and 3.0 percent, respectively. The researchers learned that transgender youth in Finland were more likely than cisgender adolescents to be victims or perpetrators of bullying. Among transgender youth, involvement in bullying was more often seen in nonbinary youth than in those identifying with the opposite gender. Transgender identities were more often associated with being a perpetrator rather than a victim of bullying. The researchers suggested that this aggressive behavior could result from being victimized or having been a witness to the victimization of other gender or sexual minorities. And being a target of bullying or being a perpetrator was more common in the younger adolescent sample than in the older group. The researchers concluded that transgender youth were at high risk for bullying, especially among nonbinary youth.[26]

Racism/Discrimination

Transgender adolescents are often presented with problems such as access to bathrooms, especially in schools and locker rooms. Gender-neutral bathrooms allow these teens to use the facilities consistent with their gender identity; however, not all schools offer these gender-affirming facilities. Researchers at the Trevor Project in West Hollywood, California, recruited 7370 transgender or nonbinary youth through targeted ads on social media; the subjects were between the ages of 13 and 24 years,

44 percent were transgender, and 82.2 percent were assigned female at birth. Measures included bathroom discrimination, gender identity–based discrimination, depressive mood, suicidality, and sociodemographic data. The researchers learned that transgender or nonbinary youth who reported bathroom discrimination had higher rates of depressive mood and suicidality, including ideation and attempts during the past year. Bathroom discrimination rates were higher among those who identified as transgender than those who identified as nonbinary. The researchers recommended offering gender-neutral bathrooms and providing private places to change in locker rooms. Such changes could potentially save lives.[27]

Researchers from New York City examined the interplay of racism and transphobia among transgender and nonbinary youth. They utilized data from a national sample of LGBTQ students who were enrolled in secondary school during the 2018–2019 academic year. The sample size was 6795, with 69 percent identifying as transgender. The majority was White (71 percent). Other races studied included Latinx, multiracial, Asian American/Pacific Islander, Black/African American, Middle Eastern/North African, and Native American. The results indicated that race-based harassment was similar for students of all color groups; it was the lowest for White transgender and nonbinary students. Among transgender and nonbinary students of color, each form of harassment (race/ethnicity, gender) was associated with greater depression and lower self-esteem. The researchers concluded that many transgender and nonbinary students of color experienced both racist and transphobic harassment. Experiencing both forms of harassment was associated with poorer mental health outcomes than experiencing one.[28]

Mortality

While it has been repeatedly shown that transgender youth are at increased risk for suicide, are some transgender subgroups at higher risk than others? Researchers in Arizona and Minnesota studied differences in suicide attempts among six adolescent gender identity groups. The researchers used data from the Profiles of Student Life: Attitudes and Behaviors survey for adolescents ages 11 to 19 years; it included responses from 120,671 teens. Gender identities were determined with the question "Which of the following best describes you?" The response options were female, male, transgender male, transgender female, transgender—do not identify as exclusively male or female, and not sure. The measures included self-reported suicidal behavior, gender identity, and demographic information. The results showed that between 30 and 51 percent of transgender adolescents engaged in lifetime suicidal behavior.

But there were variations in suicide behavior among this population. Transgender male adolescents and nonbinary adolescents had the highest rates of suicidal behavior. Approximately 51 percent of transgender male and 42 percent of nonbinary transgender adolescents attempted suicide. Cisgender female adolescents had a rate of about 18 percent, and cisgender males had a rate of 10 percent. These findings underscore the need to enhance suicide prevention efforts with transgender male adolescents and nonbinary transgender adolescents.[29]

Researchers from Pennsylvania also found suicidal variations between transgender and cisgender adolescents. Using a cross-sectional online survey, the researchers recruited 2020 cisgender and transgender adolescents from Facebook and Instagram;

of these, 1148 identified as transgender. The measures included gender identity and lifetime suicidal ideation or attempts. The researchers found that transgender adolescents had a higher risk of suicidality than cisgender youth. Thus, the adjusted odds ratio for suicidal ideation was 2.04 for cisgender female, 5.64 for transgender male, and 6.30 for transgender female. Transgender male and nonbinary adolescents assigned female at birth had the highest risk for suicidal ideation and attempts, but transgender females also had a high risk of suicidality. These findings emphasize the fact that all transgender groups are at risk and should be provided suicide prevention efforts and other mental health services.[30]

Since hormonal treatment is so frequently included in health care for transgender individuals, do these medications increase the risk of mortality or an earlier than anticipated death from cancer or cardiovascular disease? Researchers in Amsterdam designed a retrospective cohort study of all the adult transgender patients who visited the gender identity clinic of the Amsterdam University Medical Center and started hormone treatment between 1972 and 2018. Patients were excluded if they used puberty blockers or were administered hormones before the age of 17 years. Most transgender women were treated with antiandrogens and estrogens, and some had an orchiectomy, a surgical procedure to remove one or both testicles. Transgender men took a form of testosterone and, if they had persistent menses, progesterone. Transgender women had high risks of death from cardiovascular disease, HIV-related disease, lung cancer, and suicide. For transgender men, the increased mortality compared to the general public was mainly attributed to nonnatural causes of death such as suicide. It should be noted that for transgender men and women, most of the specific causes of death were not related to hormone use. An important finding from this study is that when compared to those from the general population, there was about a twofold increase in mortality risk in transgender men and women. The risk was steady over the five examined decades. The researchers concluded that it was important to monitor, optimize treatment for medical morbidities for, and improve lifestyle factors for people who are transgender. For adolescents and their families who are considering hormonal treatment, there appeared to be no lifelong risks from the hormones administered.[31]

A research team from the same clinic in Amsterdam quantified the overall death rate from suicide in adult transgender patients. They performed a retrospective chart review of clinic patients between 1972 and 2017. The cohort consisted of 8263 adults, adolescents, and children who ranged in age from 4 to 81 years when they first visited the clinic. The researcher obtained information on causes of death from multiple sources, including the National Civil Record Registry in the Netherlands. In this study, the adolescents received puberty blockers followed by estrogen or testosterone hormonal therapy. The researchers learned that 41 of the 5107 (0.0080 percent) of the trans women and 8 of the 3156 (0.0025 percent) trans men died by suicide. The mean number of suicides in the years 2013 to 2017 was three to four times higher in transgender individuals than in the Dutch population. Most suicide deaths occurred in those individuals who were still in the active phase of treatment including diagnosis, hormonal, or surgical treatments. The researchers remarked that the societal position of transgender individuals is generally less favorable compared to lesbian, gay, bisexual, and cisgender individuals, and this could be a factor in the increased suicide rate. The study confirmed suicide risk during every stage of transitioning and the need for readily available mental health services for transgender individuals. Mental health clinicians should be cognizant of these risks and attempt to create a safe environment where transgender individuals are able to openly discuss their feelings.[32]

Violence

Transgender adolescents have a high risk of being victims of violence. In 2017, the Centers for Disease Control and Prevention conducted the Youth Risk Behavior Survey, which contained questions on gender identity and victimization. The cohort consisted of 10 states and 9 large urban school districts with 131,901 high school student respondents. Overall, 1.8 percent of the students identified as transgender. Table 13.1 documents the responses of the transgender and cisgender students to questions on victimization. The various responses are noted for each reviewed topic.

Similarly, is transgender sexual victimization also a problem among college students, and if it is, when is this victimization more likely to occur? Researchers in Canada conducted surveys at six Quebec universities on students between the ages of 18 and 25 years. The surveys consisted of online questionnaires with questions about sexual violence and when it was more likely to occur. Measures included sexual violence, context of sexual violence, and sexual and gender minority status. Seventy-two of the 4262 respondents identified as transgender or nonbinary. The researchers determined that transgender and nonbinary college students reported higher levels of sexual violence than their cisgender peers. And compared to cisgender men or women, this violence was more likely to occur during athletic events, with an odds ratio of 6.34. The researchers commented that increased sexual victimization prevention efforts should be targeted at the transgender and nonbinary student population.[33] In a review from Seattle Children's Hospital, the author evaluated the literature on the intersection of LGBTQ youth and commercial sexual exploitation of children

Table 13.1 Youth Risk Behavior Survey Victimization Responses

Violence Victimization	Cisgender Males (%)	Cisgender Females (%)	Transgender Students (%)
Felt unsafe at or traveling to and from school	4.6	7.1	26.9
Threatened or injured with a weapon at school	6.4	4.1	23.8
Ever forced to have sexual intercourse	4.2	10.5	23.8
Experienced sexual dating violence	3.5	12.0	22.9
Experienced physical dating violence	5.8	8.7	26.4
Bullied at school	14.7	20.7	34.6
Electronically bullied	10.2	19.3	29.5

From Johns MM, Lowry R, Andrzejewski J, et al. Transgender identity and experiences of violence victimization, substance use, suicide risk, and sexual risk behaviors among high school students - 19 states and large urban school districts, 2017. *MMWR Morb Mortal Wkly Rep.* 2019;68(3):67–71.

(CSEC). The author concluded that transgender/gender diverse youth are disproportionately affected by CSEC, with risk factors including homelessness, polyvictim-
ization based on sexual and gender identities, and barriers to utilizing shelters and
obtaining gainful employment.[34]

There is also evidence that Black, Indigenous, and People of Color (BIPOC) transgender and/or nonbinary youth are at risk for violence. A group of researchers from
Canada studied violence and health outcomes for BIPOC compared to their White
transgender and nonbinary peers utilizing a national online survey. The study group
of transgender and nonbinary youth numbered 1519, and BIPOC youth made up
25.7 percent of the sample. The transgender and nonbinary BIPOC group reported
a significantly higher prevalence of suicide attempts and violence victimization compared to White youth. They also reported a significant difference in being threatened
or injured with a weapon or being exposed to something bad said about their race
compared to the individuals in the White sample.[35]

Treatment

As noted in the introduction, gender-affirming care for adolescents is usually performed in a multidisciplinary clinic in an academic medical center. In this model of
care, pediatric providers develop a nonjudgmental partnership with the adolescent
and their family and communicate several messages. The team conveys to the patient
and family that transgender identities and diverse gender expressions are not a mental
disorder, and gender identity variations are normal aspects of human diversity.
Furthermore, gender identity may evolve as a combination and interplay of biology,
culture, development, and socialization. In addition, if the patient does have a mental
health issue, it usually arises from stigma and negative experiences rather than being
intrinsic to the adolescent. The team may consist of medical disciplines including primary care, adolescent medicine, endocrinology, and gynecology as well as mental
health providers. These clinicians work to destigmatize gender variance, promote the
adolescent's self-worth, facilitate access to care, educate families, and advocate for safe
community spaces where the patients are free to develop and explore their gender.[36]

The medical management for transgender youth is outlined by the Endocrinology
Society practice guidelines or, as noted previously, newer guidelines formulated by
the World Professional Association for Transgender Care.[37,38] Individuals may have
different goals for treatment. For example, a transgender female may not want breast
development, so estrogen may be withheld. The treatment offered is matched to the
goals of the patient. In some individuals, management entails pausing of puberty,
followed by gender-affirming hormone therapy. If surgery is desired, then that could
include mastectomy or breast augmentation, gonadectomy, genital surgery, facial surgery, and possibly cosmetic procedures.

In some children and adolescents, gender identity is static, while in others it is a
journey. Do children who have undergone social transition then express regret
and decide to retransition to another gender identity? Researchers in New Jersey,
Washington State, and Canada studied 317 transgender children with a mean age of
8.1 years at the start of the longitudinal study. They found that at an average of 5 years

after their initial social transition, 7.3 percent of the adolescents had retransitioned at least once. The researchers concluded that retransitions are infrequent, and more commonly, transgender youth who socially transitioned at early ages continued to identify in the same way. They also observed that few youth who had begun medical interventions retransitioned to live as a cisgender individual.[39]

Researchers in the Netherlands utilized data from the Amsterdam Cohort of Gender Dysphoria to determine if adolescents who started gender-affirming medical treatment continued to do so during young adulthood. The study included 720 individuals; 31 percent were assigned male at birth and 69 percent were assigned female at birth. The mean age at the start of puberty suppression was 14.1 years for those assigned male at birth and 16.0 years for those assigned female at birth. The researchers found that 704 (98 percent) of the individuals who started gender-affirming medical treatment during adolescence continued to use gender-affirming hormones at follow-up during young adulthood.[40]

For certain individuals, there are some concerns about puberty blockers. Transgender individuals are at an increased risk for eating disorders since the effect of puberty blockers may be compounded if transgender youth are restricting their caloric intake due to image issues from an eating disorder. Researchers in Seattle studied the frequency of disordered eating in transgender and nonbinary adolescents who had established care in a gender-affirming medical clinic. The sample included 91 participants with a mean age of 15.2 years, with 61 percent transgender male, 32 percent transgender female, and 7 percent nonbinary or gender fluid. The data indicated that there were no significant changes in disordered eating in the study population after they initiated gender-affirming medical care.[41] In addition, with gender affirmation, eating disorders may improve.[42]

Furthermore, there are additional concerns about gonadotropin-releasing hormone agonists (puberty suppressors/blockers) as these medications may affect the acquisition of bone mineral density (BMD), especially in those individuals recorded as female at birth. Adolescence is the time for peak bone accrual, and inadequate bone density could lead to osteoporosis early in life and as a result subject the individual to an increased risk for fractures. To further evaluate the BMD issues, researchers in the Netherlands assessed BMD after long-term gender-affirming hormone treatment in transgender adults who used puberty suppression during adolescence. In this cohort study of 75 adults, 25 of whom were assigned as male at birth and 50 of whom were assigned as female, the BMD caught up with the pretreatment levels except for scores in the lumbar spine in participants assigned male at birth. This was thought to be due to low estradiol concentrations.[43]

Finally, there are concerns that adolescents taking puberty blockers may experience neurodevelopmental changes. Some researchers believe that pubertal hormones are needed for proper neurological development. These areas are currently being studied.

Medical treatment for transgender adults may help to transition gender dysphoria to gender euphoria. Gender euphoria is a term used by some that relates joy or satisfaction when an individual's gendered experience is aligned with their gender identity in contrast to the gender that was assigned to them at birth. Researchers in Minnesota studied 281 transgender female adults who had hair removal procedures. Utilizing an online survey, the team determined that satisfaction with the individual's current state of hair removal was negatively correlated with body image dysphoria, depressive symptoms, anxiety symptoms, and negative affect. It was positively correlated with a positive affect. This study contributes to the body of literature that gender-affirmative medical interventions can be a legitimate and effective treatment for gender dysphoria.[44]

Prevention

As previously noted, gender identity is not an individual's choice. Transphobia, which encompasses negative attitudes, ideations, or actions as well as prejudice, anger, and violence toward transgender individuals, is an area where preventive efforts would be helpful.

As a result, in part, of discrimination from cisgender individuals, transgender and nonbinary youth have an increased risk for mental health disorders, including anxiety, depression, and suicidality. Further, their risk for victimization secondary to violence is higher than cisgender people. Discrimination against transgender youth occurs during interactions among individuals, systems, and institutions. For example, limiting access to needed health care is an institutional obstacle to transgender care. In Texas, legislation and legal directives have been promulgated to stop the provision of medical care to transgender adolescents under the age of 18 years. This includes sex-change procedures, administration of treatments for gender dysphoria, and puberty blockers. The attorney general of Texas in 2022 issued an opinion that certain types of treatment provided to transgender children may constitute child abuse. Subsequently, the governor of Texas directed the state's Department of Family and Protective Services to investigate as child abuse any gender-affirming surgical procedures and administration of puberty blockers or hormones for gender dysphoria delivered to minors.[45] Governments have no role in legislating how medical care is delivered to the transgender population. These actions are potentially life threatening to some individuals.

There are other states that have limited transgender access to care. In Alabama, Arizona, Arkansas, and the legislatures have taken action to limit gender-affirming care. Prevention efforts include increased advocacy for the rights of transgender adolescents, encouraging transgender individuals to be more visible and to seek positions of power, and increasing interactions between cisgender and transgender people. Knowing individuals who are transgender has a positive influence on attitudes and beliefs toward the transgender population.[46]

Access to gender-affirming care is a global issue. Researchers from Australia and the Netherlands performed a systematic review on transgender youth accessing health care services. The review included 91 papers from 17 countries involving 884 transgender and nonbinary subjects 24 years old or younger. The subjects noted the following themes:

In health care systems, individuals reported discrimination and pervasive stigma. They experienced transphobia, felt they were stripped of personal dignity, and were invalidated by misgendering.

They felt vulnerable and uncertain in decision-making and the burden of needing to educate clinicians. There was a lack of credible information and vagueness about sexual and reproductive health. Strict gatekeeping was dehumanizing.

To overcome systematic barriers to transition, they had to take risks. In addition, they struggled to afford treatment while being restricted by limited transgender-specific services. Finally, the individuals reported that they had to deal with insurmountable legal and policy barriers.

They internalized intense fears for consequences from their actions, including powerlessness about bodily changes due to hormone therapy, apprehension about the transition process, and feeling terrified about the ramifications of HIV.

They faced prejudice in their efforts to seek help and felt marginalized by society. They censored themselves to avoid familial rejection and inertia because of gender dysphoria.

The individuals reported that they were strengthened by gender identity and finding allies in partnering with clinicians; reassured by integrated care, community outreach, and navigating online information; and bolstered by interpersonal supports and the transgender community.

The researchers concluded that barriers to health care for transgender and nonbinary youth were largely a result of legal, economic, and social deprivations. Specific strategies needed to be employed to improve access for gender-affirming care, provide support during the transition process, and manage comorbidities and social-legal stressors. Providing gender-affirming care included the use by all staff of appropriate pronouns, utilizing gender-neutral medical terminology, understanding and acknowledging gender incongruence during examinations, and avoiding as much as possible unnecessary examinations or discussion of incongruent body parts. These strategies are likely to contribute toward improved therapeutic options and quality of life for this population.[47]

A few years ago, the U.S. Congress passed the National Suicide Hotline Designation Act of 2020, which also provided specialized services for LGBTQ youth. On July 16, 2022, the 988 telephone number was activated. Americans experiencing a mental health crisis or who are at risk for suicide may call that number and receive help.

Members of the health care sector may help to improve care for sexual and gender minority youth (SGMY) by advocating for improved SGMY data from electronic medical records to inform policy discussions, programming, and research funding. They should work to ensure that health professionals support the specific needs of SGMY patients. Such actions may include instituting training programs in medical schools and residencies on SGMY health care. Finally, physicians may advocate against harmful legislation impacting SGMY and help to promote protective policies, programs, and laws concerning care delivery to SGMY.[48]

Conclusion

One to 2 percent of adolescents report that they are transgender or nonbinary. These teens are at high risk for mental health issues, including anxiety, depression, and suicidality, as well as victimization from violence. Gender-affirming health care, such as the use of puberty blockers, gender-affirming hormones, and surgical procedures, appears to improve transgender patient outcomes. Still, there are noteworthy barriers, including systematic discrimination, prejudice, and misgendering, which impact the health care of these youth. If these barriers are removed through training and prevention programming, transgender and nonbinary adolescents may have a greatly improved quality of life and healthier outcomes.

References

1   Bazelon E. The battle over gender therapy. *New York Times Magazine*. June 19, 2022; 29–57.
2   Gordon CM. Caught in the middle: The care of transgender youth in Texas. *Pediatrics*. 2022;149(6):e2022057475.
3   Shumer DE, Nokoff NJ, Spack NP. Advances in the care of transgender children and adolescents. *Adv Pediatr*. 2016;63:79–102.
4   Conrad LA, Corathers SD, Trotman G. Caring for transgender and gender-nonconforming youth. *Curr Pediatr Rep*. 2018;6:139–146.
5   Hoekzema E, Schagen SE, Kreukels BP, et al. Regional volumes and spatial volumetric distribution of gray matter in the gender dysphoric brain. *Psychoneuroendocrinology*. 2015;55:59–71.
6   Frey-Vogel A. Affirming healthcare for transgender and gender diverse youth. Pediatric Grand Rounds, Massachusetts General Hospital, Boston, MA; May 23, 2022.
7   James SE, Herman J, Rankin S, Keisling M, Mottel L, Anafi M. *The Report of the 2015 U.S, Transgender Survey*. National Center for Transgender Equality; 2016.
8   Turban JL, van Schalkwyk GI. "Gender Dysphoria" and Autism Spectrum Disorder: is the link real? *J Am Acad Child Adolesc Psychiatry*. 2018;57:8–9.e2.
9   Ehrensaft D. Double helix rainbow kids. *J Autism Dev Disord*. 2018;48(12):4079–4081.
10 Becerra-Culqui TA, Liu Y, Nash R, et al. Mental health of transgender and gender nonconforming youth compared with their peers. *Pediatrics*. 2018;141(5):e20173845.
11 Chen D, Berona J, Chan YM, et al. Psychosocial functioning in transgender youth after 2 years of hormones. *N Engl J Med*. 2023;388:240–250.
12 Turban JL, King D, Carswell JM, Keuroghlian AS. Pubertal suppression for transgender youth and risk of suicidal ideation. *Pediatrics*. 2020;145:e20191725.
13 de Vries AL, McGuire JK, Steensma TD, Wagenaar EC, Doreleijers TA, Cohen-Kettenis PT. Young adult psychological outcome after puberty suppression and gender reassignment. *Pediatrics*. 2014;134(4):696–704.
14 Coleman E, Radix AE, Bouman WP, et al. Standards of care for the health of transgender and gender diverse people, Version 8. *Int J Transgend Health*. 2022;23(Suppl 1):S1–S259.
15 Rafferty J; Committee on Psychosocial Aspects of Child and Family Health; Committee on Adolescence; Section on Lesbian, Gay, Bisexual, and Transgender Health and Wellness. Ensuring comprehensive care and support for transgender and gender-diverse children and adolescents. *Pediatrics*. 2018;142(4):e20182162. Erratum in: *Pediatrics*. 2023 Oct 1;152(4).
16 Herman JL, Flores AR, O'Neill KK. *How Many Adults and Youth Identify as Transgender in the United States?* Williams Institute, UCLA School of Law; 2022.
17 Bowen AE, Staggs S, Kaar J, Nokoff N, Simon SL. Short sleep, insomnia symptoms, and evening chronotype are correlated with poorer mood and quality of life in adolescent transgender males. *Sleep Health*. 2021;7:445–450.

18 Tommey RB. Advancing research on minority stress and resilience in trans children and adolescents in the 21st century. *Child Dev Perspect.* 2021;15:95–102.

19 Eisenberg ME, Gower AL, McMorris BJ, Rider GN, Shea G, Coleman E. Risk and protective factors in the lives of transgender/gender nonconforming adolescents. *J Adolesc Health.* 2017;61(4):521–526.

20 Hisle-Gorman E, Schvey NA, Adirim TA, et al. Mental healthcare utilization of transgender youth before and after affirming treatment. *J Sex Med.* 2021;18:1444–1454.

21 de Vries AL, Doreleijers TA, Steensma TD, Cohen-Kettenis PT. Psychiatric comorbidity in gender dysphoric adolescents. *J Child Psychol Psychiatry.* 2011;52(11):1195–1202.

22 Riddle M, Silverstein S, Wassenaar E. The care of transgender and gender diverse adolescents with eating disorders. *Curr Pediatr Rep.* 2023;11:148–156.

23 Doss B. Exploring the role of social media in the identity development of trans individuals. Missouri State University Graduate Thesis; 2018.

24 Kosenko K, Bond B, Hurley R. An exploration into the uses and gratification of media for transgender individuals. *Psychol Pop Media Cult.* 2018;7:274–288.

25 Selkie E, Adkins V, Masters E, Bajpai A, Shumer D. Transgender adolescents' uses of social media for social support. *J Adolesc Health.* 2020;66:275–280.

26 Heino E, Ellonen N, Kaltiala R. Transgender identity is associated with bullying involvement among Finnish adolescents. *Front Psychol.* 2021;11:612424.

27 Price-Feeney M, Green AE, Dorison SH. Impact of bathroom discrimination on mental health among transgender and nonbinary youth. *J Adolesc Health.* 2021;68:1142–1147.

28 Zongrone AD, Truong NL, Carl CM. Transgender and nonbinary youths' experiences with gender-based and race-based school harassment. *Teach Coll Rec.* 2022;124:121–144.

29 Toomey RB, Syvertsen AK, Shramko M. Transgender adolescent suicide behavior. *Pediatrics.* 2018;142:e20174218.

30 Thoma BC, Salk RH, Choukas-Bradley S, Goldstein TR, Levine MD, Marshal MP. Suicidality disparities between transgender and cisgender adolescents. *Pediatrics.* 2019;144(5):e20191183.

31 de Blok CJ, Wiepjes CM, van Velzen DM, et al. Mortality trends over five decades in adult transgender people receiving hormone treatment: a report from the Amsterdam cohort of gender dysphoria. *Lancet Diabetes Endocrinol.* 2021;9:663–670.

32 Wiepjes CM, den Heijer M, Bremmer MA, et al. Trends in suicide death risk in transgender people: results from the Amsterdam Cohort of Gender Dysphoria study (1972–2017). *Acta Psychiatr Scand.* 2020;141:486–491.

33 Martin-Storey A, Paquette G, Bergeron M, et al. Sexual violence on campus: differences across gender and sexual minority status. *J Adolesc Health.* 2018;62:701–707.

34 Georges E. Review of the literature on the intersection of LGBTQ youth and csec: more than a monolith. *Curr Pediatr Rep.* 2023;11:105–115.

35 Chan A, Pullen Sansfaçon A, Saewyc E. Experiences of discrimination or violence and health outcomes among Black, Indigenous and People of Colour trans and/or nonbinary youth. *J Adv Nurs.* 2023;79(5):2004–2013.

36 Rafferty J; Committee on Psychosocial Aspects of Child and Family Health; Committee on Adolescence; Section on Lesbian, Gay, Bisexual, and Transgender Health and Wellness. Ensuring comprehensive care and support for transgender and gender-diverse children and adolescents. *Pediatrics.* 2018;142(4):e20182162. Erratum in: *Pediatrics.* 2023 Oct 1;152(4).

37 Hembree WC, Cohen-Kettenis PT, Gooren L, et al. Endocrine treatment of gender-dysphoric/gender-incongruent persons: an Endocrine Society clinical practice guideline. *J Clin Endocrinol Metab.* 2017;102:3869–3903. Erratum in: *J Clin Endocrinol Metab.* 2018;103:699. Erratum in: *J Clin Endocrinol Metab.* 2018;103:2758–2759.

38 Coleman E, Radix AE, Bouman WP, et al. Standards of care for the health of transgender and gender diverse people, Version 8. *Int J Transgend Health.* 2022;23(Suppl 1):S1–S259.

39 Olson KR, Durwood L, Horton R, Gallagher NM, Devor A. Gender identity 5 years after social transition. *Pediatrics.* 2022;150:e2021056082.

40 van der Loos MATC, Hannema SE, Klink DT, den Heijer M, Wiepjes CM. Continuation of gender-affirming hormones in transgender people starting puberty suppression in adolescence: a cohort study in the Netherlands. *Lancet Child Adolesc Health.* 2022;6:869–875.

41 Pham AH, Eadeh HM, Garrison MM, Ahrens KR. A longitudinal study on disordered eating in transgender and nonbinary adolescents. *Acad Pediatr.* 2023;23:1247–1251.

42 Riddle MC, Safer JD. Medical considerations in the care of transgender and gender diverse patients with eating disorders. *J Eat Disord.* 2022;10:178.

43 van der Loos MATC, Vlot MC, Klink DT, Hannema SE, den Heijer M, Wiepjes CM. Bone mineral density in transgender adolescents treated with puberty suppression and subsequent gender-affirming hormones. *JAMA Pediatr.* 2023;177:1332–1341.

44 Bradford NJ, Rider GN, Spencer KG. Hair removal and psychological well-being in transfeminine adults: associations with gender dysphoria and gender euphoria. *J Dermatolog Treat.* 2021;32:635–642.

45 Gordon CM. Caught in the middle: The care of transgender youth in Texas. *Pediatrics.* 2022;149(6):e2022057475.

46 Silva K, Nauman CM, Tebbe EA, Parent MC. Policy attitudes toward adolescents transitioning gender. *J Couns Psychol.* 2022;69:403–415.

47 Chong LSH, Kerklaan J, Clarke S, et al. Experiences and perspectives of transgender youths in accessing health care: a systematic review. *JAMA Pediatr.* 2021;175:1159–1173.

48 Liu M, Sandhu S, Keuroghlian AS. Achieving the triple aim for sexual and gender minorities. *N Engl J Med.* 2022;387:294–297.

14
Poverty

Introduction

Around 20 percent of American children live in poverty, a state of being extremely poor, and about 40 percent are poor or near poor. The federal poverty level for a family of four in 2023 was $30,000.[1] That means that millions of American children and adolescents live at the economic fringes of society. Why is that such an important public health problem? There is an association between a lack of economic resources and health disparities, especially when indicators of children's mental health are studied. Children who live in households with income levels less than 100 percent of the federal poverty level had the highest prevalence of attention-deficit/hyperactivity disorder, behavior or conduct problems, depression, and mental health services use.[2]

Poverty has a significant impact on the provision of medical care to adolescents, especially in lower-income countries. Some issues resulting from poverty include lack of medical insurance and proximal medical facilities, poor transportation systems, utilizing the emergency room for medical care, and lack of appropriate medical information.

It is possible that poverty induces material deprivation and toxic stressors that impact brain development, including the volume of the prefrontal cortex. Functionally, family material deprivation may affect an infant's cognitive stimulation at home, leading to diminished educational opportunities and a weakened language environment. Stress placed on parents from poverty may affect parental quality, behaviors, and capacities. These issues may then impact the developing infant brain, particularly in language- and reading-related areas, the hippocampus, amygdala, and prefrontal cortex. The neurocognitive outcomes resulting from the stress on the developing child may be apparent in reading/language abilities and executive functions, as the hippocampus supports learning and memory; the amygdala is involved in emotional learning, motivation, and processing of threats and emotions; and the prefrontal cortex supports higher-order planning, reasoning, and decision-making. When a child reaches adolescence, these changes may present as psychosocial issues.[3]

The Great Smoky Mountains Study of Youth was a longitudinal study of the mental health of children in rural North Carolina. The sample included Native American and non-Native American children. During the study, a casino opened on the Eastern Cherokee reservation, and profits from the casino were distributed every 6 months to adult members of the tribe regardless of their wealth or employment status.

In 2000, Native Americans there had a poverty rate in excess of 37 percent, with a real per capita income of $8000. Just prior to the onset of casino operations, there was a $10,000 difference in average household income between the Native American and non-Native American families in the study. Randall Akee from Tufts University in Massachusetts and his colleagues observed the permanent effects on children of a $4000 annual cash transfer from the casino earnings to the impoverished Native American households. There were improvements in adolescent outcomes in terms of educational attainment at ages 19 and 21 years and reduced criminal behavior at ages 16 and 17 years. This is in contrast to the non–Native American households that did not receive cash payments from the casino, where no such improvements were noted. While the researchers were unable to identify the exact cause of the improvements in the adolescents, they believed that after the additional household payments began, the parents developed an overall better relationship with their children. Though the extra money represented one-fourth or one-third of the family income, neither the mothers nor the fathers appeared to leave the workforce. By lifting the families out of the depths of poverty, the additional income appeared to have resulted in improved outcomes for the adolescents.[4]

Early childhood poverty has significant negative outcomes for individuals, including lower school achievement, educational attainment, and adult earnings. During adolescence, higher family income is associated with better scores on assessments for language, memory, self-regulation, and social emotional processing. Poverty seems to negatively impact the structural development and functional activity of the brain, which support these skills.

Poverty is linked to differences in the brain's electrical activity. Researchers in New York designed a randomized controlled study to determine if several years of predictable, monthly, unconditional cash transfers to low-income families would affect the brain activity of the children. Members of the control group received $20 per month, while those in the intervention group received $333 per month; these payments began shortly after the birth of a newborn. After baseline brain activity measurements, the infants were tested at 1 year of age for resting brain activity. The results demonstrated that the infants of the families that received the higher cash payments demonstrated more high-frequency brain activity than those in the lower cash payment group. This was especially apparent in the frontal and central brain regions. These changes reflect neuroplasticity (the ability of the neural network in the brain to change through growth and reorganization) in the first year of life as well as environmental adaptations; such patterns of change have been correlated with the development of subsequent cognitive skills.[5]

Persistent childhood poverty and family adversity may significantly impact adolescents' physical, mental, cognitive, and behavioral outcomes. Utilizing data from the UK Millennium Cohort Study, researchers in the United Kingdom followed a cohort of 11,564 children from age 9 months to 14 years. The measures included parental mental health, parental alcohol use, and domestic violence and abuse. There were six waves over the study when the main caregiver completed the Strengths and Difficulties questionnaire. In part, this questionnaire assessed the child/adolescent for emotional, mental, and conduct problems. Those adolescents with persistent poverty had more than 2.4 times the odds of child mental health problems such as hyperactivity, emotional symptoms, and conduct disorders. The researchers noted that those children with persistent poverty and poor parental mental health up to age 14 had over six times the odds of child mental health problems and double the odds of obesity and cognitive disability.[6]

Epidemiology

According to the Pew Research Center, in 2019, before the COVID-19 pandemic, the rates of poverty in the United States had reached record low levels. At that point, 26 percent of Black children, 21 percent of Hispanic children, 8 percent of White children, and 7 percent of Asian children lived in poverty.[7]

Between 2019 and 2020, the overall poverty rate in the United States increased by 1 percentage point, and, according to the U.S. Census Bureau, the median household income decreased by 2.9 percent. In 2020, the official poverty rate was 11.4 percent, placing 37.2 million people in poverty; the poverty threshold income for a family of four was $26,496. After 5 consecutive years of declining rates of poverty, this was the first increase. For children and adolescents under the age of 18, the poverty rate increased from 14.4 percent in 2019 to 16.1 percent in 2020. Compared to 2018, more children under the age of 19 in poverty were uninsured in 2020, with the uninsured rates for children in poverty rising from 7.7 percent in 2018 to 9.3 percent in 2020. See Tables 14.1 and 14.2.[8]

According to a World Bank/UNICEF analysis, in 2020 one in six children lived in extreme poverty before the pandemic. This means that individuals lived on less than $1.90 per day.[9] Poverty is associated with shorter lifespans and other health issues. The World Bank also noted that the severe effects of the COVID-19 pandemic triggered a worsening of extreme poverty in sub-Saharan Africa by 1.3 percentage points.[10]

Biopsychosocial Issues and Poverty

Biological Issues and Poverty

Sleep
It is well known that the stress in daily life may affects an adolescent's sleep patterns, especially resulting in shorter sleep duration. Researchers in Norway and New Zealand wanted to learn if the deterioration of a family's financial circumstances would cause changes in patterns of adolescents' sleep. They designed a population-based study to

Table 14.1 Percentage of Americans Living Below United States Poverty Level

	2019	2020
White	9.1	10.1
Black	18.8	19.5
Asian	7.3	8.1
Hispanic (any race)	15.7	17.0
< 18 years old	14.4	16.1

Source: https://www.census.gov/library/publications/2021/demo/p60-273.html

Table 14.2 Poverty Rates (%) for Youth Under 18
Years Old in the United States

Year	Percent Poverty Rate
2020	16.1
2019	14.4
2018	16.2
2017	17.4
2016	18.0
2015	19.7
2014	21.1
2013	21.5
2012	21.8
2011	21.9
2010	22.0
2009	20.7
2008	19.0
2007	18.0
2006	17.4
2005	17.6
2004	17.8
2003	17.8
2002	16.7
2001	16.3
2000	16.2

Source: https://www.census.gov/library/publications/2021/
demo/p60-273.html

determine how the trajectories of poverty related to sleep duration and sleep efficacy
in adolescents. They used data from the youth@hordaland-survey, which assessed
mental health problems, including sleep, among adolescents ages 16 to 19 years.
A questionnaire was completed by 8873 adolescents with a mean age of 17.4 years
from western Norway; 53.5 percent were female. The measures included the official
family income, which was obtained from a central Norwegian registry for the years
2004 to 2010 using students' identification numbers, and sleep variables, including
self-reported bedtimes and rise times. The researchers learned that compared to the
reference group (those who were never poor), adolescents moving into poverty displayed worse sleep across most measures. However, adolescents who were chronically
in poverty or who moved out of poverty did not differ significantly from the reference
group with respect to sleep indicators. The findings support the belief that new family
financial stressors may negatively impact adolescent sleep.[11]

Adolescents who live in disadvantaged neighborhoods are more likely to face exposure to violence, harbor feelings of hopelessness, and deal with food insecurity. Researchers from Arcadia, Penn State, and Stony Brook Universities examined the relationship between residence in a disadvantaged neighborhood and sleep issues in a national sample of adolescents. They used data from the Fragile Families and Child Wellbeing Study, a longitudinal cohort study of children born in large U.S. cities between 1998 and 2000. With five waves of collection, including one when the subjects were 15 years old, the study sample had 3055 adolescents from wave 5, as well as 1090 randomly sampled adolescents. From this randomly selected group, 923 returned valid actigraphy data. The measures were neighborhood characteristics including families below the poverty level as determined by the U.S. Census Bureau, sleep duration, sleep efficiency, and others as assessed by actigraphy. The researchers learned that when compared to adolescents in less disadvantaged neighborhoods, there was a significant association between disadvantaged neighborhoods and sleep quality. The data demonstrated that adolescents had greater wake time after sleep onset and before rising. They also had lower sleep efficiency, which is the percentage of a sleep interval spent asleep rather than awake. Lower household income was linked to more variability in sleep duration; the most variability was noted in households earning less than half of the designated poverty line for household size.[12]

Psychological Issues and Poverty

Poverty is a significant social determinant of physical as well as mental health. It has many negative consequences including homelessness and lack of access to medical care. Poverty is related to such mental health issues as anxiety, depression, and substance abuse.

Depression
In adolescents, it is generally believed that social class is a predictor of mental health. Adolescents and young adults with a low socioeconomic status (SES) are thought to be at greater risk for depression than peers with higher SES. Several studies on the association between depression and poverty are reviewed in Chapter 5.

Researchers from Ohio wanted to learn if material hardship as a measure of economic deprivation was correlated with depression. Material hardship was defined to include food and housing insecurity and the inability to pay bills or utilities or seek medical services. In essence, this definition of economic disadvantage is the inability to meet basic needs. The researchers used data from the Fragile Families and Child Wellbeing Study; there were 3222 adolescents. As was previously noted, there were five waves of data collection from baseline to age 15 years, and there were measures for depression, anxiety, and material hardship when the subjects were ages 1, 3, 5, 9, and 15 years. When the data were controlled for material hardship at age 15 years, the researchers observed a strong relationship between early childhood hardship and depressive symptoms at age 15 years. They commented that insecurity during mid-childhood and the stress of lacking basic needs during a critical age may influence mental health in adolescence.[13]

Social Issues and Poverty

Social Media

For some disadvantaged adolescents who live in historically disadvantaged neighborhoods with high levels of crime, violence, and poverty, a digital divide may be quite dramatic. These adolescents may lack access to home networks, computers, or even smartphones. Undoubtedly, some of these teens may have a third space (after home and school), such as a church or community center, where they may use computers. Researchers from Pennsylvania and New Jersey joined with a primary school teacher from New Orleans to conduct a series of interviews with 60 adolescents and young adults (50 percent male) between the ages of 13 to 24 years. They were majority Black and Hispanic participants, and the childhood poverty rate was 19 percent. The researchers learned that the teens who turned to social media as a third space found a place apart from an environment plagued by poverty, violence, and high rates of crime. On the other hand, social media became an avenue for some teens to instigate aggression, violence, and sexual harassment. This may be seen as a second digital divide. The researchers concluded that developers of social media sites should focus on creating tools for social connection and community building and minimize the possibility for misuse.[14]

With the onset of the COVID-19 pandemic, another already well-established digital divide became more apparent. Many medical appointments were held online (telemedicine), especially in primary care and mental health. Important information on all aspects of the pandemic was also listed online. Adolescents living in disadvantaged circumstances were homebound and may not have had access to smartphones or the internet. And because the mental health appointments with these patients had to be held on regular telephones, mental health clinicians were unable to observe visual cues.

In England, medical care is free at the point of delivery through the National Health Service. However, about 37 percent of children from working-class families have no internet access at home. Poverty rates vary by ethnicity, with 29 percent of children from Bangladeshi households, 24 percent of children from Pakistani households, and 22 percent of children from Black households living in material deprivation. For telemedicine to be effective, they need to have access to online sites that provide trusted health information, confidential digital third spaces, or community resources to eliminate this divide.[15]

Racism/Discrimination

Racism, poverty, and adolescent health are interrelated.[16] Structural racism, which is defined as differential access to societal goods, services, and opportunities by race, means that certain adolescents have unequal access to resources, rights, power, and protection. The inequality in their lives impacts how they live, learn, and play. This in turn affects their health, as well as the health of their families and communities.

A type of structural racism, redlining was a system in which certain neighborhoods were designated as mortgage lending risks. Areas with racial minorities were often redlined, which led to higher interest rates and predatory lending practices. Accordingly, Black families in America in particular were often excluded from owning homes, leading to a diminished ability to accumulate even modest levels of wealth. Redlined neighborhoods became deserts for local health care resources, recreational facilities, and healthy food. Much of the housing stock was substandard, and minority renters were at the mercy of landlords, who tended to care more about generating income and less about the safety of their residents.

During the housing boom of the early 2000s, banks marketed subprime mortgages to many people with lower credit scores and lower incomes, who tended to be minorities. When the Great Recession hit in 2008, many of these new homeowners could no longer afford their mortgages, leading to increases in foreclosures and a further loss of wealth. Poverty rates then were highest among Black (26 percent) and Hispanic (25 percent) individuals.[17]

Given the historically disproportionate percentage of African American families below the poverty line, researchers in Illinois and Georgia investigated the relationship between the health of Black adolescents and the economic trajectories of their families during the Great Recession (2007–2009). The families lived in rural Georgia, where some of the communities had the highest poverty rates in the country at that time. The adolescents were followed from fifth grade, with a mean age of 11.2 years, until they were 18 years old. Five hundred families participated in the biological data collection; they were working poor with 45.8 percent living below the federal poverty level. Measures included family economic hardship, epigenetic aging (how behaviors and environment affect genes), allostatic load (cortisol, epinephrine, systolic and diastolic blood pressure), C-reactive protein (index of inflammation), body mass index, and self-reported health. The epigenetic aging, allostatic load, and self-reported health findings indicated that the longer the amount of time that Black adolescents experienced economic hardship during the Great Recession, the worse their health profiles became. When compared to adolescents who had stability and little economic hardship, the adolescents who had economic decline had greater increases in allostatic load. The researchers concluded that negative economic conditions such as poverty alter biological and health trajectories over time in adolescents, and these changes may be seen early in life and persist into adulthood.[18]

Transgender/Gender Dysphoria

Although data on the prevalence of poverty in the younger adolescent transgender population are not available, researchers at the Williams Institute at the UCLA School of Law did study its prevalence in older adolescents and young adults. The data were obtained from the Behavioral Risk Factor Surveillance System, a telephone survey of more than 400,000 people ages 18 years and older, which was funded by the Centers for Disease Control and Prevention. Thirty-five states used an optional module with the survey to provide sexual orientation and gender identity questions that yielded the data in Table 14.3. For example, the poverty rate for all transgender participants in the survey was 35.6 percent.[19]

The high poverty rates in the transgender older adolescents and young adults placed them at higher risk for associated mental health issues. As detailed in Chapter 13, transgender people are at higher risk for anxiety, depression, suicidal ideation, and suicidal attempts than their cisgender counterparts. Transgender youth faced with poverty are thus at very high risk for mental health problems.

Table 14.3 Poverty Rates by Sexual Orientation and Gender Identification

Sexual Orientation and Gender Identity	18–24 Years Old % Poverty Rate	Number of Individuals in the Sample
Cis-straight men	23.0	2620
Cis-straight women	31.2	2951
Cis-gay men	20.3	73
Cis-lesbian women	34.3	67
Cis-bisexual men	19.9	106
Cis-bisexual women	37.3	345
Transgender	35.6	70

Divorce

Divorce may trigger significant economic consequences due to the loss of joint income. A major reduction in income may lead to material deprivation and a range of other adversities for adolescents, including poverty. Researchers in the Netherlands studied the relationship between divorce and poverty. They reviewed data for the years 2003 to 2005 from a study population of first marriages for individuals between the ages of 18 and 35 years ($N = 179,018$). The measures included marital status, divorce, educational attainment, and disposable income. The researchers learned that for divorced mothers (but not fathers), lower education levels and increased economic consequences both contributed to higher levels of poverty. According to the study, adolescents with divorced mothers were at increased risk for poverty and consequent material deprivation and possible psychological consequences.[20]

The U.S. Census Bureau provides poverty data based on a number of demographics. From 2013 to 2016, 15.2 percent of the U.S. population lived in poverty. In their analysis of the average monthly poverty rates, the data demonstrated that married couples had a 7.1 percent poverty rate, families with a male householder and no spouse had a 17.2 percent poverty rate, and families with a female householder and no spouse had a 32.8 percent poverty rate. While the data do not provide a reason the single householders had no spouse, they do present important information on the increased risk for poverty (and corroborate the Netherlands study), especially in families with a female head. Since there were more than 53 million people living in this status, this prevalence of poverty clearly had an impact on a significant number of adolescents.[21]

Mortality

As was discussed in Chapter 8, higher countrywide concentrations of poverty have been associated with increased rates of completed suicides among youth from ages 5 to 19 years. The World Health Organization stratified other causes of adolescent deaths from ages 10 to 19 years by the income of the country in which they resided. They compared data from lower- to middle-income countries with the same data from higher-income countries. They noted that the death rate per 100,000 adolescents in higher-income countries was 12.5 compared to 90.0 per 100,000 in lower- to middle-income countries.

They provided further information on the top three causes of death in adolescents who resided in lower- to middle-income African countries: meningitis, diarrheal disease, and lower respiratory infections. These causes accounted for 60 per 100,000 deaths. On the other hand, self-harm, leukemia, and congenital abnormalities accounted for 6 per 100,000 adolescent deaths in higher-income countries. In these countries, adolescents had access to vaccines and medications that prevented or treated the infections suffered by adolescents in the African countries.[22]

With respect to lack of access to medical care, researchers at multiple academic medical centers in the United States examined the relationship between poverty and the risk of relapse and death among neuroblastoma patients who received targeted immunotherapy. They conducted a retrospective cohort study of 371 children and focused on the association between poverty and event-free survival and overall survival for children with this illness. Household poverty was defined as the child being on public insurance such as Medicaid. Neighborhood poverty was characterized as living in a zip code with a median household income within the lowest quartile for the cohort. The researchers determined that the children living in *household* poverty had significantly fewer event-free survivals and overall survivals than those not living in poverty. But *neighborhood* poverty was not related to event-free survival or overall survival for children with this cancer and treatment modality.[23] While this study was performed in children, the concepts should apply to adolescents.

Climate Change

Climate change is a social determinant of health and has the potential to impact the biopsychosocial health of adolescents.[24] As poverty reduction is driven by asset accumulation, climate change may also affect the ability of individuals to escape poverty. For example, lower agricultural productivity and loss of assets from natural disasters reduce family income. As a result, the accumulation of assets slows. If climate change is increasing the risk of drought, farmers may decide to plant fewer crops, making it more difficult to escape poverty.[25] Adolescents and their families, who are already living in poverty, may sink to an even deeper level of impoverishment due to climate change.[26]

According to economists at the Massachusetts Institute of Technology and Harvard University, both in Cambridge, Massachusetts, climate change threatens the mental health of individuals, especially those in low-income countries.[27] For example, during the growing season in agricultural regions in India, extreme temperatures have been reported to increase the incidence of suicides.[28] Presumably, due to lower crop yields and loss of life, this may exacerbate poverty. Clearly, loss of a parent to suicide and worsening poverty due to climate change have broad implications for the mental health of adolescents.

A group of researchers at Columbia University in New York City developed a model that explains how energy insecurity may impact adolescents' health. In this model, climate change may lead to energy insecurity, defined as the inability of a family to afford adequate energy to meet household needs. This may result in the family's inability to heat a home in cold weather or cool it in hot conditions due to lack of financial resources. The resulting temperature extremes in the home can lead to family maladaptive coping. Health outcomes may include heat/cold physical stress, poor sleep quality, emotional stress, maladaptive behaviors, and mental health issues such as anxiety in adolescents.[29]

Immigration

Immigrant children are defined as having at least one foreign-born parent. First-generation immigrant children were born outside the United States, and second-generation immigrant children were born in the United States. Researchers at Pennsylvania State University used the official poverty measures from the U.S. government and an additional poverty measurement to study poverty rates among the immigrant generation between 1993 and 2016. The researchers determined that poverty rates were highest among first-generation children, followed by second-generation children who had two foreign-born parents. Between 1993 and 2016, the poverty rate for both groups of children fell from 34.4 percent to 28.6 percent. In separate stratified analyses, Hispanic children encountered disproportionately high levels of poverty regardless of generation, while Asian children faced below-average poverty rates. Approximately 40 percent of first-generation Hispanic children live in poverty, as do 25 percent of first-generation Asian children.[30] This is in comparison to an overall poverty rate of 14 percent for children residing in the United States.[31] Immigrant adolescents living in poverty face biopsychosocial disparities compared to those not living in poverty.

One of these disparities appears to be brain development. Researchers in Michigan, North Carolina, and Wisconsin examined the relationship between atypical patterns of structural brain development, household poverty, and impaired academic performance in children and adolescents. According to these researchers, in 2013, 51 percent of the students in U.S. public schools came from low-income families. Children living in poverty had lower scores on standardized tests of academic achievement, lower grades in school, and lower educational attainment that persisted into adulthood. Since it is known that early life stressors may affect brain structure and functioning, growing up in poverty may expose children to stress, increased family instability, and less parental nurturance. Focusing on the gray matter tissue of the brain, which is more vulnerable to early life stress, the researchers used data from the National Institutes of Health Magnetic Resonance Imaging Study of Normal Brain Development. The sample included 389 children between the ages of 4 and 22 years, with a mean age of 12 years. The family income ranged from well below the federal poverty level to more than eight times the federal poverty level. Subjects were screened at baseline and every 24 months for a total of three periods with neuroimaging and neurobehavioral testing. The researchers learned that low SES was related to atypical gray matter development. There were structural differences in the frontal and temporal lobes as well as the hippocampus. The volumes of regional gray matter in children living below 1.5 times the federal poverty level averaged 3 to 4 percentage points below the developmental norms for their sex and age. The estimated gap increased to 7 to 10 percentage points in children living below the federal poverty level. On average, children from low-income households scored four to seven points lower on standardized tests ($p <$ .05). The researchers concluded that the influence of poverty on children's learning and achievement is mediated by structural brain development.[32] Immigrant and nonimmigrant children living in poverty should be targeted for additional resources aimed at remediating their early childhood environments. Academic deficits persist into adulthood, contributing to a lifetime reduction of occupational attainment.

Another biopsychosocial disparity faced by immigrant children was studied by researchers in California, New York, and Illinois who wanted to learn more about the psychosocial issues and challenges of Chinese immigrant youth. They designed a study with 10 focus groups; there were 4 student groups, 3 teacher groups, 2 parent groups, and 1 school counseling group from a public high school in a large metropolitan city in the United States that primarily served recent immigrant youth. The student population was low income, and the graduation rate was about 25 percent. Thirty-two students (50 percent female) with a mean age of 18.97 years made up the student focus group. The researchers found that poverty from immigrant status had multiple impacts, including occupational status, career aspirations, academic performance, relationship dynamics, and available social support systems for the students and their families. Their immigrant status resulted in a loss of socioeconomic security. Devoid of economic resources, the adolescents could no longer afford to attend college, and they revised their career aspirations. Poverty created tensions in their daily lives, relationships, and academic performance.[33]

Violence

Exposure to violence and low family income may possibly be correlated with changes in the adolescent brain. Modeling suggests that exposure to violence alters an individual's emotional processing, so environmental threats are more rapidly identified. In violence-exposed youth, increased amygdala reactivity has been observed in response to threatening social stimuli. To study this further, researchers from the Boys Town National Research Hospital and Northwestern and Harvard Universities recruited 277 eighth-grade youth who were highly diverse with respect to race, ethnicity, and SES. While viewing various degrees of angry facial expressions, they were administered a functional magnetic resonance imaging (fMRI) test. The researchers hypothesized that the teens with increased exposure to violence and lower SES would have a greater amygdala response to the angry faces. Measures included a history of medical or psychiatric illness, SES, exposure to violence, and data from the fMRI. The researchers observed a negative association between income and amygdala response to angry faces. Likewise, violence exposure was related to heightened amygdala response. The link between amygdala responsiveness and SES was only via income. The researchers concluded that low-income levels were linked with an increased responsiveness to angry faces (within the amygdala) only in those youth not exposed to violence. Thus, there are other aspects of the low SES beyond violence that may lead to increased sensitivity to threats.[34]

Adolescents who have lived in poverty during early childhood appear to have higher risk for violent behavior during adolescence. Researchers from several universities but based in New Jersey examined the early-life individual, family, and community influences that were associated with the future violent behaviors of adolescents. They created a study to identify specific risk factors during a child's first 3 years of life that might predict adolescent behaviors that result in juvenile arrest records of violent, nonviolent, and nonoffending males. The study participants were part of the Pitt Mother & Child Project (Department of Psychology, University of Pittsburgh), which was an ongoing longitudinal study of vulnerability and resilience in boys from low socioeconomic backgrounds. The study used data from home visits or laboratory assessments when the children were ages 18, 24, and 42 months. At the assessments, mothers completed questionnaires, and parent-child interactions were videotaped. When the boys were between the ages of 15.9 and 18 years, juvenile court records were collected. Complete data were available on 272 of the subjects. Measures included child oppositional behavior, child emotion regulation, mothers' depressive symptomatology, rejecting parenting, demographics, court petitions, and juvenile court records. The researchers found that compared to the adolescents with no juvenile arrests, the adolescent violent offenders were more likely to have lived in poverty and been a minority. They were also more often rated oppositional by their parents and had less ability to regulate their emotions. And compared to the adolescents arrested only for nonviolent crimes, the adolescents arrested for violent crimes were more likely to have experienced harsh parenting, and they had lower emotion regulation skills during their early childhood years.[35]

A team of researchers from Indiana, New York, and Alabama wanted to learn if parents had the ability to shield youth from exposure to the violence in high-poverty settings. The researchers used data from the Mobile Youth Survey, an adolescent risk behavior study that included five waves of self-reported data collected annually between 1998 and 2002. The subjects, who were between the ages of 9 and 19 years, lived in 12 high-poverty neighborhoods in Mobile, Alabama. Though there were 360 respondents who participated in the five waves, the researchers focused their analyses on the 348 youth. The subjects answered questions without the presence of their parents. The first measure consisted of five trajectories of exposure to violence: high declining, middle declining, sharply increasing, middle increasing, and stable-low. The second measure was trajectories of parental monitoring: high-stable, middle-level stable, and declining. The researchers found that about half of the adolescents had a trajectory of hypervigilant parental monitoring and that these adolescents were 109 percent more likely to have middle-declining exposure to violence. Half of the parents responded and adapted to exposure to violence at wave 1 for youth in the middle-declining trajectory by tightening their control over these youth with hypervigilant parenting. This was a key factor accounting for the steadily declining exposure to violence over the 5-year time period. In summary, families played a key role in violence prevention and intervention efforts among high-risk adolescents.[36]

Prevention

It is well established that poverty has multiple impacts on the mental, emotional, and behavioral lives of adolescents, and these are cumulative. The poverty-related stress felt by parents naturally affects their children and adolescents through biological and psychosocial pathways. Family poverty mediators may be associated with parental depression and marital conflict, which may be observed by other family members. Impoverished neighborhoods and poorly funded schools only exacerbate the situation.

Myriad different programs have been created to lessen the effects of poverty on adolescents. These programs have focused on many areas including early child interventions, parenting attachment issues, and parental depression. At the school level, efforts have targeted social-emotional learning processes with the delivery of these interventions by teachers in preschool, elementary school, middle school, and high school.[37]

Researchers in North Carolina and Texas developed a randomly controlled study, the New Hope Program, where they increased parent employment and reduced poverty by income supplementation sufficient to raise family income above the poverty threshold. Subsidies for childcare and health insurance were also provided to the families. The program was 3 years in duration, and the children were followed for up to 5 years after the study and assessed at ages 9 to 19. Compared to the control population, the male adolescents in the study worked for longer periods during the school year and had more positive attitudes toward work.[38] In addition, the program had significant positive impacts on youth's overall progress in school and school achievement.[39,40]

Other approaches to poverty prevention include those that directly reduce poverty and may include childhood allowances and tax credits, cash transfers, and income supplementation. The income supplementation program on the Eastern Cherokee reservation resulted in a reduction of minor offenses and self-reported drug dealing in adolescents at age 16 years and improved rates of high school graduation.[41] In addition, in the Adolescent Brain and Cognitive Development Study, where 10,633 adolescents ages 9 to 11 were followed, lower income was associated with smaller hippocampal volume and higher internalizing psychopathology. In those states with a high cost of living that provided more generous cash benefits for low-income families, the socioeconomic disparities in hippocampal volume were reduced by 34 percent. And internalizing problems in the adolescents were also lower in those states providing more cash benefits.[42]

Given the potentially serious consequences on the health of adolescents of poverty and neighborhood poverty, there are many reasons to try to elevate families from this condition. A number of interventions to reduce the effects of poverty or directly lessen the degree of poverty have received research support and should be continued. Programs aimed at early childhood may have positive impacts on the individual during adolescence and adulthood. Since one strategy has not proven to be successful in reducing poverty, interventions need to be quite intensive and continue for several years.

Conclusion

Poverty impacts the biopsychosocial domains of adolescents and may have negative effects later in their lives. By limiting access to clinical resources, poverty may also affect the medical care available to youth. Strategies to reduce poverty, such as through increased parental education or employment or cash payments to families, may help prevent these serious consequences. Such preventive efforts should be coordinated through local, state, and federal governments.

References

1   2023 poverty guidelines for the 48 continuous states and the District of Columbia. *Federal Register.* 2023;88(12):3424–3425, January 19, 2023. Washington, DC.

2   Bitsko RH, Claussen AH, Lichstein J, et al. Mental health surveillance among children—United States, 2013–2019. *MMWR Suppl.* 2022;71:1–42.

3   Johnson SB, Riis JL, Noble KG. State of the art review: poverty and the developing brain. *Pediatrics.* 2016;137:e20153075.

4   Akee RKQ, Copeland WE, Keeler G, Angold A, Costello EJ. Parents' incomes and children's outcomes: a quasi-experiment using transfer payments from casino profits. *Am Econ J Appl Econ.* 2010;2:86–115.

5   Troller-Renfree SV, Costanzo MA, Duncan GJ, et al. The impact of a poverty reduction intervention on infant brain activity. *Proc Natl Acad Sci USA.* 2022;119:e2115649119.

6   Adjei NK, Schlüter DK, Straatmann VS, et al. ORACLE Consortium. Impact of poverty and family adversity on adolescent health: a multi-trajectory analysis using the UK Millennium Cohort Study. *Lancet Reg Health Eur.* 2021;13:100279.

7   Thomas D, Fry R. Prior to COVID-19, child poverty rates had reached record lows in U.S. Pew Research Center, November 30, 2020.

8. Shrider EA, Kollar M, Chen F, Semega J. Income and Poverty in the United States: 2020. United States Census Bureau, Report Number P60-273, September 14, 2021.

9   United Nations. One in six children living in extreme poverty, with figure set to rise during pandemic. UN News, October 20, 2020.

10 Yonzan N, Cojocaru A, Lakner C, Mahler DG, Narayan A. The impact of COVID-19 on poverty and inequality: evidence from phone surveys. *World Bank Blogs,* January 18, 2022.

11 Sivertsen BT, Bøe T, Skogen JC, Petrie KJ, Hysing M. Moving into poverty during childhood is associated with later sleep problems. *Sleep Med.* 2017;37:54–59.

12 Nahmod NG, Master L, McClintock HF, Hale L, Buxton OM. Neighborhood disadvantage is associated with lower quality sleep and more variability in sleep duration among urban adolescents. *J Urban Health.* 2022;99:102–115.

13 Edmunds C, Alcaraz M. Childhood material hardship and adolescent mental health. *Youth Soc.* 2021;53:1231–1254.

14 Sevens R, Gilliard-Matthews S, Dunaev J, Woods M, Brawner B. The digital hood: social media use among youth in disadvantaged neighborhoods. *New Media Soc.* 2017;19:950–967.

15 Aisbitt GM, Nolte T, Fonagy P. Editorial perspective: the digital divide—inequalities in remote therapy for children and adolescents. *Child Adolesc Ment Health.* 2022;28:105–107.

16 Heard-Garris N, Boyd R, Kan K, Perez-Cardona L, Heard NJ, Johnson TJ. Structuring poverty: how racism shapes child poverty and child and adolescent health. *Acad Pediatr.* 2021;21:S108–S116.

17 Heard-Garris N, Boyd R, Kan K, Perez-Cardona L, Heard NJ, Johnson TJ. Structuring poverty: how racism shapes child poverty and child and adolescent health. *Acad Pediatr.* 2021;21:S108–S116.

18 Chen E, Miller GE, Yu T, Brody GJ. The great recession and health risks in African American youth. *Brain Behav Immun.* 2016;53:234–241.

19 Badgett MVL, Choi SI, Wilson BDM. *LGBT Poverty in the United States: A Study of Differences Between Sexual Orientation and Gender Identity Groups.* Williams Institute; 2019.

20 Hogendoom B, Leopold T, Bol T. Divorce and diverging poverty rates: a risk-and-vulnerability approach. *J Marriage Fam.* 2020;82:1089–1109.

21 Mohanty A. *Dynamics of Economic Well-Being: Poverty 2013–2016.* P70-BR-172. U.S. Census Bureau; August 2021.

22 World Health Organization. *Global Accelerated Action for the Health of Adolescents (AA-HA!): Guidance to Support Country Implementation*. World Health Organization; 2017.

23 Bona K, Li Y, Winestone LE, et al. Poverty and targeted immunotherapy: survival in children's oncology group clinical trials for high-risk neuroblastoma. *J Natl Cancer Inst.* 2021;113:282–291.

24 Ragavan MI, Marcil LE, Garg A. Climate change as a social determinant of health. *Pediatrics.* 2020;145:e20193169.

25 Hallegatte S, Fay M, Barbier E. Poverty and climate change: introduction. *Environ Dev Econ.* 2018;23:217–233.

26 Goldstein M. Climate change and its effects on children and adolescents: a call to action. *Curr Pediatr Rep.* 2022:10:55–56.

27 Ridley M, Rao G, Schilbach F, Patel V. Poverty, depression, and anxiety: causal evidence and mechanisms. *Science.* 2020;370(6522):eaay0214.

28 Carleton TA. Crop-damaging temperatures increase suicide rates in India. *Proc Natl Acad Sci USA.* 2017;114:8746–8751.

29 Jessel S, Sawyer S, Hernández D. Energy, poverty, and health in climate change: a comprehensive review of an emerging literature. *Front Public Health.* 2019;7:357.

30 Thiede B, Brooks MM. Child poverty across immigrant generations in the United States, 1993–2016: evidence using the official and supplementary poverty measures. *Demographic Res.* 2018;39:1065–1080.

31 Kearney M. Child poverty in the U.S. *Econofact*, February 5, 2021.

32 Hair NL, Hanson JL, Wolfe BL, Pollak SD. Association of child poverty, brain development, and academic achievement. *JAMA Pediatr.* 2015;169:878.

33 Yeh CJ, Kim AB, Pituc ST, Atkins M. Poverty, loss, and resilience: the story of Chinese immigrant youth. *J Couns Psychol.* 2008;55:34–48

34 White SF, Voss JL, Chiang JJ, Wang L, McLaughlin K, Miller GE. Exposure to violence and low family income are associated with heightened amygdala responsiveness to threat among adolescents. *Dev Cogn Neurosci.* 2019;40:100709.

35 Sitnick SL, Shaw DS, Weaver CM, et al. Early childhood predictors of severe youth violence in low-income male adolescents. *Child Dev.* 2017;88:27–40.

36 Spano R, Rivera C, Bolland JM. Does parenting shield youth from exposure to violence during adolescence? A 5-year longitudinal test in a high-poverty sample of minority youth. *J Interpers Violence.* 2011;26:930–949.

37 Yoshikawa H, Aber JL, Beardslee WR. The effects of poverty on the mental, emotional, and behavioral health of children and youth: implications for prevention. *Am Psychol.* 2012;67:272–284.

38 McLoyd VC, Kaplan R, Purtell KM, Huston AC. Assessing the effects of a work-based antipoverty program for parents on youth's future orientation and employment experiences. *Child Dev.* 2011;82:113–132.

39 Huston A, Walker J. Dowsett C, Imes AE, Ware A. *Long-Term Effect of New Hope on Children's Academic Achievement and Achievement Motivation.* MDRC; 2008.

40 Huston AC, Duncan GJ, Granger R, et al. Work-based antipoverty programs for parents can enhance the school performance and social behavior of children. *Child Dev.* 2001;72:318–336.

41 Akee RKQ, Copeland WE, Keeler G, Angold A, Costello EJ. Parents' incomes and children's outcomes: a quasi-experiment using transfer payments from casino profits. *Am Econ J Appl Econ.* 2010;2:86–115.

42 Weissman DG, Hatzenbuehler ML, Cikara M, Barch DM, McLaughlin KA. State-level macro-economic factors moderate the association of low income with brain structure and mental heal in U.S. Children. *Nat Commun.* 2023;14:2085.

Life Events

15
Divorce

Introduction

Parental divorce impacts adolescents in the biological, psychological, and social domains. When faced with the divorce of their parents, immediate responses from teens include anger, feelings of sadness, and anxiety. They are anxious about how the divorce will alter their lives and their place and role in the changing family unit. Children and adolescents are growing up with divorce.[1]

Although divorce has been a part of American society for a long time, its impact on adolescents has only been well studied for about four decades. Judith Wallerstein from the California Children of Divorce Project completed a landmark study of children of divorce in 1971. She and her team explored the experiences of 60 Northern California families whose 131 children were between 2.5 and 18 years at the time of the divorce. She did not have a control group of children not undergoing divorce. While much of their research focused on the psychological and social functioning of 38 subjects, most were male adolescents who were between 6 and 8 years old at the time of the divorce. Ten years after the divorce, Wallerstein reported that most of the 131 adolescents were in school full time, living at home, holding part-time jobs, and considered law abiding. The majority had remained with their mothers; about one-quarter moved in with their fathers during adolescence. They tended to express sadness, neediness, and a sense of their own vulnerability, and they spoke with sorrow about their loss of an intact family. A central concern was a fear of betrayal in relationships, being hurt, and abandonment. Female adolescents were more likely to be involved in a relationship; the males tended to refrain from opposite gender involvement. During adolescence, 40 percent of the female adolescents had three or more relationships; between the ages of 13 and 16 years, one-quarter had abortions. The male adolescents had low levels of drug use, alcoholism, and school truancy. Depression was noted among the group, as well as suicide attempts between the ages of 13 and 16. The findings underscored the fact that the effects of divorce on children and adolescents were significant and continued for many years.[2] In an article published in 1991, when the subjects were in their 20s and 30s, Wallerstein concluded that children of divorce were forced to deal with the normal challenges of adolescence as well as many additional psychological burdens. Whether children of divorce do well or poorly or in between, they may experience psychological consequences that manifest themselves at the threshold of adulthood when the major life decisions of love, commitment, and marriage are being made.[3]

Acknowledging that adolescents have an increased risk for emotional and behavioral problems (EBPs) after parental divorce, a team of researchers from the Netherlands wanted to learn if these issues occurred before or after the divorce. They performed a prospective study of the Tracking Adolescents' Individual Lives

Survey (TRAILS), a large cohort of adolescents living in the northern section of the Netherlands. When the study began, the mean age of the sample was 11.1 years. Measures were noted from T1 to T4, every 2 or 3 years beginning in 2001. The measures included the occurrence of parental divorce and internalizing and externalizing problem scales, using the Youth Self-Report. When the researchers' work was published in 2022, the sample size was 1881, with slightly more female than male adolescents. The mean age at T4 was 19.1 years. The adolescents, who were primarily Dutch, had diverse backgrounds. While there were no increases in EBPs before the divorce, the researchers found that after a divorce, there were significant increases, which enlarged over time. The researchers learned that the effects of divorce did not diminish. In fact, after the divorce, EBPs increased for an additional 4 years. Female adolescents demonstrated increasing internalizing problems 2 years after the divorce, but externalizing (behavioral problems) did not differ by gender. After divorce, female adolescents may exhibit internalizing problems, such as anxiety and depression, while male and female adolescents may have behavioral problems. These different presentations should be taken into account when developing psychological support and appropriate programming for adolescents experiencing parental divorce.[4]

During adolescence, the brain has heightened plasticity, which may lead to a more pronounced response from an adverse childhood experience (ACE). A parental divorce, which is a known ACE, could therefore have a major and long-lasting effect on brain circuitry, which may lead to adult EBP issues.[5] Researchers from Finland wondered if a parental divorce during adolescence had long-term consequences on an adult's psychological well-being, life situation, health behavior, social networks and support, negative life events, and interpersonal problems. Did those who experienced parental divorce before the age of 16 years differ in psychosocial well-being or life trajectories at age 32 from those who had nondivorced, two-parent families? They designed a prospective study of all ninth-grade pupils in a city in southern Finland ($N = 2269$). At T1, in 1983, when students had a mean age of 15.9 years, 96.7 percent completed a self-administered questionnaire. At T2, in 1999, when they were 32 years old, 70.3 percent of the 2091 subjects still in the cohort completed a follow-up questionnaire. The measures in both questionnaires included questions on psychological and somatic health, health behavior, family background, personal characteristics, social relationships, and life events. The second questionnaire had additional measures on psychological well-being. The researchers discovered that parental divorce was an indicator of significant stress that continued to manifest itself well into adulthood. Compared to female adolescents from nondivorced families, at age 32 years, female adolescents from families with parental divorce had significantly higher psychosomatic symptoms and a higher incidence of depression. Male adolescents who came from divorced or nondivorced families had similar psychological well-being. Both male and female adolescents from families with divorce before their 16th birthdays had lower rates of college education, higher rates of marriage, and an increased use of substances. Female adolescents from divorced families had fewer social networks and fewer relationships with important family members, relatives, and friends. And the toll of negative life events, such as financial difficulties, job loss, severe illness, relationship breakups, and death of a family member, was higher and statistically significant in the subjects from divorced families. Though the researchers acknowledged that divorce may have a detrimental effect on the life course of children, in their study the majority of the adolescents with divorced parents demonstrated good psychosocial adaptation as adults. The impact of the divorce was directly related to the adolescent's resilience, interpersonal relationships, and social support. In some cases, community resources were useful in modifying stress. It was evident that during and after a divorce, the specific needs of children should be addressed to minimize or prevent intractable long-term problems.[6]

Given the litany of potential difficulties, it should not be surprising that the *Diagnostic and Statistical Manual of Mental Disorders*, fifth edition added a new diagnostic term called "child affected by parental relationship distress." This term describes the anxiety and/or depression felt by a child when parents continuously argue or the somatic symptoms caused by intense loyalty conflict—trying to maintain affection for both conflicting parents.[7]

To help children and their families deal with separation and divorce, a clinical report from the American Academy of Pediatrics recommended that pediatricians advocate for the physical and emotional needs of children and communicate that concern to parents. This may include pediatrician-parent conferences to discuss how the divorce process affects children and possible referrals to mental health and child-oriented services and resources with expertise in separation and divorce.[8]

Epidemiology

Since the 1970s, there has been an increase in divorce rates. According to data from the United Nations, throughout the world, the proportion of divorced adults between the ages of 35 and 39 years has increased from 2 percent in the 1970s to 4 percent in the 2000s. For many countries, the divorced rates increased significantly between the 1970s and 1990s, and the rates seemed to subsequently stabilize. However, the United States was an outlier, with divorce rates now higher than most other countries. Although the divorce rates in the United States peaked in the 1980s and then declined steadily in the first two decades of the 21st century, they are still higher than most countries. The decline in divorce rates may have been due to delay in marriage across different cohorts. For example, 48 percent of the 1970s cohort of marriages ended in divorce within 25 years. On the other hand, for the 1980s cohort, the divorce rate was 40 percent by 25 years; for the 1990s cohort, it was about 25 percent.[9]

A closer look at data provided by the Centers for Disease Control and Prevention shows that the national divorce rate per 1000 total population was 4.0 in 2000 and 2.5 in 2021. In 2021, Wyoming was the state with the highest divorce rate at 3.7, and Massachusetts had the lowest at 1.0.[10] Meanwhile, to study the cohort of people born during the 1957–1964 period, the U.S. Bureau of Labor Statistics examined divorce data from the National Longitudinal Survey of Youth 1979. They found that approximately 42 percent of marriages that took place with individuals who were 15 to 46 years old ended in divorce by the age of 46. For both genders, higher levels of education were associated with lower divorce rates.[11]

Biopsychosocial Issues and Divorce

Biological Issues and Divorce

Stress

Parental divorce is a cause of significant stress for adolescents. In addition, marital conflict and its severity are predictors of adolescent adjustment. With good support networks, many teens who are resilient handle the stress without adverse outcomes. However, sometimes there are tragic outcomes. Finnish investigators studied stress in adolescents due to parental divorce and its relationship to completed suicide. They performed a psychological analysis, also known as a psychological autopsy, on all completed suicides in adolescents from April 1, 1987, to March 31, 1988; there were a total of 53 subjects with a mean age of 17.4 years, and 83 percent were male. The psychological analysis consisted of interviews with family members, reviews of medical records, and medicolegal or forensic testing. A suicide victim was considered to have experienced major stress during the year preceding the suicide if they had one or more of the following stressors: parental divorce, severe parental illness, death of a significant other, severe somatic or psychiatric illness, abortion, psychiatric hospitalization, or imprisonment. The deceased adolescents were placed into three categories: history of alcohol abuse (26.4 percent), history of depressive disorder (34.0 percent), or other (39.6 percent). The researchers discovered that every adolescent with a completed suicide had at least one stressor during the final month before their death. Family discord, which included divorce, was noted as a stressor in 50 percent of those abusing alcohol, 39 percent in those with a depressive disorder, and 29 percent in the other group. Thus, family discord is a major stressor in adolescents who die by suicide, especially those with a history of alcohol abuse. The alcohol abuse may be related to the family discord. Since those who abused alcohol were not necessarily depressed, they may not have shown mood symptoms prior to their completed suicide. This study demonstrated the importance of ongoing surveillance of adolescents whose parents are undergoing divorce, and there should be a very low threshold for referral to a therapist.[12]

Psychological Issues and Divorce

Anxiety

It has been well established that many adolescents deal with EBPs after a parental divorce. Researchers in Norway compared the development and psychological adjustment of adolescents whose parents did and did not divorce as well as the effect of parental remarriage. In addition, they looked for gender differences between the two groups. The researchers used data from the Nord-Trondelag Health Study—Young-HUNT I (T1) and Young-HUNT II (T2). T1 was conducted from 1995 to 1997, and T2 from 2000 to 2001. The mean age of T1 was 14.4 years and the mean age of T2 was 18.4 years. A total of 2270 adolescents participated in both time periods, and there were slightly more female than male adolescents; by T1, 18.2 percent had parents who had divorced. Divorces between T1 and T2 were excluded. The measures included symptoms of anxiety and depression, subjective well-being, self-esteem, and school functioning. The researchers learned that the adolescents who had already undergone divorce at T1 had symptoms of problems with anxiety, depression, subjective well-being, self-esteem, and school at T2 greater than those whose parents were still together. Gender differences were noted. While the predominant problems with male adolescents were school related, female adolescents had issues with anxiety, depression, subjective well-being, and school. The absence of a father seemed to have a significant effect on relative change in symptoms of anxiety, depression, and well-being. The findings demonstrated that after a divorce, anxiety may develop and progress, especially in female adolescents, and the absence of a father may be a mediating factor.[13]

Does the anxiety and depression experienced by female adolescents when their parents divorce persist into young adulthood? Researchers in Luxembourg and Germany recruited 121 women with a mean age of 23. Half of these women had parents who divorced during their childhoods; their mean age when the parents divorced was 10 years. Each woman was interviewed for Axis I (major mental health) disorders and Axis II (personality) disorders. There were measures for depression, childhood trauma, chronic stress, social connectedness, and parental bonding. The single interviewer was blinded to the parental marriage situation. The researchers learned that a higher percentage of women with divorced parents had symptoms of anxiety and depression than the women without divorced parents. Those with divorced parents had higher childhood trauma scores including physical, emotional, and sexual abuse and significantly higher levels of chronic stress. This study provided clear evidence that young adult females whose parents divorced when they were children were vulnerable to mental health issues. To help prevent long-term problems, it may be useful to offer professional mental health counseling to children and adolescents during and after divorce.[14]

Depression
When compared to children of married parents, children of divorced parents have a greater risk for depression and suicidality. Yet, most children from divorced families do not have negative outcomes. To understand moderators for the association between parental separation/divorce and children's depressive symptoms and divorce, researchers from Australia performed a systematic review to assess the familial and individual characteristics associated with a higher risk for depression or depressive symptoms, as well as the factors that increase resilience against these medical problems. The researchers located 14 relevant studies that included moderating factors such as offspring gender, age, age at onset of depression, IQ, and socioeconomic status. One study of 648 prepubertal to late adolescent males and adolescent females demonstrated that males had a 5.19 times greater risk for major depression. Another study of adults aged 36 to 43 years found that women who experienced parental divorce had higher depression scores. Hoping to learn if age played a pivotal role, two studies examined middle and late adolescents and early and middle adolescents who had parental divorce. No moderation was noted. One study examined offspring age at the time of the divorce and depressive symptoms. While statistical significance was not reached, there were higher depressive scores when the divorce occurred at ages 0 through 16 years compared to 17 to 33 years. Another study, which evaluated the

importance of the age at which depression begins, found that children with depression diagnosed at age 14 or younger had a significantly increased risk for lifetime major depression when the parental divorce occurred before the child was age 7. Interestingly, the findings from one study showed that higher IQ was protective against depression, and two studies found no support for parental socioeconomic status as a moderator against divorce-related offspring depression. The implications of this study are that there are significant moderators of the relationship between parental divorce and offspring depression or depressive symptoms, and these moderators include the child's gender, IQ, history of emotional problems, and age at depression onset.[15]

In 2017, divorce rates were rising rapidly in Lebanon; in recent years, the rates had risen by 25 percent. Some studies found that up to half of the adolescents in Lebanon who had parents who were separated, divorced, or deceased had psychiatric disorders. Researchers explored the correlation between divorce and mental health outcomes, especially depression, anxiety, and suicidal ideation. They designed a cross-sectional study and enrolled 1810 adolescents between the ages of 14 and 17 years from five Lebanese governorates. From a school-based survey, the researchers learned that the mean age of the sample was 15.4 years, 53.3 percent female, and 11.9 percent had parents living separately. Measures included demographics, social anxiety, depression, and suicidality. The researchers discovered that there was a significant association between adolescent social anxiety and parents living separately ($p < .001$), adolescent depression and parents living separately ($p = .030$), and adolescent suicidal ideation and parents living separately ($p < .001$). The researchers emphasized that adolescents and their divorced parents need additional supportive programming.[16]

Research studies have determined that marital conflict and the severity of the conflict and fighting are more important predictors of offspring adjustment than an actual divorce. Buffers to this include having a good relationship with at least one parent or caregiver, parental warmth, sibling support, and having good self-esteem and peer support. Interventions for divorcing families that may be useful include divorce education programs that are often connected to the court. They teach parents how children respond to separation and divorce, as well as the problems linked to continued high levels of conflict. Divorce mediation is an effective alternative to the adversarial process. This may lead to more joint legal custody agreements and reduce conflict. The long-term outcome for divorce with most adolescents is resiliency rather than dysfunction. Nonetheless, some adolescents are a higher risk for problems, including substance abuse.[17]

Substance Use

Parental separation or divorce can be a significant trigger to the onset of substance abuse in adolescents. Noting rising divorce cases in Lebanon, researchers from Lebanon and France investigated the association between the divorce of parents and the rates of smoking and alcohol and internet addiction among Lebanese adolescents. Cross-sectional in design and with a proportionate random sample of Lebanese private schools, the study was conducted between January and May 2019. Two thousand questionnaires were distributed, and 1810 (90.5 percent) were completed and collected. The students ranged in age from 14 to 17 years, with a mean age of 15.42 years; 53.3 percent were female, 74.1 percent were nonsmokers, and 11.9 percent had separated or divorced parents. To avoid input from parents, students completed the questionnaire in their classrooms. The questionnaire included demographic inquiries and measures for internet, alcohol, waterpipe, and nicotine addiction. The researchers learned that the teens whose parents were separated or divorced had higher rates of alcohol (hazardous alcohol disorder), waterpipe, or nicotine addiction; no such differences were seen in the internet addiction test. The researchers underscored the need for health managers and policymakers to develop evidence-based interventions to reduce the risk and consequences of divorce. And parents who have separated or divorced need to learn how to communicate better with their teens to reduce their emotional upset and loneliness.[18]

Could parental separation or divorce affect the timing of an adolescent's first drink? Researchers from Rhode Island and Connecticut examined whether parental separation or divorce accelerated the timing of the first full drink consumed by an adolescent. The cohort consisted of 931 middle school students who were enrolled in a prospective study on drinking initiation and progression; 52 percent of the subjects were female. At baseline, the mean age of the students was 12.2 years. Students noted whether and at what age they consumed a full drink of alcohol. Parental separation or divorce was coded from a parent-reported life events inventory. Other measures included perceived stress, family history of drinking problems, parent drinking, and child psychopathology. The researchers found that the students whose parents were separated or divorced initiated drinking and consumed their first drink earlier than those whose parents were still together. With each year of age, the odds increased. For the female adolescents, the odds were 49 percent higher; for male adolescents, the odds were 31 percent higher. In fact, among all the constructs that they examined, parental separation or divorce in childhood was the strongest predictor of the age of the onset of drinking. While perceived stress and child psychopathology were also related to initiation, neither a family history of drinking problems nor current parental drinking reached a level of significance. Interestingly, separation and divorce had the strongest effects on drinking initiation when the parents drank higher amounts, which supports the belief that the children fare worse when exposed to both separation and divorce and parental modeling of substance use. In addition, prior to the separation or divorce, 92.7 percent of the students had not consumed a full drink.[19]

Would parental separation or divorce affect the early use of a broad number of substances? A team of researchers from the United States, the United Kingdom, and Australia studied the link between early substance involvement and parental separation during childhood and parental alcohol and cannabis dependence. During telephone interviews, data were obtained from 1318 adolescent children from monozygotic or dizygotic Australian twin parents. The children were asked questions about the use of alcohol, cigarettes, and cannabis, including the first and lifetime use of alcohol, history of intoxication, and regular smoking. Measures were also taken to assess parental substance use and a history of parental separation or divorce prior to the offspring's 18th birthday. The researchers determined that having a substance-dependent parent was generally predictive of earlier onset of alcohol use, drinking to intoxication, smoking, regular smoking, and cannabis use. When they controlled for both genetic and environmental risks from parental substance dependence, the researchers noted that parental separation was correlated with early initiation across substance classes, with the effects most notable from ages 10 through 13 years. The researchers commented that in their various approaches, the effects of parental separation remained strong, suggesting that it brings unique risks apart from demographic, familial, and individual-level influences. There is a need to implement prevention programs for very young adolescents whose parents are separated.[20]

Suicidality and Self-Harm

Since divorce increases an adolescent's vulnerability to psychopathology, including depression, some researchers believe that divorce may also increase suicide risk. Researchers from New York designed a study to determine which factors underlie, amplify, or reduce the association between divorce and adolescent completed suicide. They performed a psychological autopsy or analysis on 120 completed suicides of children under the age of 20 years in New York, Connecticut, and New Jersey and compared their findings to a random sample of 147 age-, gender-, and ethnic-matched controls. A subsample of 58 suicide victims and 40 community controls came from nonintact families. The psychological autopsy of those who died by suicide consisted in part of information obtained from a parent, another adult in the household, a sibling, a friend, and one to three teachers. Measures included demographic variables, parent-child relationships, parental psychopathology, and child/adolescent psychiatric diagnoses. The mean age of the victims of suicide in nonintact families was 16.8 years, with over 95 percent between the ages of 10 and 19 years, and majority male. The researchers learned that parental divorce significantly increased suicide risk. Adolescents with completed suicides from intact families were more likely to have a poor relationship with their fathers. The impact of divorce was a significant risk factor for suicide when the father had mood symptoms, substance problems, and/or a history of psychiatric treatment. Nevertheless, the researchers concluded that the impact of separation/divorce on adolescent suicide risk was small; rather, it was more related to parental psychopathology. They felt that the rise in the youth suicide rate in the late 1990s was likely not caused by the rise in the divorce rate.[21]

Still, since parental separation/divorce appears to mildly elevate adolescent suicidality risk, it is important to know if this risk is raised during specific periods of time during childhood and/or adolescence. In 2012, Swedish researchers administered a cross-sectional survey to a stratified random sample of Swedish adults and received 28,028 responses to questions on suicidality, parental separation/divorce, and the respondent's age at the separation/divorce. The children were divided into four categories according to age: 0 to 4 years, 5 to 9 years, 10 to 14 years, and 15 to 18 years. The researchers learned that 12.1 percent of the male adolescents and 15.5 percent of the female adolescents had ever had suicidal ideation, and 3.2 percent of the male adolescents and 5.3 percent of the female adolescents had a suicide attempt. For male and female adolescents, the odds ratio for ever having a suicidal ideation was higher in all subcategories, but this was especially true for those in the 0- to 4-year-old group.[22]

Mortality

Double bereavement refers to the loss of a parent through divorce as well as death. When this occurs, there is a high risk for an adolescent to experience a complicated and prolonged grief and stress overload. A group of researchers from Denmark, Norway, Australia, New Zealand, and Greenland examined how children, adolescents, and young adults react to double bereavement after losing a divorced parent. They observed nine support groups, three of which had six children and adolescents ages 7 to 15 years. Three main themes emerged. First, the children and teens expressed significant concern about navigating through multiple transitions, including the new living arrangements and possibly a new school and friends. The second theme was the potential mental health consequences, such as stress overload from being in two different family worlds and the potential disruptions to their well-being. The third theme was a need for support from two families and a lack of sufficient support from either. It was not clear if the families would offer to include professional support, which was obviously needed. The researchers concluded that when children, adolescents, and young adults must deal with double bereavement, they may have a stress overload and their coping capacity may exceed its limit. Mental health problems and mental health consequences may follow. To promote mental health and coping for adolescents experiencing double bereavement, it is suggested that interventions that provide a broad approach of support for the family be initiated.[23]

Further, researchers from Denmark and Norway found that double bereavement in children is impacted by age, gender, feelings, multiple losses, and custodial loss. There are challenges related to custodial or noncustodial loss. For example, if the custodial parent dies, then the adolescent must seek other living arrangements preferentially from the noncustodial parent. The new custodial parent may not fully understand the distress resulting from the adolescent's bereavement. If the noncustodial parent dies, there may be some lack of understanding of the bereavement issues from the custodial parent. This could result in the adolescent grieving in silence. Thus, there is a higher risk of mental health problems, such as mood disorders, psychosis, depression, and posttraumatic stress disorder, in adolescents experiencing double bereavement. Support interventions, such as family support programs, therapeutic relationships, multidisciplinary support, and surviving parent support, are crucial.[24]

Violence

Researchers from Lebanon, France, and Cyprus examined the association between parental divorce and anger, aggression, and hostility in Lebanese adolescents. Their cross-sectional study used a proportionate random sample to enroll 1810 private school students, aged 12 to 17 years, between January and May 2019. The students were administered a questionnaire in their classrooms; it required about 60 minutes to complete. Measures included sociodemographic questions and the Buss-Perry Scale, which assessed four elements of aggression—physical and verbal aggression, anger, and hostility. The total aggression score was calculated by adding up the four scores. The researchers learned that the mean age of the students was 15.42 years, with 53.3 female, 74.1 percent nonsmokers, and 11.9 percent with divorced parents. Compared to female adolescents, significantly higher mean verbal aggression scores were found in male adolescents. Adolescents who had divorced parents had higher total aggression scores than those who had married parents. The researchers commented that this finding reinforces the theory that stress contributes to anger in young adolescents with divorced parents.[25]

Researchers from the United Kingdom and Denmark evaluated the association between child-parent separation and later risk for violent criminality. They used data from the Danish Civil Registration System, which included people born in Denmark between 1971 and 1997 ($N = 1,346,772$). From birth until the age of 15, child-parent status was noted annually, and the subjects were followed from their 15th birthday until the date of their first violent offense conviction, death, emigration from Denmark, or December 12, 2012, whichever came first. This represented a total of 16.3 million person-years. Analyses were conducted from 2016 to 2017. Danish residents are required by law to inform the authorities of any changes in their permanent address. Child-parent separation status was classified as no separation, paternal separation, maternal separation, and paternal and maternal separation regardless of death or divorce. Information on convictions for violent crimes was obtained from the National Crime Register. A total of 37,415 people (2.8 percent of the cohort) were convicted of a first violent offense, with 33,671 (90 percent) of the offenders being male. More than 93 percent of the study population lived with both parents at the time of birth; that fell to 71 percent at age 15 years. Being separated from a parent at age 15 years was linked to a greater elevation in violent offending risk; the highest risk was seen among those who were separated from both parents at age 15. The only situation in which no elevated risk was observed was among those who never lived with a parent from birth to their 15th birthday. The researchers noted that violence prevention programming, such as professional counseling, mediation services, and intervention programs that promote positive parenting behaviors and tackle the adverse impact of separation, may be useful.[26]

Researchers from the United Kingdom and the United States also examined the correlation between "broken homes" and adult violence. They used data from the Cambridge Study of Delinquent Development, a prospective longitudinal survey of 411 male adolescents born in South London around 1953 and followed for over 40 years. Repeated searches first from the Criminal Records Office and then from the Police National Computer provided information on the number of convictions of the men, their parents, and their siblings. Forty-one percent were convicted of an offense between the ages of 10 and 50 years. Of the 44 men who experienced their parents' marital breakdown up to the age of 14, 31.8 percent had a violent conviction between the ages of 15 and 50. Of those who had parents who remained together, 15.6 percent had a violent conviction. The researchers observed a significant relationship between a child living in a "broken home" up to the age of 14 years and a violent conviction between the ages of 15 and 50 years, and they suggested that these children should have greater access to family counseling and support services.[27]

Treatment and Prevention

Clinicians can play a key role in preventing issues for adolescents dealing with parental separation/divorce. Primary care providers for adolescents should serve as their advocates and carefully consider biopsychosocial issues in their treatment. On occasion, when an adolescent is demonstrating psychosocial issues, such as substance use, mental health changes, or academic problems, issues of marital discord or stress are uncovered. These present an opportunity to refer parents and their teens for counseling that could include individual, family, or group sessions.

Although adolescents are able to understand divorce-related issues, it is natural for them to have difficulty accepting divorce, and they may self-blame and act out with such externalizing problems as substance abuse and/or inappropriate sexual activity or internalizing issues such as anxiety and depression. Participation in peer support groups may be helpful, and both parents should set clear and consistent behavior expectations. This could include similar rules of conduct around the custodial and the noncustodial parent.[28,29]

The New Beginnings Program (NBP) is a theory- and evidence-based preventive intervention that was designed to improve developmental outcomes and protective factors and modify the risks for children whose parents are divorced. Researchers from Arizona used data from a 6-year longitudinal follow-up sample of 240 families who participated in a randomized trial of prevention interventions for divorced families with children ages 15 to 19 years. The program focused on improving the mother-child relationship and, in so doing, led to decreases in the symptoms of internalizing and externalizing problems and improvements in self-esteem in the children and adolescents. The families were divided into three groups: mother-only program (11 sessions on adolescent's postdivorce mental problems, effective discipline, interparental conflict, and father's access to adolescent), mother and child program (11 sessions on improving coping, reducing negative thoughts about divorce-related stressors, and improving mother-adolescent relationship quality), and control group (literature only on divorce adjustment and syllabi). The families were interviewed at pretest (T1), posttest (T2), 3-month follow-up (T3), 6-month follow-up (T4), and 6-year follow-up (T5). The measures included mother-child relationship quality, effective discipline, internalizing and externalizing problems, adolescent substance use, risky sexual behavior, self-esteem, and academic performance. The researchers learned that the NBP improved the quality of the mother-child relationship, which decreased internalizing problems and increased adolescent self-esteem. Likewise, the program increased effective discipline, leading to decreases in adolescent substance use and better academic performance. The researchers concluded that improving the mother-child relationship in divorced families has lasting positive effects, even 6 years later.[30]

After a parental divorce, an adolescent's sense of belonging may be an important protective factor. The sense of belonging is associated with positive outcomes particularly during adolescence. After divorce, there may be changes in an adolescent's family, school, peer group, or neighborhood. These changes can impact the adolescent's sense of belonging and postdivorce adjustment. Both parents should work on facilitating a smooth transition between the adolescent's overlapping worlds by maintaining a cooperative coparenting role.[31]

Conclusion

Parental divorce may have a profound effect on the biopsychosocial domains of adolescents. These include changes in stress levels, internalizing and externalizing symptoms, risky behaviors, and academic performance issues. Parents and clinicians need to be vigilantly aware of these changes and promptly refer the adolescent to the appropriate therapist or health professional.

References

1   Lebowitz ML. Divorce and the American teenager. *Pediatrics.* 1985;76:695–698.
2   Wallerstein JS. Children of divorce: report of a ten-year follow-up of early latency-age children. *Am J Orthopsychiatry.* 2087;57:199–211.
3   Wallerstein JS. The long-term effects of divorce on children: a review. *J Am Acad Child Adolesc Psychiatry.* 1991;30:349–360.
4   Tullius JM, De Kroon MLA, Almansa J, Reijneveld SA. Adolescents' mental health problems increase after parental divorce, not before, and persist until adulthood: a longitudinal TRAILS study. *Eur Child Adolesc Psychiatry.* 2022;31:969–978.
5   Casey BJ, Jones RM, Hare TA. The adolescent brain. *Ann N Y Acad Sci.* 2008;1124:111–126.
6   Huurre T, Junkkari H, Aro H. Long-term psychosocial effects of parental divorce: a follow-up study from adolescence to adulthood. *Eur Arch Psychiatry Clin Neurosci.* 2006;256:256–263.
7   Bernet W, Wamboldt MZ, Narrow WE. Child affected by parental relationship distress. *J Am Acad Child Adolesc Psychiatry.* 2016;55:571–579.
8   Cohen GJ, Weitzman CC. Helping children and families deal with divorce and separation. *Pediatrics.* 2016;138:e20163020.
9   Estaban O, Rosen M. Marriages and divorces. *Our World in Data.* July 25, 2020.
10 Centers for Disease Control and Prevention, National Center for Health Statistics. National marriage and divorce rate trends for 2000–2022. March 7, 2024.
11 Aughinbaugh A, Robies O, Sun H. Marriage and divorce: patterns by gender, race, and educsitonal attainment. *Monthly Labor Review,* Bureau of Labor Statistics. October 2013.
12 Marttunen MJ, Aro HM, Henriksson MM, Lönnqvist JK. Psychosocial stressors more common in adolescent suicides with alcohol abuse compared with depressive adolescent suicides. *J Am Acad Child Adolesc Psychiatry.* 1994;33:490–497.
13 Størksen IE, Røysammb E, Moum T, Tambs K. Adolescents with a childhood experience of parental divorce: a longitudinal study of mental health and adjustment. *J Adolesc.* 2005;28:725–739.
14 Schaano VK, Schulz A, Schächinger H, Vögele C. Parental divorce is associated with an increased risk to develop mental disorders in women. *J Affect Disord.* 2019;257:91–99.
15 Di Manno L, MacDonald JA, Knight T. Family dissolution and offspring depression and depressive symptoms: a systematic review of moderation effects. *J Affect Disord.* 2015;188:68–79.
16 Obeid S, Karaki G, Haddad C, et al. Association between parental divorce and mental health outcomes among Lebanese adolescents: results of a national study. *BMC Pediatr.* 2021;21:455.
17 Kelly JB. Children's adjustment in conflicted marriage and divorce: a decade review of research. *J Am Acad Child Adolesc Psychiatry.* 2000;39:963–973.
18 Jabbour N, Rached V, Haddad C, et al. Association between parental separation and addictions in adolescents: results of a national Lebanese study. *BMC Public Health.* 2020;20:965.
19 Jackson KM, Rogers ML, Sartor CE. Parental divorce and initiation of alcohol use in early adolescence. *Psychol Addict Behav.* 2016;30:450–461.

20 Waldron M, Grant JD, Bucholz KK, et al. Parental separation and early substance involvement: results from children of alcoholic and cannabis dependent twins *Drug Alcohol Depend.* 2014;134:78–84.

21 Gould MS, Shaffer D, Fisher P, Garfinkel R. Separation/divorce and child and adolescent completed suicide. *J Am Acad Child Adolesc Psychiatry.* 1998;37:155–162.

22 Lindström M, Rosvall M. Parental separation in childhood, social capital, and suicide thoughts and suicide attempts: A population-based study. *Psychiatry Res.* 2015;229:206–213.

23 Marcussen J, Thuen F, O'Connor M, Wilson RL, Hounsgaard L. Double bereavement, mental health consequences and support needs of children and young adults when a divorced parent dies. *J Clin Nurs.* 2020;29:1238–1253.

24 Marcussen J, Thuen F, Bruun P, et al. Parental divorce and parental death—an integrative systematic review of children's double bereavement. *Clin Nurs Stud.* 2015;3:103–111.

25 Zakhour M, Haddad C, Salameh P, et al. Association between parental divorce and anger, aggression and hostility in adolescents: results of a national Lebanese study. *J Fam Issues.* 2023;44:587–609.

26 Mok PLH, Astrup A, Carr MJ, Antonsen S, Webb RT, Pedersen CB. Experience of child-parent separation and later risk of violent criminality. *Am J Prev Med.* 2018;55:178–186.

27 Theobald D, Farrington, D, Piquero A. Childhood broken homes and adult violence: an analysis of moderators and mediators. *J Crim Justice.* 2013;41:44–52.

28 Kleinsorge C, Covitz LM. Impact of divorce on children: developmental considerations. *Pediatr Rev.* 2012;33:147–154.

29 Cohen GJ, Weitzman CC, Committee on Psychosocial Aspects of Child and Family Health; Section on Developmental and Behavioral Pediatrics. Helping children and families deal with divorce and separation. *Pediatrics.* 2016;138:e20163020.

30 McClain DB, Wolchik SA, Winslow E, Tein JY, Sandler IN, Millsap RE. Developmental cascade effects of the New Beginnings Program on adolescent adaptation outcomes. *Dev Psychopathol.* 2010;22:771–784.

31 Rajaan Z, van der Valk I, Schrama W, et al. Adolescents' post-divorce sense of belonging: an interdisciplinary review. *Eur Psychol.* 2022;27:277–290.

16

Bereavement and Mortality

Introduction

The World Health Organization estimated that more than 10 million children world-wide lost a parent or caregiver to COVID-19 through May 1, 2022, and 7.5 million became orphans during the same time period.[1] The loss of a parent or a primary caregiver such as a grandparent is not an uncommon occurrence for children and adolescents. It has been estimated by the U.S. Census Bureau that 4.3 percent of children and adolescents lose a parent or guardian by the age of 17 years.[2] The loss challenges those adolescents with short-term grief and long-term emotional and economic support that may require significant adaptation. That said, most adolescents are resilient and do well.

Approximately one-fifth of American children live in a multigenerational household, defined as having a grandparent, parent, and child.[3] In about one-third of multigenerational households, grandparents are the adults who assume most of the responsibility for the basic needs of their grandchildren since the parents are employed and childcare is expensive. The death of a grandparent in these households, especially if the grandparents offered significant support to the adolescent, is similar to a parental loss.[4]

It is normal for adolescents to grieve after parental loss for at least 1 year. While they may have symptoms of depression, they do not necessarily have diagnosable depression. Eventually, 1 year after a death, most adolescents will have accepted the loss of a parent or grandparent. However, about 5 to 10 percent may experience grief that persists for longer than 12 to 18 months. Prolonged grief may increase the risk of subsequent problems, including anxiety, depression, suicidality, substance use, and/or the symptoms of posttraumatic stress disorder (PTSD).[5-7]

While the loss of either parent will have a negative effect on adolescent health, most research studying the loss of a parent in adolescence focuses on paternal loss. In many families, paternal death may negatively influence the family's socioeconomic status, and this may impact where the family lives, the schools the children attend, and the pursuit of a higher education. Moving may disconnect adolescents from their peers, schools, coaches, and teachers, who may be important resources for adolescents dealing with an adverse event. Such cascading negative events may present still more challenges to the adolescent. And families who had preexisting inequality, such as poverty or the lack of a higher education, have less ability to adapt to parental loss. In those families, the adolescent has a higher chance of future problems.[8]

Researchers from Sweden and England examined the association between childhood parental death and school outcomes for adolescents who were 15 and 16 years old. They obtained their data from a population-based sibling cohort from the Swedish Medical Birth Register that included all children born in Sweden between

1991 and 2000. The data on these children were linked to data of their parents. Since the researchers were able to connect the children to parents who died before the child was 17 years, they compared their educational level to older siblings who were not bereaved while still in school as well as to nonbereaved children. The researchers learned that the bereaved adolescents had lower average school grades and an increased risk of being ineligible for higher education compared to nonbereaved adolescents. And when they were evaluated with their older siblings, the younger siblings had lower mean school grade averages. The researchers concluded that losing a parent at a younger age was associated with lower academic grades.[9]

The deceased parent's mental health may be a contributing factor to the adolescent's risk for mental health issues. Researchers in Pennsylvania evaluated psychiatric issues that increased the risk of sudden parental death and how this death affected the psychiatric health of the children. They recruited 140 bereaved families in which a parent died suddenly by suicide, accident, or natural causes. Each family had biological offspring between the ages of 7 and 25 years, with 76 percent between 12 and 17 years. The control group consisted of 99 families with parents and offspring living at home. Interviews were conducted with both groups; the interviews with the deceased parent group were conducted about 9 months after the death. The offspring also completed questionnaires. When they compared the parents who died from suicide, accident, or sudden natural death to the control group parents, the researchers learned that the parents who died had a significantly higher ($p < .001$) prevalence of bipolar disease, alcohol/substance abuse, and personality disorder. Their offspring had significantly higher rates of new-onset depression, PTSD, or another psychiatric disorder. The researchers noted that bereaved offspring were at increased risk for adverse mental health outcomes after a sudden parental death in part because of factors that may have contributed to the parent's death.[10]

Given the psychological toll on adolescents from parental death, researchers from Denmark, Sweden, Finland, and the United States wondered if early parental death increased the risk of premature death of offspring. Using data from the three Nordic countries, they examined the association between parental death during an offspring's childhood and adolescence and subsequent mortality risk for the offspring. They established a population-based cohort of over 7 million people born between 1968 and 2008. Over 189,000 children in the cohort lost a parent before the age of 18 years; this was termed the exposed cohort. Those that did not lose a parent before the age of 18 were termed the unexposed cohort. The researchers discovered that 29,683 children and adolescents of both cohorts died during the follow-up period, which was up to 42 years. Compared to the unexposed cohort, the exposed cohort had a 50 percent higher risk of all-cause mortality. The higher risk for mortality in the exposed cohort persisted into early adulthood. The researchers believed that genetics played only a small role in this increased risk for mortality. Rather, biological-genetic susceptibility and psychosocial behavioral mechanisms and early life adversities, such as the death of a parent, appeared to negatively impact the future health and social well-being of children and adolescents. For example, the increased risk of death could be caused by shared social or economic disadvantages. These findings suggested that after a parental death, bereaved children and adolescents should receive health and social support, and this could be necessary for an extended period of time.[11]

Adolescents also face issues that arise when a nonparent custodial caregiver dies. As has been noted, in the United States, a significant number of children and adolescents are being raised in households headed by grandparents, who are older and may well have their own physical and/or mental health issues. Researchers at the U.S. Department of Health and Human Services were interested to determine if children in these households received timely preventive and specialty care. Using data from the National Survey of Children's Health across 4 years, they assembled a sample of 3464 children from grandparent-led households and 113,907 children from parent-led households. In grandparent-led households, most of the caregivers were female; the mean age of the grandparents was 59.9 years, compared to 41.6 years in the parent-led households. Compared to parent-led households, children in grandparent-led households had increased health problems, including oral health, overweight/obesity ($p = .0002$), and emotional, mental, and developmental health conditions, such as depression, behavioral issues, and attention-deficit/hyperactivity disorder ($p \leq .0001$). Further, they had statistically fewer visits for preventive checkups, preventive dental visits, and specialty care. It is not clear if the grandparents' health conditions impacted their ability to bring the adolescents to medical care. Therefore, adolescents with these health issues who are cared for in a grandparent-led household may be at risk for adequate care.[12]

Looking at mortality, there is a disturbing trend for children and adolescents. All causes of mortality in this age group increased by 10.7 percent between 2019 and 2020; mortality increased by 8.3 percent between 2020 and 2021. Most of the upsurge was due to mortality in the 10 to 19 age range. Most of the increased mortality was due to injuries, not COVID-19. Suicides in the 10 to 19 age range began to increase in 2007, and homicide rates started to increase in 2013. By 2019, suicide rates had increased by 69.5 percent and homicide rates by 32.7 percent. From 2019 to 2020, injury mortality in the 10 to 19 age group increased by 22.6 percent and was especially increased by homicides and deaths from drug overdoses. Racial and ethnic disparities were noted across the injuries. The causes for the increasing mortality in the adolescent age range included depression, suicidality, opioid use, systemic racism, widening inequities, and societal conflict and violence. These issues are discussed in other chapters.[13]

Epidemiology

The U.S. Census Bureau reports that fathers die earlier in their children's lives than mothers. By the age of 19 years, about 5 percent of adolescents have lost their fathers and 2 percent have lost their mothers. There are differences in the timing of parental mortality across racial groupings. For those under 18 years, adolescents who are non-Hispanic Black and Hispanic are more likely to have lost one or both parents than those adolescents who are non-Hispanic Asian and non-Hispanic White. These disparities in mortality can impact adolescents in the biopsychosocial domains. Social-economic status, including poverty status, may influence the timing of parental loss. The more impoverished the family, the greater the likelihood that an adolescent under age 18 years will have lost one or both parents. The reasons include but are not limited to the following: lower-income individuals experience health care inequity, tend to be sicker, and may be subject to increased stressors. These issues are discussed in Chapter 14. Those living in more prosperous households lose their parents later in life.[14]

The Childhood Bereavement Estimate Model projects the percentage of children by ethnic group who will lose a parent by the age of 18. The data indicate the following percentages for adolescent offspring: Black, 7.9 percent; Native American/Alaska Native, 6.9 percent; White, 6.0 percent; Asian or Pacific Islander, 2.9 percent. These data document mortality disparities that, combined with other issues such as poverty, can further impact the biopsychosocial domains in certain groups of adolescents.[15]

Biopsychosocial Issues and Bereavement/Mortality

Biological Issues and Bereavement/Mortality

Obesity

There appears to be a relationship between elevated body mass index (BMI) and bereavement in adolescents. Researchers from Pennsylvania studied the correlation between parental bereavement and BMI in 123 bereaved offspring and 122 nonbereaved children. They hypothesized that the bereaved children would have higher BMI levels and that the offspring who had depression before or after the death or who had caregivers with depression would be more likely to have obesity, compared to bereaved offspring without these psychiatric issues. At baseline, the offspring were 6 to 20 years old; at the 5-year follow-up, they were 11 to 25 years old. Measures included psychiatric diagnosis status and BMI at follow-up. The researchers determined that the bereaved offspring were more likely than the nonbereaved to have a BMI in the obese range ($p < .01$). The cause of death did not make a significant difference. Of note, in the nonbereaved group, offspring with caregivers who had a history of depression were more likely to have a BMI in the obese range. It is evident that bereaved adolescents have an increased risk for obesity. To prevent excessive weight gain, these teens should be monitored for their diet and physical activity. It may be useful for bereaved offspring to have preventive education about stress, negative emotions, and eating behaviors.[16]

The finding that obesity may be linked with bereavement in adolescents was confirmed in a larger study published 3 years later in 2016. A team in Minnesota proposed the theory that there is an association between obesity in adolescents and adverse childhood experiences (ACEs). They used data from the 2011–2012 National Survey of Children's Health, a cross-sectional survey of U.S households with at least one child or adolescent under age 18. The study group included 43,863 children aged 10 years or older. Data obtained included the child's height and weight. One of the ACEs was the death of a parent. The results suggested that after the death of a parent, an adolescent should be monitored for biopsychosocial changes including increases in BMI. The researchers determined that in the study subjects, the death of a parent (odds ratio 1.59; 95 percent CI 1.18–2.15) was independently linked with obesity after adjustment for other ACEs and sociodemographic factors.[17]

Psychological Issues and Bereavement/Mortality

One can expect psychological issues after an adolescent experiences the death of a parent. Researchers in Alabama studied children and adolescents who had lost a parent, experienced a tornado disaster, or were coping with an ongoing social or academic stressor. The subjects completed measures for anxiety, depression, and PTSD. The results indicated that parentally bereaved children and adolescents demonstrated significantly more symptoms than the other two groups. In particular, bereaved girls whose surviving parent scored high on a PTSD measure were at greater risk for PTSD symptoms. This study suggests that bereaved adolescents may be at increased risk for PTSD.[18]

A paper published a decade later confirmed psychological issues in adolescents after parental bereavement. The Great Smoky Mountains Study was a longitudinal epidemiological study of psychiatric disorders in youth; it had an initial random sample of 4390 adolescents who lived in western North Carolina. Using data from this study, researchers in Michigan, California, and North Carolina investigated the psychiatric symptoms in youth ages 11 to 21 years who were parent bereaved or not parent bereaved. For the parent-bereaved youth, psychiatric symptoms were appraised by the Child and Adolescent Psychiatric Assessment during the wave before death, during the death, and during the wave after death. The waves were about 2 years apart. For the nonbereaved adolescents, a year was selected randomly for symptom review. The researchers found that the loss of a parent was related to psychiatric symptoms above and beyond sociodemographic variables and previous psychiatric symptoms. Compared to the nonbereaved group, during the death wave, the bereaved adolescents had symptoms of separation anxiety but were not more likely to show symptoms of depression. However, during the wave after death, parent-bereaved adolescents were more likely to have symptoms of a conduct disorder, exhibit substance use problems, and have greater functional impairment. The researchers concluded that even controlling for preexisting risk factors, parent-bereaved adolescents were at increased risk for psychological and behavior health problems for several years after parental death.[19]

Eating Disorders

The death of a parent is one of the most traumatic events that can occur to an adolescent. Like other profoundly transformative events, such trauma has the potential to trigger an eating disorder. Researchers in Norway wanted to determine if parental death by an external cause, such as suicide, accident, drowning, or falling, during an offspring's childhood or adolescence increased the risk of the offspring's psychiatric disorders. Using data from four longitudinal Norwegian registers that provided links with parents, causes of death, and their offspring, they sampled Norwegian residents born between 1970 and 2012 who had links to both parents in the registers. The cohort comprised 655,477 individuals. Since the researchers had information on psychiatric diagnoses, they could connect the offspring, their diagnoses, parents and their causes of death, and specific dates for events. The researchers found that the children and adolescents who had lost a parent to an external cause had a significantly increased risk for a wide range of psychiatric disorders, but not eating disorders, specifically anorexia nervosa, bulimia, and overeating disorder. So at least in this study, there was no association between parental death by external causes and the specified eating disorders.[20]

Suicidality

It is believed that between 7000 and 12,000 children and adolescents lose a parent by suicide each year in the United States: Are these youth at risk for their own psychiatric issues, including their own suicidality?[21] To understand the correlation between parental death and the risks of offspring for suicide, hospitalization for a suicide attempt, and/or a major psychiatric disorder, researchers in Maryland, Sweden, and Pennsylvania used a Swedish national total population cohort with data from 1969 to 2004. The cohort consisted of 503,000 offspring of parents who died by suicide, accident, or other cause. Matched to these offspring were 3.8 million children whose parents were alive. The offspring of the decedents were divided into three age groups: 0 to 12 years, 13 to 17 years, and 18 to 25 years. For the 13 to 17 group, the children of a parent who died by suicide had an incidence rate ratio of 3.1 (95 percent CI 2.1–4.6); that means that the offspring in this group were three times more likely to die from suicide than the offspring in the same age group in which the parents were alive. For the 18 to 25 age group, that figure was 1.9. In contrast, for the 13 to 17 age group, the offspring whose parents died by accident had a risk of 1.1 for their own suicide, and for those whose parents died by other causes, the risk was 0.9. The data also indicated that the children whose parents died by suicide had a significantly elevated risk for their own hospitalization for a suicide attempt and depression and warranted close observation during adolescence.[22]

Are there long-term suicidal risks for offspring when a parent dies during their childhood? Researchers in Denmark, Finland, and Sweden used population-based cohorts from all three countries for the period 1968 to 2008 to identify children who lost a parent by death before the age of 18 years. Each of the 189,094 children were matched with 10 children who did not have a parent die before 18. The researchers, who followed both groups for up to 25 years, measured the incidence of suicides among these children. During the 25 years, 265 of the bereaved (0.14 percent) and 1342 of the nonbereaved (0.07 percent) died from suicide. The risk was highest for those who lost a parent before the age of 6 years, and the risk remained high for at least 25 years. The absolute risk of suicide was 4 in 1000 persons for bereaved males and 2 in 1000 persons for nonbereaved males; for females, the absolute risk of suicide was 2 for bereaved and 1 for nonbereaved. Adolescent survivors of suicide decedents were at a threefold greater risk for suicide, while young adults were at no increased risk. This study underscores the need for public health strategies and initiatives that focus on families with a history of suicidality and the need to monitor distress in bereaved children and adolescents.[23,24]

Social Issues and Bereavement/Mortality

Social Media

Facebook provides a unique platform for adolescents who are mourning the loss of a peer as it can serve as a community for grieving individuals. These adolescents develop a connection through the platform that helps to facilitate relationships between one another. In addition, the digital space of the decedent's profile page remains the same in appearance after death as it did while they were living. Adolescents produce memorial posts that tend to speak directly to the deceased, respond to other group members.[25]

While the death of a parent or grandparent deeply affects adolescents, the death of a friend or peer can also have negative outcomes. Given the important role that social media plays in the lives of adolescents, social media may be able to help bereaved adolescents process their emotions. Researchers from Oklahoma examined how online social networking affected adolescent grieving following the sudden death of a peer. The researchers studied 20 online social networking profiles authored by adolescents between the ages of 15 and 19, 70 percent male, who had died suddenly, as well as the online responses from their friends. For the 20 profiles, there were 3721 listed friends and 1167 adolescents posting 4780 comments over 12 months. The researchers observed that the adolescents directed their comments to their deceased friend. They wrote memorial statements, talked about current events or reminisced, and demonstrated indicators of coping strategies. The researchers commented that by allowing the adolescents to prolong their attachment to the decreased person, the online networking sites appeared to facilitate the adolescents' ability to reflect on their relationship with the deceased, thereby helping them to cope with bereavement.[26]

Refugees and Immigration

The World Health Organization estimates that between the years 2030 and 2050, there will be 250,000 annual deaths in the elderly from heat exposure caused by climate change. There will be additional deaths due to infectious diseases such as malaria and due to flooding. Many of these deaths can occur in lower-income countries, where climate change can bring on migration and refugee status.[27] Due to reductions in the availability of food by 2050, there may be an additional 736,000 adult deaths. Many of these people may well be parents or grandparents of adolescents. Aggressive effects to mitigate climate change must become far more widespread.[28]

As mentioned in the introduction to this chapter, recently there has been an increasing rate of mortality among adolescents in the 10-to-19-year age group. Hoping to learn more about the association between immigration status in childhood and adolescence and mortality, researchers from Michigan used data from the Swedish Work and Mortality Database, which contains a rich array of demographic information. Using the database, they were able to compare Swedish-born children of immigrants and non-Swedish-born children of immigrants on measures including family characteristics, such as mother's level of education, birth region, birth year, and generational status disaggregated by arrival age. The researchers learned that compared to Swedish-born children, the foreign-born children had a 16 to 17 percent higher death risk through adulthood; analysis indicated that the higher mortality risk was due to a number of external and nonexternal causes of death. This higher mortality rate included all ages of children including adolescence, but it was particularly notable in infants to age 7 years. The researchers concluded that for children under the age of 19 years, being foreign born was correlated with increased rates of death.[29]

Violence

Parental death can cause long-term issues for adolescents, including anxiety, depression, PTSD, substance use, and even violence. Researchers in the United Kingdom and Denmark hypothesized that the greatest risk for violence is found among the offspring of a parent who died from suicide or if both parents died during the adolescent's childhood. They used interlinked Denmark national registries to study residents born between 1970 and 2000, as well as information on the cause of death of the parents and self-harm or criminality. All of the children who were age 15 years or older who had a parent die were included in the cohort, and they were followed from their 15th birthday. The researchers discovered that 52,589 children and adolescents (3.1 percent of the children/adolescent population) had lost a parent by the age of 15. Suicide was the cause of death for 0.5 percent of the parents. With an adjusted hazard ratio of 1.0 for adolescents with both parents living, there was an elevated adjusted hazard ratio of 1.43 to 1.95 for adolescent self-harm if they lost one or both parents, with the highest ratio for those who lost both parents by any cause. Moreover, the researchers observed that the adjusted hazard ratios were elevated to 1.46 to 2.18 for violent criminality. It appeared that the self-harm and violent criminality risks between mid-adolescence and early middle age were elevated for all categories of people who experienced parental death during childhood. The associations were stronger among younger people who had to deal with an unnatural death such as suicide. The researchers commented that early intervention is indicated to help affected children and adolescents develop coping strategies to deal with the immediate crisis and recognize that the impact of parental death could be delayed for years. They also suggested that there be an enhanced level of cooperation between health, social service, and criminal justice agencies to help mitigate the elevated risks for detrimental behaviors as adolescents transition into adulthood.[30] In a previously cited study from Scandinavia, researchers found that parental death of any cause before the child's 26th birthday increased the risk for violent criminal convictions in the offspring. The researchers noted that the death of a parent is often associated with socioeconomic disruption and less care or supervision for the offspring.[31]

Intervention and Prevention

Since there is an increased risk for mental health and psychosocial issues for adolescents who lose a parent, intervention and prevention programs are of great importance. Researchers from Sweden performed a systematic review of such programs that included 17 studies published between 1985 and 2015; most of these were randomized controlled trials of children from school age to 18 years. There were group meetings for children, family interventions, parental guidance, and camp activities. Most studies focused on the child and the remaining caregiver and tended to be brief, such as two sessions over three days. One program continued for a year. Two studies demonstrated efficacy between the experimental and control groups, while four studies showed moderate results. The researchers concluded that relatively brief interventions may help prevent children from developing more severe problems after the loss of a parent.[32]

Researchers from Arizona reviewed the Family Bereavement Program (FBP), a 12-month intervention for parentally bereaved children between the ages of 8 and 16 years. It included 184 families living in the Phoenix area with children who lost a biological parent or parent figure 4 to 30 months before the study. The child and surviving parent were assessed at baseline, at the end of the study, and at an 11-month follow-up. The experimental arm included a parent guidance group that attempted to increase the positive qualities of the parent-child relationship, decrease mental health problems of the caregiver, lower the child's exposure to negative events, and improve effective discipline. The control arm consisted of parent telephone monitoring. The researchers determined that the FBP quickly improved family and individual risk and protective factors. At the 11-month follow-up, the FBP led to reduced internalizing and externalizing problems in female adolescents and for those who had poorer scores at baseline. There were improvements in parenting, coping, and caregiver mental health. Clearly, as this study shows, there are ways to mitigate the profound problems associated with parental loss.[33]

The Writing for Recovery group intervention is a treatment approach developed by the Children and War Foundation to assist traumatized and bereaved adolescents after disasters. Researchers from Iran, the United Kingdom, and Norway studied the efficacy of this intervention in 12- to 18-year-old bereaved Afghani refugees. These adolescents were screened using the Traumatic Grief Inventory for Children (TGIC); 61 were randomly assigned to either an experimental group ($n = 29$) or a control group ($n = 32$). The 15-minute Writing for Recovery program was administered in school, two times a day for 3 consecutive days. The adolescents were asked to write about their innermost feelings and thoughts on their traumatic losses, or they were told to reflect on what advice they would have given another person in the same situation. The control group had no interventions. The range of time from the loss was 2 to 19 years, with a mean of 10.77 years (SD = 3.710). Scores on the TGIC in the posttest experimental group decreased significantly from 56.3 to 44.9 ($p < .001$) and increased in the control group from 49.9 to 53.9. According to the researchers, these findings confirmed the underlying hypothesis that writing about traumatic experiences may alleviate grief symptoms in these bereaved adolescents over the short term.[34]

Conclusion

The death of a parent, grandparent, sibling, or peer is a devastating experience for adolescents. Although most teens do well and recover, 5 to 10 percent may have persisting emotional problems for years and may be at risk for self-harm. Adolescents who are bereaved need close observation by parents, teachers, and clinicians for biopsychosocial issues related to their loss.

With respect to increasing mortality in adolescents, the underlying causes need to be examined; policy and preventive efforts are urgently needed. Firearm deaths led to a substantial increase in overall adolescent mortality in 2020, so it is critical for all groups to understand gun violence and to work together to develop sensible firearm policies.

References

1   Hillis S, N'konzi JN, Msemburi W, et al. Orphanhood and caregiver loss among children based on new global excess COVID-19 death estimates. *JAMA Pediatr.* 2022;176:1145–1148.

2   Hayward GM. New 2021 data visualization shows parent mortality: 44.2% had lost at least one parent. United States Census Bureau, Washington DC. March 21, 2023.

3   Cohn D, Horowitz JM, Minkin R, Fry R, Hurst K. The demographics of multigenerational households. Pew Research Center, Washington, DC. March 24, 2022.

4   Teglia D, Cutuli J, Arasteh K, et al. *Hidden Pain: Children Who Lost a Parent or Caregiver to COVID-19 and What the Nation Can Do to Help Them.* COVID Collaborative; 2021.

5   Berg L, Rostila M, Hjern A. Parental death during childhood and depression in young adults—a national cohort study. *J Child Psychol Psychiatry.* 2016;57:1092–1098.

6   Keyes KM, Pratt C, Galea S, McLaughlin KA, Koenen KC, Shear MK. The burden of loss: unexpected death of a loved one and psychiatric disorders across the life course in a national study. *Am J Psychiatry.* 2014;171:864–871.

7   Simbi CMC, Zhang Y, Wang Z. Early parental loss in childhood and depression in adults: a systematic review and meta-analysis of case-controlled studies. *J Affect Disord.* 2020;260:272–280.

8   Herbers JE, Hayes KR, Cutuli JJ. Adaptive systems for student resilience in the context of COVID-19. *Sch Psychol.* 2021;36:422–426.

9   Liu C, Grotta A, Hiyoshi A, Berg L, Rostila M. School outcomes among children following death of a parent. *JAMA Netw Open.* 2022;5:e223842.

10 Melhem NM, Walker M, Moritz G, Brent DA. Antecedents and sequelae of sudden parental death in offspring and surviving caregivers. *Arch Pediatr Adolesc Med.* 2008;162:403–404.

11 Li J, Vestergaard M, Cnattingius S, et al. Mortality after parental death in childhood: a nationwide cohort study from three Nordic countries. *PLOS Med.* 2014;11:e1001679.

12 Joshi DS, Lebrun-Harris LA. Child health status and health care use in grandparent- versus parent-led households. *Pediatrics.* 2022;150:e2021055291.

13 Woolf SH, Wolf ER, Rivara FP. The new crisis of increasing all-cause mortality in US children and adolescents. *JAMA.* 2023;329:975–976.

14 Scherer Z. Parental mortality is linked to a variety of socio-economic and demographic factors. United States Census Bureau, Washington, DC. May 6, 2019.

15 Burns M, Briese B, King S, Talmi A. Childhood bereavement: understanding prevalence and related adversity in the United States. *Am J Orthopsychiatry.* 2020;90:391–405.

16 Weinberg, RJ, Dietz LJ, Stoyak S, et al. A prospective study of parentally bereaved youth, caregiver depression, and body mass index. *J Clin Psychiatry.* 2013;74:834–840.

17 Lynch BA, Agunwamba A, Wilson PM, et al. Adverse family experiences and obesity in children and adolescents in the United States. *Prev Med.* 2016;90:148–154.

18 Stoppelbein L, Greening L. Posttraumatic stress symptoms in parentally bereaved children and adolescents. *J Am Acad Child Adolesc Psychiatry.* 2000;39:1112–1119.

19 Kaplow J, Saunders J, Angold A, Costello EJ. Psychiatric symptoms in bereaved versus non-bereaved youth and young adults: a longitudinal epidemiological study. *J Am Acad Child Adolesc Psychiatry.* 2010;49:1145–1154.

20 Burrell LV, Mehlum L, Qin P. Parental death by external causes during childhood and risk of psychiatric disorders in bereaved offspring. *Child Adolesc Ment Health.* 2022;27:122–130.

21 Cerel J, Jordan JR, Duberstein PR. The impact of suicide on the family. *Crisis.* 2008;29:38–44.

22 Kuramoto SJ, Stuart EA, Runeson B, Lichtenstein P, Langstrom N, Wilcox HC. Maternal or paternal suicide and offspring's psychiatric and suicide-attempt hospitalization risk. *Pediatrics.* 2010;126:e1026–e1032.

23   Wilcox HC, Kuramoto SJ, Lichtenstein, Langstrom N, Brent DA, Runeson B. Psychiatric morbidity, violent crime, and suicide among children and adolescents exposed to parental death. *J Am Acad Child Adolesc Psychiatry.* 2010;49:514–523.

24   Guldin MB, Li J, Pedersen HS, et al. Incidence of suicide among persons who had a parent who died during their childhood: a population-based cohort study. *JAMA Psychiatry.* 2015;72:1227–1234.

25   Frost M. The grief grapevine: Facebook memorial pages and adolescent bereavement. *Aust J Guid Couns.* 2014;24:256–265.

26   Williams A, Merten M. Adolescents' online social networking following the death of a peer. *J Adolesc Res.* 2009;24:67–90.

27   Goldstein MA. Climate change and its effects on children and adolescents: a call to action. *Curr Pediatr Rep.* 2022;10:55–56.

28   Haines A, Ebi K. The imperative for climate action to protect health. *N Engl J Med.* 2019;380:263–273.

29   Mehta NK, Martikainem P, Cederström A. Age of immigration, generational status, and death among children of immigrant mothers: a longitudinal analysis of siblings. *Am J Epidemiol.* 2019;188:1237–1244.

30   Carr MJ, Mok PLH, Antonsen S, Pedersen CB, Webb RT. Self-harm and violent criminality linked with parental death during childhood. *Psychol Med.* 2020;50:1224–1232.

31   Wilcox HC, Kuramoto SJ, Lichtenstein P, Langstrom N, Brent DA, Runeson B. Psychiatric morbidity, violent crime, and suicide among children and adolescents exposed to parental death. *J Am Acad Child Adolesc Psychiatry.* 2010;49:514–523.

32   Bergman AS, Axberg U, Hanson E. When a parent dies—a systematic review of the effects of support programs for parentally bereaved children and their caregivers. *BMC Palliat Care.* 2017;16:39.

33   Sandler IN, Ayers TS, Wolchik SA, et al. The family bereavement program: efficacy evaluation of a theory-based prevention program for parentally bereaved children and adolescents. *J Consult Clin Psychol.* 2003;71:587–600.

34   Kalantari M, Yule W, Dyregrov A, Neshatdoost N, Ahmadi SJ. Efficacy of writing for recovery on traumatic grief symptoms of Afghani refugee bereaved adolescents: a randomized control trial. *Omega (Westport).* 2012;65:139–150.

PART IV
CURRENT EVENTS

17

COVID-19

Introduction

As of June 28, 2023, over 1.136 million people had died from COVID-19 in the United States. Although COVID-19 is not fatal for the majority of adolescents, with the number of deaths of children and adolescents between the ages of 5 and 18 years in the United States at 1,071, the disease can still have profound effects on adolescent health.[1]

Most adolescents who test positive for COVID-19 have either mild or no symptoms. Some develop what is called long COVID, which may involve multiple organ systems with symptoms that include fatigue, shortness of breath, headache, heart palpitations, chest pain, abdominal pain, and diarrhea. Mental health symptoms may include memory loss, depression, concentration problems, visual hallucinations, and confusion.[2] It is not clear why some develop long COVID, but it is evident that the COVID-19 pandemic and the responses of society may cause biological, psychological, and social issues in adolescents, whether they test positive or negative.

In response to the COVID-19 pandemic, the American Academy of Pediatrics declared a national emergency in children's mental health. The rate of mental health issues among adolescents had been increasing for a decade even before the pandemic, but with the pandemic-related school closures, social distancing, economic issues, uncertainty, fear, and grief, matters have only worsened. Compared to the same period in 2019, visits to emergency departments by females ages 12 to 17 years for suspected suicide attempts were up by 51 percent in 2021.

COVID-19 has also been linked to adverse mental health effects for adolescents, including anxiety and depression. In 2021, Canadian researchers estimated the global prevalence of child and adolescent anxiety and depression symptoms during the pandemic and compared them to prepandemic estimates. Using published and unpublished studies, they calculated from pooled estimates obtained in the first year of the pandemic that one in four youth globally experienced clinically elevated depression symptoms, while one in five youth had clinically elevated anxiety symptoms. These estimates were double those of prepandemic values.[3] A year later, researchers in California studied 163 adolescents (63.2 percent female) who were in a larger longitudinal study assessing the effects of early life stress on psychobiology across puberty with data collected before and after the pandemic shutdowns. For this study, they evaluated the youth for anxiety and internal and external symptoms. A subset (128) had a magnetic resonance imaging scan. They found that the youth studied after the pandemic shutdowns had more severe internalizing mental health problems, reduced brain cortical thickness, larger hippocampal and amygdala volume, and more advanced brain age. They concluded that the pandemic had adversely affected the mental health of the subjects, and the youth had neuroanatomical changes that were more typical of individuals who were older and had experienced significant adversity in childhood. It appeared that the pandemic had accelerated their brain maturation. It is still too early to understand the clinical implications of these changes in their brain growth.[4]

Epidemiology

Given the prevalence of COVID-19 and the relaxation of pandemic restrictions, it is reasonable to assume that most adolescents have been exposed to this virus. The Centers for Disease Control and Prevention (CDC) reported that as of February 2022, approximately 75 percent of children and adolescents had serologic evidence of a previous infection with the virus causing COVID-19, with about one-third becoming newly positive between December 2021 and February 2022.[5] The CDC has epidemiological data on death of children and adolescents ages 5 to 18 years. Of the reported deaths from COVID-19, a disproportionately higher percentage were in Black and Hispanic children and adolescents than White children and adolescents.[6] Some of the drivers for these racial/ethnic disparities are social determinants of health. In addition, access to quality inpatient and outpatient care, nutrition, and medical vulnerabilities should be considered.[7]

Biopsychosocial Issues and COVID-19

Biological Issues and COVID-19

Sleep

Researchers in Ohio performed a prospective study of the sleep changes in adolescents that occurred during the COVID-19 pandemic. They investigated certain sleep behaviors, including sleep patterns and duration, delayed sleep/wake times, and daytime sleepiness, in 122 adolescents between the ages of 15 and 17 years. The study was divided into two sections: prepandemic (September 2019 to February 2020) and during the pandemic (May to June 2020). The study included input from parents, who noted that their teens had more difficulty initiating and maintaining sleep during the pandemic than they had before the pandemic began. The adolescents also reported later shifts in bedtime and wake time. However, the teens observed that they had longer sleep durations and less daytime sleepiness during the pandemic. Thus, the pandemic had positive and negative impacts on sleep, though the researchers commented that just because the teens slept longer did not mean the quality of their sleep improved.[8]

Another sleep study was performed by a group of researchers in Canada who examined the effect of school shutdowns on adolescent sleep. Their cohort consisted of 45 teens who lived in Canada during the pandemic; their remote learning began at 10 AM. The researchers found improvements in the quality and/or duration of sleep and a 2-hour shift in the sleep pattern of the teens. The researchers suggested that delaying the start time of high school may be a useful way to increase the quality and duration of sleep, reduce daytime sleepiness, and lower adolescent stress.[9]

Obesity

The COVID-19 pandemic helped to structure an obesogenic environment for adolescents with mandatory school closings, limited physical activity offerings, and increased stress. In addition, the absence of healthy food from the school lunch programs and increased home stress from problems such as parental unemployment helped to promote weight gain.[10]

Researchers based in Michigan performed a retrospective cohort study of 191,509 California youths between the ages of 5 and 17 years who had body mass index (BMI) measurements before and during the pandemic. Prepandemic BMI measurements were obtained before January 2020, and the pandemic BMI measurements were obtained from March 2020 to January 2021. The study group was racially and ethnically diverse. According to the data, the youth gained more weight during the pandemic than during the prepandemic period. Prior to the pandemic, 19.06 percent of the 12- to 15-year-olds had obesity, compared to 23.2 percent during the pandemic. For the youth who were 16 or 17 years old, 17.97 percent had obesity before the pandemic, and 20.07 percent had obesity during the pandemic.[11] These increases in weight were significant.

Adolescents with obesity were at higher risk for COVID-19 complications. A group of researchers in New York studied 494 COVID-19-positive patients between ages newborn and 21 years. Of these, 280 were adolescents. The researchers learned that adolescents with obesity were more likely than adolescents without obesity to have severe respiratory complications, including pneumonia and respiratory failure. The researchers concluded that obesity was an independent risk factor for critical COVID-19 illness in adolescents.[12]

Stress

In Switzerland, researchers studied adolescents during the country's first COVID-19 lockdown. The cohort consisted of 1146 adolescents between the ages of 12 and 17 years and their parents, who both completed an online questionnaire that included a measure of perceived stress from the pandemic and inquiries concerning the teens' regular and problematic use of the internet. According to the adolescents, their most perceived stressors during the first lockdown were caused by their inability to participate in social activities and normal routines. They were also stressed by the cancellation or postponement of events. While 30 percent of the teens met the criteria for problematic internet use (PIU), the researchers were unable to learn if the PIU was related to increased or decreased stress among the teens.[13]

During the COVID-19 pandemic, adolescents, their parents, and those functioning in a supportive role, including teachers and coaches, were stressed. Resilience, or the ability to maintain well-being under stressful conditions, was taxed. Everyone could have benefited from resources to support resilience, and the following tips may enhance it:[14]

- Stay socially connected and talk to your friends.
- Cut yourself some slack if something bad happens to you.
- Work to take care of yourself physically, mentally, and spiritually.
- Place things in perspective.
- Help someone.

Psychological Issues and COVID-19

Anxiety

The COVID-19 pandemic had a substantial impact on the mental health of adolescents. The added stress from such factors as lack of social contact, remote learning, fear of interaction, and economic difficulties was particularly difficult for teens. Both before and during the pandemic, researchers in Oklahoma and California performed a longitudinal case-controlled study that included healthy adolescents and adolescents who had a history of early life stress. Hoping to learn more about the effects the pandemic had on symptoms of anxiety and depression, the cohort included 15 healthy teens and 9 with early life stress exposures such as child abuse, neglect, domestic violence, or parental psychopathology. Anxiety and depression were assessed using the Patient-Reported Outcome Measurement Information System. The baseline visits began in August 2019, well before the pandemic, and continued until June 2020. The researchers discovered that after the pandemic began, the healthy adolescents exhibited large increases in self-reported anxiety and depression. Interestingly, the teens with a history of early life stress did not report any changes in their symptoms from the pandemic. The researchers commented that the subjects with early life stress may have been connected to therapy, may have already been taking selective serotonin reuptake medications, and/or may have had other resources enabling them to better deal with pandemic stress.[15]

Depression

As noted in the introduction, the pandemic had significant effects on the mental health of adolescents. Before and during the pandemic, researchers from New York and Florida studied depression and anxiety in adolescents and young adults who lived on Long Island. These assessments occurred between December 2014 and July 2019 and between March 27, 2020, and May 15, 2020. The screening measures included administration of the Children's Depression Inventory and the Screen for Child Anxiety Related Symptoms. During the pandemic, additional pandemic-related questions were added. While the original study had 713 subjects, 505 participated in the pandemic survey. The final sample consisted of subjects between the ages of 12 and 22 years, with a mean age of 17.49 years. Regardless of their ages, the researchers discovered that the psychiatric symptoms of the subjects, including depression and anxiety, had increased during the pandemic. Prepandemic, the Children's Depression Inventory scores for both genders was 5.93; during the pandemic it rose to 9.61, which was statistically significant. The researchers noted that the increase was unlikely to be secondary to normal developmental processes. Female adolescents were more affected than males, and school-related problems, fear of contracting COVID-19, and home confinement were linked to worsening psychiatric symptoms.[16]

The pandemic brought on school closures, disruption of social networks, and loneliness for adolescents. Researchers from multiple institutions in the United States examined the effects of the pandemic on adolescent mental health and social media use before the shutdown (T1), 8 weeks after the initial shutdown (T2), and about 8.5 months after the shutdown (T3). Prepandemic data had been collected an average of 2 years prior to the shutdown. When the shutdown began, there were 175 subjects; they had a mean age of 16.01 years. Depression was measured at T1, T2, and T3; loneliness and time spent per day engaging in social media were assessed at T2 and T3; social activity participation was evaluated only at T3. Prior to the pandemic, there was no significant difference between male and female adolescent depression scores. During the shutdown, female adolescents experienced a significant increase, while the male adolescents did not until T3. Higher degrees of loneliness were associated with higher levels of depressive symptoms for female and male adolescents at T2 and T3. Further, female adolescents who spent more time on social media during the pandemic had higher depressive symptoms than female adolescents with lower social media use. According to the researchers, their findings highlighted the need to address depression in adolescents and the importance of social support, especially during a pandemic. Social supports may include family, peers, schools, communities, and government. For example, the federal government passed the American Rescue Plan, which had a number of provisions applicable to adolescents, one of which was improving the connection and coverage of children and adolescents with medical care. This was enabled through the Connecting Kids to Coverage program, with a particular focus on mental health.[17,18]

Eating Disorders

The COVID-19 pandemic had a number of significant negative impacts on adolescents with eating disorders. School closures and remote learning dramatically changed daily routines for these youth, diminishing social connections and increasing social isolation. School sports were mostly eliminated, and the computer-based learning that replaced in-person learning led many to the social media that exacerbated their eating disorder. Their connections to care, especially in-person medical, nutrition, and therapy visits, were initially stopped and then transitioned to telemedicine, which does not allow for optimal examinations and measurements of weights and vital signs. There were also youth suffering from an eating disorder who did not have access to care due to limited office hours or lack of technological equipment to connect to telemedicine. Researchers from Canada performed a retrospective chart review on adolescents with eating disorders who were evaluated from April 1, 2020, to October 31, 2020 (during the pandemic). They also reviewed the charts of those seen 1 year earlier during the same months in 2019. The chart review included medical and psychological measures. Both groups had an average age of 14 years. During the pandemic, 48 patients were evaluated and 19 noted that the pandemic triggered their eating disorder, most often anorexia. When compared to a group studied before the pandemic began, the pandemic patients had significantly lower BMI and were more than two times as likely to be medically unstable at assessment and two times as likely to be admitted to the hospital within 4 weeks. The patients also had a higher level of restriction and overexercising that was enabled by pandemic-related closures and increased solitary time at home.[19]

Researchers in Massachusetts wanted to learn if the pandemic increased the number of adolescent patients seeking eating disorder–related care. Using a time series regression, they examined the data on a monthly basis prior to and during the pandemic. The researchers learned that when compared to the prepandemic levels, by the 10th month of COVID-19 the number of hospitalizations for adolescents with

eating disorders had doubled. Likewise, the researchers observed a significant increase in the number of family inquiries for care during the pandemic, signifying a
rising need for regional services related to eating disorders in adolescents.[20]

Looking at both inpatient and outpatient activities, another group of researchers
from 15 sites across the United States used an observational case series design to study
changes in volume in eating disorder–related care during the pandemic. They found a
significant pandemic-related increase in the number of patients with eating disorders
across the sites, particularly during the first year of the pandemic.[21]

Substance Use
The COVID-19 pandemic caused a significant disruption in the lives of adolescents, leading to increased stress that could have affected the prevalence of substance
use. Researchers from multiple centers in the United States studied the use of substances in a nationwide, diverse sample of younger adolescents and followed them
for 6 months after the COVID-19 stay-at-home orders were first issued at the study
sites from March 19, 2020, to April 6, 2020. The subjects were initially enrolled in
2018 in the Adolescent Brain Cognitive Development Study; the cohort consisted of
11,880 youth, 48 percent female, 20 percent Hispanic, 15 percent Black, and 2 percent
Asian. Before the pandemic, the researchers had obtained substance use information
on the subjects in 2018, 2019, and January 2020. They obtained three waves of similar data after the pandemic stay-at-home orders were in place: May 2020, June 2020,
and August 2020. The measures included drinking alcohol, smoking cigarettes, using
an electronic nicotine delivery system, using cannabis or other drugs, and smoking
cigars/hookahs/pipes. After the lockdown began, fewer teens were using alcohol.
However, more were using nicotine or misusing prescription drugs. Pandemic-related
uncertainty, an increased prevalence of anxiety and depression, and family dealing
with material hardship were each risk factors for adolescent substance use. That said,
during lockdown, there was relative stability in the overall rate of substance use by this
cohort. This may be explained by the increased time spent with parents and presumably more supervision, as well as decreased face-to-face contact with peers. And the
social distancing mandated during the stay-at-home orders may have prevented the
onset of early substance use in some adolescents, which may then decrease the risk of
these teens developing a substance abuse disorder during adulthood.[22]

COVID-related restrictions may have also discouraged substance use in other
countries. The Youth in Iceland study is a survey administered every other year to
all 13- to 18-year-old adolescents who attend school in Iceland. The main outcomes
of the survey, which was administered in 2016, 2018, and November 2020, after the
pandemic lockdown, were substance use, depression, and mental well-being. With
substance use, the adolescents rated their use of cigarettes, e-cigarettes, and alcohol
intoxication during the previous 30 days. Responses from same-aged peers as well as
all age groups were evaluated for the three cohorts of data. The researchers learned
that while the rates of alcohol intoxication among all ages were similar in 2016 and
2018, they were significantly lower in 2020. Compared to 2016, e-cigarette use rose in
2018 but decreased in the teens who were 16 to 18 years old in 2020 ($p < .0001$). A significant decrease from previous cohorts was also noted for cigarette smoking in adolescents between 15 and 18 years old. In 2020, when compared to previous surveys, all

age groups had increases in depressive symptoms and worsening mental well-being. Females had even greater increases in depressive symptoms and decreases in mental well-being. The researchers commented that the social restrictions implemented to prevent the spread of COVID-19 led to less peer pressure and social rewards for exploring the use of substances. Furthermore, there was a public health campaign about the health risks of e-cigarettes conducted within the national school system.[23]

Suicidality/Self-Harm

Pandemic-related stressors such as social isolation and social distancing may have increased suicide-related behaviors. Researchers in Texas hypothesized that during the first part of the pandemic in 2020, suicidal behaviors would be higher than they were in 2019. The cohort consisted of 12,827 subjects between the ages of 11 and 21 years who were screened for suicide risk at three pediatric hospitals in the Houston area from January to July 2019 and January to July 2020. The subjects, who had a mean age of 14.5 years and were 59 percent female, completed the Columbia-Suicide Severity Rating Scale. As the researchers anticipated, when compared to February, March, April, and July of 2019, those months in 2020 had significantly higher rates of suicidal ideation. The researchers commented that the months with significantly higher rates of suicide-related behaviors appeared to correspond to the times when COVID-19-related stressors were higher, periods when adolescents were likely experiencing elevated distress.[24]

The best way to prevent suicide in adolescents is to identify those who are at risk and refer them to the appropriate provider(s). Children's Mercy Hospital in Missouri had a program where all patients between the ages of 12 and 24 years were screened for suicide risk, generally with a four-item screening tool. (Those seen in mental health clinics were screened with another tool.) The researchers reviewed the demographics and screening results from April to June 2020 (T2) and compared them to screens from April to June 2019 (T1). During T1, 24,863 patients were seen, thousands more than the 17,986 seen during T2. The adjusted odds level of a positive screen was 1.24 in T2 as compared to T1. In T2, the odds of a positive screen were higher for older patients, female patients, and those on public insurance. Overall, 11.1 percent of the screens were positive in T1 compared to 12.2 percent in T2. These data indicated that the rate of positive suicide risk screens among adolescents increased in the early months of the COVID-19 pandemic.[25]

Through a partnership with 14 state departments of public health, researchers at the Massachusetts Institute of Technology assessed pandemic-period changes in suicide for adolescents aged 10 to 19 years. They were able to compare data for prepandemic suicides (2015 to 2019) and pandemic suicides (2020). The researchers aggregated the data across all 14 states and noted that the proportion of overall suicides among adolescents compared to other ages increased during the pandemic. There was also an increase in the absolute number of suicides in the youth age group. The researchers suggested that suicide risk assessments should be more readily available. This would be consistent with the previous study from Missouri.[26]

Data released recently from the CDC determined that suspected suicide attempts by self-poisoning among individuals ages 10 to 19 years increased 30 percent in 2021 compared to prepandemic rates noted in 2019. The rate increases were significantly higher in adolescents ages 10 to 12 years (73.0 percent) and 48.8 percent among individuals ages 13 to 15 years. This study confirmed a potential impact of the COVID-19 pandemic on suspected suicide attempts by self-poisoning in adolescents. The researchers noted that similar increases in suicide attempts are commonly seen among individuals affected by crises such as wars and natural disasters.[27]

Social Issues and COVID-19

Social Media

Peer relationships are especially important during adolescence, when adolescents strive to become more independent from their parents through building relationships with peers. However, the early pandemic lockdowns, online schooling, and social distancing disrupted the daily in-person activities of teens, with greater amounts of time spent online. In fact, national findings from the Adolescent Brain Cognitive Development Study showed that during the first part of the pandemic, the mean total daily screen time for adolescents between the ages of 10 and 14 years was 7.7 hours per day, over twice the prepandemic estimate of 3.8 hours per day.[28] Obviously, the increased use of social media had both positive and negative effects for the adolescents. For example, while teens were able to connect online with their teachers during the pandemic, the online connection was less valuable in an educational sense than in-person classes.

Researchers in Switzerland performed a systematic review and meta-analysis of studies to determine whether digital media use positively or negatively impacted adolescent mental health during the COVID-19 pandemic. They located 30 papers published up to and including September 2021 for the systematic review and a subset of 23 for the meta-analysis. Their findings are summarized in Box 17.1.

Parents and other adults should promote the supportive aspects of online activities for adolescents, and they should be aware of the adverse consequences of such activities. These adverse events include PIU, fear of missing out, and body comparison.[29]

Researchers in Belgium wondered if social media during the lockdown period of the pandemic helped adolescents cope with anxiety and loneliness. The researchers surveyed 2165 Belgian adolescents between the ages of 13 and 19 years; 66.6 percent were female. There were measures for happiness, anxiety, and loneliness, as well as a calculation of how the adolescents used social media to cope with the pandemic lockdown. The vast majority of the subjects (76.2 percent) noted having many more social interactions during the lockdown. The reports were consistent with mood management theory, which argues that media use is driven by a need to regulate and improve negative emotions in an attempt to feel better. The adolescents said that they used social media to have less distress and anxiety and to improve mood. Feelings of loneliness seemed to have more impact on the teens than feelings of anxiety. The subjects who were anxious used social media more often to help them adapt to the lockdown, thus affecting their happiness in a positive way. These findings confirmed a beneficial consequence of increased social media usage during the pandemic.

A group of researchers from Massachusetts General Hospital performed a systematic review of research on social media and provision of health care to adolescents and

Box 17.1 Consequences of Digital Media Use by Adolescents During the COVID-19 Pandemic

- Most studies reported that digital media use was associated with diminished well-being; this was related to worry, fear of the pandemic, and fear of missing out.
- Older adolescents were more affected by the negative consequences of social media content exposure.
- Social media was used as a coping mechanism to avoid boredom, displace time from homework, and seek entertainment without direct involvement. This led to feelings of anxiety, depression, and low self-esteem, as well as body-related concerns.
- Increased screen time displaced activities that promoted mental health, including physical activity and regular sleep patterns.
- Increased screen time led some adolescents to develop media addiction symptoms, thus reducing the feelings of well-being; this was seen especially in younger adolescents who had relative immaturity of the frontal cortex and instant gratification from social media sites.
- Positive consequences included improved social and mental well-being when social media use included one-to-one communication, online mutual relationships, and experiencing positive content.

Adapted from Marciano L, Ostroumova M, Schulz PJ, Camerini AL. Digital media use and adolescents' mental health during the Covid-19 pandemic: a systematic review and meta-analysis. *Front Public Health*. 2022 Feb 1;9:793868.

young adults. They concluded that social media provides a vehicle where adolescents and young adults can be engaged by medical personnel, and it is a method to provide health information. This study, which was conducted prior to the pandemic, should inform the medical profession on the potential of digital sources of communication with this age group.[30]

Problematic Internet Use

The COVID-19 pandemic significantly disrupted the lives of adolescents, especially with respect to their education. Stay-at-home orders and remote schooling led to isolation, limited movement, and increased use of the internet for both education and leisure activities. Studies have demonstrated that disasters and terrorist incidents have led to higher levels of addictive behaviors, including PIU; the COVID-19 pandemic had a similar effect. Due to their stage of development, adolescents appear to be especially vulnerable.

Researchers from Massachusetts wanted to learn if the pandemic triggered an increase in PIU in certain youth. They assembled a sample of 69 subjects between the ages of 12 and 23 years who received outpatient mental health treatment in a community hospital setting. The subjects provided 6 weeks of data through an ecological momentary assessment, a smartphone protocol that collected daily information about the participants' qualitative digital media use, PIU, and symptoms of anxiety and depression. From the data, the researchers were able to determine how the use of digital media and the mental health status of the subjects may have changed during the pandemic, and it explained how the personal or familial exposure to the novel coronavirus may have impacted their digital media use habits and mental health. Twenty-seven adolescents, with a mean age of 15.3 years, provided prepandemic data, and 42 adolescents, with a mean age of 16.95 years, had data collected during the pandemic. Compared to the prepandemic subjects, the subjects with data from the pandemic were significantly more likely to meet the criteria for PIU and to spend more time using social media each day. Further analysis of the data demonstrated that there was a significant increase in average daily screen time among subjects who were exposed to COVID-19 either personally or through their family. The researchers recommended that mental health clinicians screen for PIU in these adolescents to prevent potential psychiatric crises.[31]

On a broader scale, researchers from Germany evaluated the prevalence of PIU in German adolescents after the third wave of the pandemic. Adolescents ($N = 1268$) with a mean age of 14.37 years completed the Short Compulsive Internet Use Scale and two additional items to capture their digital media usage time while obtaining their COVID vaccine. The average prevalence of PIU was 43.7 percent. The research team reported this was a significant increase compared to the prepandemic prevalence rate. They reported a 10 to 24 percent prepandemic prevalence rate based on other studies.[32]

Racism/Discrimination

Discrimination involving adults, some of whom are parents to adolescents, could directly or indirectly impact youth. Researchers from the National Institutes of Health and the University of California, San Francisco studied the prevalence of COVID-19-related discrimination among adults in major U.S. racial/ethnic groups and looked for associations between this discrimination and other sociodemographic characteristics. The team utilized an online survey of a nationally representative group of 5500 Native American/Alaska Native, Asian, Black/African American, Hawaiian/Pacific Islander, Latino, White, and multiracial adults between December 2020 and February 2021. In this adult population, 22.1 percent reported experiencing discriminatory behaviors. All racial/ethnic minorities encountered higher levels of COVID-19-related discrimination than White adults, with Native American/Alaska Native, Asian, Hawaiian/Pacific Islander, and Latino adults having the highest prevalence. Limited English proficiency, lower education, lower income, and residing in a big city or the East South Central census division also increased the prevalence of discrimination.[33]

Many have observed that racism against Chinese American populations appeared to increase during the pandemic, and this contributed to health disparities. Researchers from Maryland studied direct and vicarious online and in-person racial discrimination during the pandemic. Likewise, they reviewed Sinophobia in the media and assessed the link between Sinophobia and mental health indices in youth. The researchers recruited a sample of 543 Chinese American parents and their children ($N = 230$), mean age 13.83 years, 48.3 percent female. The adolescents and parents completed their own surveys from March 2020 to the end of May 2020. The measures included questions about various types of COVID-19-related racial dis-crimination and Sinophobia and questions about psychological well-being, anxiety, and internalizing and externalizing issues. The researchers determined that a signif-icant percentage of Chinese American adolescents and their parents personally wit-nessed or experienced anti-Asian or anti-Chinese discrimination online or in person due to the COVID-19 pandemic. For example, 91.9 percent of the adolescents noted that they had witnessed vicarious in-person racial discrimination. Many of the youth thought that Americans considered Chinese people and their culture to be a threat to public health. These feelings were related to higher levels of anxiety and depres-sive symptoms in the adolescents. The researchers underscored the need for effective public health and education strategies to decrease the stigmatization of and discrimi-nation against Chinese Americans.[34]

LGBTQ

Pandemics and other disasters lead to population-level increases in psychopathology and other mental health outcomes in adolescents. When compared to heterosexual adolescents, LGBTQ peers were more likely to experience food insecurity, homeless-ness, unstable housing, and poverty during the COVID-19 pandemic, which only worsened existing mental health problems. As a result of pandemic-related school and university closures, adolescents and young adults were forced to return home to live, thereby losing at least some autonomy and peer and adult support. If they had not shared their LGBTQ status with their families, these youth may have struggled with their inability to live authentically in their daily lives. For the LGBTQ population, the pandemic not only caused sexual minority stress but also severed ties to supportive and affirming resources such as teachers, coaches, and/or structured mental health services. Access to medical care during the earlier part of the pandemic was limited or, sometimes, unavailable. Social media may have played a role in helping to alleviate some of these stressors. Such supports included online mental health services through telemedicine, other digital support groups, online chat spaces, text-based mental health services, and social and crisis support programs.[35]

Researchers from Canada noted that LGBTQ individuals were overrepresented among homeless youth, accounting for between 20 and 40 percent of the homeless youth in North America. So the researchers evaluated the impact of the pandemic on 61 LGBTQ youth who were homeless or at risk for homelessness in the greater Toronto area. The youth, with a mean age of 21 years, participated in one-on-one interviews and completed online surveys. The subjects had diverse ethnicities and racial backgrounds; the majority were cisgender, and their sexual orientations were LGBTQ. The researchers determined that since the pandemic began, most of the subjects had multiple mental health difficulties and challenges, such as anxiety and depression. Approximately 81 percent engaged in nonsuicidal self-injury, and 36 per-cent had attempted suicide. They reported increases in their use of substances and al-cohol, and most had changes in access to their medical care, although 66 percent were able to obtain mental health care virtually. The researchers commented that essential health supports, including social services and housing services, previously available to the LGBTQ homeless or those at risk for homelessness had curtailed or stopped their services during the pandemic. And there was a significant need for those services to address the preexisting social and health issues in the LGBTQ community that were exacerbated by the pandemic.[36]

Transgender and Gender Dysphoria

The COVID-19 pandemic posed risks for all adolescents, but especially to those in more vulnerable subgroups, such as gender minority adolescents. With social distancing measures, home quarantine, and economic shutdowns, the pandemic caused increased psychological symptoms in youth. Hypothesizing that transgender and gender nonconforming (TGN) adolescents were more severely affected by the pandemic than their cisgender peers, researchers from Israel developed an online COVID-19 health impact survey. They recruited 18 TGN males, 29 cisgender males, and 29 cisgender females between the ages of 9 and 18 years and their principal caregivers through social media, mailings, and referrals. The participants in the TNG group were similar to those in the cisgender group, except the former had poorer physical and emotional health before the pandemic. All of the participants completed the survey, which had six parts: COVID-19 exposure status, life changes, emotions/feelings, daily behavior patterns, media use, and substance use. There was also a second measure, an emotion regulation questionnaire. The majority of the participants completed a follow-up survey 2 or 3 weeks later. The researchers learned that the effects of the pandemic on the mental health of the adolescents were similar for the TNG group, cisgender males, and cisgender female adolescents. All of the groups had increases in negative emotions and feelings. However, the cisgender youth used more adaptive emotion regulation strategies than the TGN youth, which may have been the reason that the TGN youth had elevated levels of mental health symptomatology. The researchers concluded that adolescents in high-risk subgroups should be offered counseling on effective emotional regulation strategies such as cognitive reappraisal. This refers to changing the way one thinks about an emotion-eliciting situation.[37]

Poverty

Approximately 150 million additional children were living in multidimensional poverty as a result of the COVID-19 pandemic. UNICEF considers child poverty to have six dimensions: education, health, housing, nutrition, sanitation, and water. The two areas of poverty that changed the most quickly from COVID-19 were education and health. During the COVID-19 pandemic, most governments set up various forms of long-distance teaching for children and adolescents to continue their education. However, while telemedicine was made available to improve access to health care during the pandemic, many in poverty lacked computers or internet connections to benefit from this modality of health care.[38]

In the United States, most school districts used remote learning for at least some of the pandemic. Researchers from the Center for Education Policy Research at Harvard studied the consequences of remote and hybrid learning on children and adolescents during the pandemic. The researchers used testing data from 2.1 million students in 10,000 schools in 49 states and the District of Columbia; the students were in grades 3 to 8. The researchers compared student achievement levels from the fall of 2019 to the fall of 2021 with data from the fall of 2017 to the fall of 2019 on the role of remote and hybrid learning and achievement by race and school poverty level. The researchers learned that schools that were considered high poverty spent about 5.5 more weeks in remote instruction during 2020 to 2021 than low- and middle-poverty schools. In the states with high remote instruction, such as California and New Jersey, high-poverty schools spent an additional 9 weeks in remote instruction compared to low-poverty schools. Furthermore, high-poverty schools were more likely to go remote, and when they did, they suffered larger declines in achievement. In school districts that were remote for most of the 2020–2021 school year, high-poverty schools had a 50 percent higher loss of math achievement than low-poverty schools. The researchers concluded that based on test results, students attending high-poverty schools that went to remote learning during the pandemic suffered a significant lag in educational achievement, widening the gap. This is estimated to be about 50 percent of math learning during a typical school year.[39]

Mortality

Worldwide, over 10.5 million children and adolescents have lost a parent or caregiver to COVID-19.[40] In the United States, more than 50,000 adolescents between the ages of 14 and 17 years lost a parent or grandparent, with non-White adolescents losing caregiving adults at a higher rate than their White peers. Although the vast majority of adolescents will experience a normal course of grief, the consequences of losing a parent or other caregiver may persist throughout an adolescent's lifetime. They may have a higher risk for anxiety, depression, PTSD, lower academic achievement, failure to complete educational programs, substance use, and suicidal behavior, which is further discussed in Chapter 16. Recommended clinical interventions may include the expansion of access to mental health care in schools and outpatient centers and reducing the costs of this care.

According to the COVID Collaborative, more than 203,500 children had lost a parent or other in-home caregiver to the pandemic as of the end of February 2022. About 30 percent of the children were between ages 14 and 17 years. Some adolescents lost multiple relatives to COVID, further complicating the grieving process. Following the loss of a parent or caregiver, between 5 and 10 percent of adolescents will have more complicated grief. For the majority, positive parenting and supportive teachers, mentors, and peers may help the healing process. Further, there are specialized services, such as grief camps, which are short-term interventions for bereaved adolescents. These camps concentrate on normalizing death, grief, and the responses, which may reduce the sense of isolation and angst. Mentoring through Big Brothers Big Sisters of America provides role models and positive relationships to adolescents. There are peer-supported programs that match adolescents with similar backgrounds, interests, and life circumstances. And there are family bereavement programs for adolescents and their caregivers that enhance resilience. Those having a harder time may wish to consider cognitive behavioral therapy, which usually includes 3 to 6 months of clinician-directed and focused talk therapy.[41]

Early in the pandemic, the social isolation, lockdowns, and physical distancing made adolescent grief from parental loss even more difficult. There was little if any programming for the grief associated with COVID-19 deaths. Some adolescents were forced to say their last goodbyes to parents or grandparents via an electronic device. Because losses from COVID-19 were so much higher in disadvantaged communities, clinicians who provide care for these communities should carefully screen those adolescents for associated symptoms of grief.[42]

Treatment and Prevention

Immunization with COVID-19 vaccines is the primary preventive measure for adolescents. As recommendations for this vaccine change periodically, the website for the CDC (https://www.cdc.gov) should be consulted. Local health departments may provide other measures to prevent the spread of the disease.

Researchers in the Netherlands and Oklahoma noted the wide-reaching implications of the pandemic on adolescent emotional, social, and academic adjustment. They suggested three avenues for intervention and prevention of maladjustment during this pandemic. The first is to target those adolescents with higher mental health problems prior to the pandemic as these youth are at higher risk for mental health problems during a crisis. Second, policymakers need to understand the risks of social isolation and the benefits of in-person interactions for youth during the pandemic, parents need to provide virtual and safe social interactions to maintain their adolescents' social connections. Finally, it is important to have training for emotion regulation skills before and during a pandemic. Adolescents then may be able to buffer some of the negative effects of a pandemic on their mental health and academic engagement.[43]

Up-to-date information on the treatment of COVID infections in adolescents is also available on the CDC website as well as from local health departments and primary care clinicians. As noted in this chapter, adolescents have experienced biopsychosocial issues from the pandemic. For information on the treatment of such problems, please refer to the appropriate chapter.

Conclusion

For most adolescents, COVID-19 is a relatively mild infection, and fortunately, thus far, the mortality rate has been relatively low compared to adults and seniors. Still, the pandemic has had profound effects on the biopsychosocial domains for adolescents, with increasing numbers of adolescents developing mental health symptoms. In addition, those students attending high-poverty schools likely lost more ground in academic achievement during the pandemic compared to low-poverty schools. While health care providers generally agreed with the need for remote learning, social isolation, and lockdowns, few anticipated the profound overall functioning and mental health effects of these measures on adolescents. In the midst of all these associated problems, there emerged one positive development. Increasingly, patients and their medical providers communicated via telemedicine, which enabled care to be delivered under very difficult circumstances and in different locations, including homes and schools.

References

1 Provisional COVID-19 deaths: focus on ages 0–18 years. Centers for Disease Control and Prevention, Atlanta, GA. July 12, 2023.

2 Thallapureddy K, Thallapureddy K, Zerda E, et al. Long-term complications of COVID-19 infection in adolescents and children. *Curr Pediatr Rep.* 2022;10:11–17.

3 Racine N, McArthur BA, Cooke JE, Elrich R, Zhu J, Madigan S. Global prevalence of depressive and anxiety symptoms in children and adolescents during COVID-19: a meta-analysis. *JAMA Pediatr.* 2021;175:1142–1150.

4 Gotlib IH, Miller JG, Borchers LR, et al. Effects of the COVID-19 pandemic on mental health and brain maturation in adolescents: implications for analyzing longitudinal data. *Biol Psychiatry Glob Open Sci.* 2022; 3:912–918.

5 Clarke KEN, Jones JM, Deng Y, et al. Seroprevalence of infection-induced SARS-CoV-2 antibodies—United States, September 2021–February 2022. *MMWR Morb Mortal Wkly Rep.* 2022;71:606–608.

6 McCormick DW, Richardson LC, Young PR, Viens LJ, Gould CV, Kimball A. Deaths in children and adolescents associated with COVID-19 and MIS-C in the United States. *Pediatrics.* 2021;148(5):e2021052273.

7 Pathak EB, Garcia RB. Racial and ethnic disparities in COVID-19 mortality among children and teens. Perspectives in Primary Care, Center for Primary Care, Harvard Medical School, Boston, MA. October 6, 2020.

8 Becker SP, Dvorsky MR, Breaux R, Cusick C, Taylor KP, Langber JM. Prospective examination of adolescent sleep patterns and behaviors before and during COVID-19. *Sleep.* 2021;44:zsab054.

9 Gruber R, Gauthier-Gagne G, Voutou D, Somerville G, Saha S, Boursier J. Pre-pandemic behavior and adolescents' stress during COVID-19: a prospective longitudinal study. *Child Adolesc Psychiatry Ment Health.* 2021;15:43.

10 Browne NT, Snethen JA, Greenberg CS, et al. When pandemics collide: the impact of COVID-19 on childhood obesity. *J Pediatr Nurs.* 2021;56:90–98.

11 Woolford SJ, Sidell M, Li X, et al. Changes in body mass index among children and adolescents during the COVID-19 pandemic. *JAMA.* 2021;326:1434–1436.

12 Guzman BV, Elbel B, Jay M, Messito MJ, Curado S. Age-dependent association of obesity with COVID-19 severity in paediatric patients. *Pediatr Obes.* 2022;17(3):e12856.

13 Mohler-Kuo M, Dzemaili S, Foster S, Werlen L, Walitza S. Stress and mental health among children/adolescents, their parents, and young adults during the first COVID-19 lockdown in Switzerland. *Int J Environ Res Public Health.* 2021;18:4668.

14 Alvord MK, Gurwitch R, Martin J, Palomares RS. Resilience for teens: 10 tips to build skills on bouncing back from rough times. American Psychological Association, Washington, DC. June 1, 2020.

15 Cohen ZP, Cosgrove KK, DeVille DD, et al. The impact of COVID-19 on adolescent mental health: preliminary findings from a longitudinal sample of healthy and at-risk adolescents. *Front Pediatr.* 2021;9:622608.

16 Hawes MT, Szenczy AK, Klein DN, Hajcak G, Nelson BD. Increases in depression and anxiety symptoms in adolescents and young adults during the COVID-19 crisis. *Psychol Med.* 2021;13:1–9.

17 Liu SR, Davis EP, Palma AM, Sandman CA, Glynn LM. The acute and persisting impact of COIVD-19 on trajectories of adolescent depression: sex differences and social connectedness. *J Affect Disord.* 2021;299:246–255.

18 Fact sheet: improving access and care for youth mental health and substance use conditions. The White House, Washington, DC. October 19, 2021.

19 Spettigue W, Obeid N, Erbach M, et al. The impact of COVID-19 on adolescents with eating disorders: a cohort study. *J Eat Disord*. 2021;9:65.

20 Lin JA, Hartman-Munick SM, Kells MR, et al. The impact of the COVID-19 pandemic on the number of adolescents/young adults seeking eating disorder-related care. *J Adolesc Health*. 2021;69:660–663.

21 Hartman-Munick SM, Lin JA, Milliren CE, et. al. Association of the COVID-19 pandemic with adolescent and young adult eating disorder care volume. *JAMA Pediatr*. 2022;176:1225–1232.

22 Pelham WE 3rd, Tapert SF, Gonzalez MR, et al. Early adolescent substance use before and during the COVID-19 pandemic: a longitudinal survey in the ABCD study cohort. *J Adolesc Health*. 2021;69:390–397.

23 Thorisdottir IE, Asgeirsdottir BB, Kristjansson AL, et al. Depressive symptoms, mental well-being, and substance use among adolescents before and during the COIVD-19 pandemic in Iceland: a longitudinal, population-based study. *Lancet Psychiatry*. 2021;8:663–672.

24 Hill RM, Rufino K, Kurian S, Saxena J, Williams L. Suicide ideation and attempts in a pediatric emergency department before and during COVID-19. *Pediatrics*. 2021;147:e2020029280.

25 Lantos JD, Yeh HW, Raza F, et al. Suicide risk in adolescents during the COVID-19 pandemic. *Pediatrics*. 2022;149:e2021053486.

26 Charpignon ML, Ontiveros J, Sundaresan S, et al. Evaluation of suicides among US adolescents during the COVID-19 pandemic. *JAMA Pediatr*. 2022;176:724–726.

27 Farah R, Rege SV, Cole RJ, Holstege CP. Suspected suicide attempts by self-poisoning among persons aged 10-19 years during the COVID-19 pandemic—United States, 2020–2022. *MMWR Morb Mortal Wkly Rep*. 2023;72:426–430.

28 Nagata JM, Cortez CA, Cattle CJ, et al. Screen time use among US adolescents during the COVID-19 pandemic: findings from the Adolescent Brain Cognitive Development (ABCD) study. *JAMA Pediatr*. 2022;176:94–96.

29 Marciano LM, Ostroumova M, Schulz PJ, Camerini AL. Digital media use and adolescents' mental health during the Covid-19 pandemic: a systematic review and meta-analysis. *Front Public Health*. 2022;9:793868.

30 Yonker LM, Zan S, Scirica CV, Jethwani K, Kinane TB. "Friending" teens: systematic review of social media in adolescent and young adult health care. *J Med Internet Res*. 2015;17(1):e4.

31 Gansner M, Nisenson M, Lin V, Pong S, Torous J, Carson N. Problematic internet use before and during the COVID-19 pandemic in youth and outpatient mental health treatment: app based ecological momentary assessment study. *JMIR Ment Health*. 2022;9:e33114.

32 Paulus FW, Joas J, Gerstner I, et al. Problematic internet use among adolescents 18 months after the onset of the COVID-19 pandemic. *Children (Basel)*. 2022;9:1724.

33 Strassle PD, Stewart AL, Quintero SM, et al. COVID-19-related discrimination among racial/ethnic minorities and other marginalized communities in the United States. *Am J Public Health*. 2022;112:453–466.

34 Cheah CSL, Wang C, Ren H, Zong X, Cho HS, Xue X. COVID-19 racism and mental health in Chinese American families. *Pediatrics*. 2020;146:e2020021816.

35 Salerno JP, Devadas J, Pease M, Nketia B, Fish JN. Sexual and gender minority stress amid the COVID-19 pandemic: implications for LGBTQ young persons' mental health and well-being. *Public Health Rep*. 2020;135:721–727.

36 Abramovich A, Pang N, Moss A, et al. Investigating the impacts of COVID-19 among LGBTQ2S youth experiencing homelessness. *PLoS One*. 2021;16:e0257693.

37 Perl L, Oren A, Klein Z, Shechner T. Effects of the COVID19 pandemic on transgender and gender non-conforming adolescents' mental health. *Psychiatry Res*. 2021;302:114042.

38 Irwin M, Lazarevic B, Soled D, Adesman A. The COVID-19 pandemic and its potential en-during impact on children. *Curr Opin Pediatr.* 2022;34:107–115.

39 Goldhaber D, Kane T, McEachin A, Morton E, Patterson T, Staiger DO. *The Consequences of Remote and Hybrid Instruction During the Pandemic.* Research Report. Center for Education Policy Research, Harvard University; May 2022.

40 Hillis S, N'konzi JN, Msemburi W, et al. Orphanhood and caregiver loss among children based on new global excess COVID-19 death estimates. *JAMA Pediatr.* 2022;176:1145–1148.

41 Teglia D, Cutuli J, Arasteh K, et al. *Hidden Pain: Children Who Lost a Parent or Caregiver to COVID-19 and What the Nation Can Do to Help Them.* COVID Collaborative; 2021.

42 Weinstock L, Dunda D, Harrington H, Nelson H. It's complicated—adolescent grief in the time of COVID-19. *Front Psychiatry.* 2021;12:638940.

43 Branje S, Morris AS. The impact of the COVID-19 pandemic on adolescent emotional, so-cial, and academic adjustment. *J Res Adolesc.* 2021;31:486–499.

18
War

Introduction

The impact of war on children and adolescents may be life altering—ranging from immediate stress responses to increased risk for such mental health disorders as anxiety, depression, and posttraumatic stress disorder (PTSD). In addition, there are broad consequences to their biopsychosocial functioning, which may range from physical injuries to mental disorders to separation from or death of their parents. The risk inflicted by war, living in conflict zones, flight, and forced migration or relocation may have lifelong impacts on the adolescent's physical, mental, social, and developmental domains, especially since there may be sensitive periods of brain development in early adolescence when the effects of experiences are particularly impactful on the brain. The kidnapping of Israeli child and adolescent age hostages by Hamas during the Israel-Hamas war is an event that will likely induce serious lifelong changes for those individuals. The social, economic, and educational systems of a nation are disrupted by war, and this disruption will broadly impact adolescents.[1,2]

A war occurring in a neighboring country can affect adolescents in their home country. Researchers in Romania studied the effects of the war in Ukraine on adolescents in Romania. Adolescents were directly involved in helping refugees from Ukraine, and in addition, they interacted with social media content concerning the war. The research team noted that the war in Ukraine is "the most online war of all time until the next one." Both parties were using social media to convey information about the war, which may contain photos of atrocities. The researchers studied 90 Romanian adolescents ages 11 to 15 years by having them complete self-report questionnaires. Some of the measures included anxiety, social media engagement, and resilience. They concluded that even though social media was a source of information about the war, it also seemed to increase the vulnerability in the adolescents to unwanted emotional states such as anxiety symptoms.[3]

Researchers at the Pratt Institute in New York studied how the war was affecting adolescents in Ukraine. The investigators noted that war is a traumatic event that could affect adolescents' mental health by impacting basic needs such as shelter, food, and school; disrupting family relationships due to loss or separation; and encountering stigma and discrimination. They were particularly interested in how the war affected the adolescents' emotional reactions to the disruptions, their coping strategies, and the role played by information technology. The study group was 27 Ukrainian adolescents ages 10 to 18 years who underwent semistructured interviews. The results indicated that the adolescents had multiple signs of trauma. Their resilience was supported by information technology including social media, schools, families, communities, and friends.[4]

Adolescents may also fight in wars as child soldiers, defined as any person under 18 years of age who is or has been recruited by the armed forces or an armed group to be used in any capacity, such as combatant, cook, sex worker, or spy. There are significant risks for a child soldier's physical and mental health.[5] In addition, child soldiers may have incomplete maturation of judgment processes, which makes them more likely to take unnecessary risks.

Many adolescents living in Ukraine have been forced to deal with physical injuries from bombings, burns, acute stress reactions, nutritional deficiencies, mental health challenges from parental absence or death, and social issues including loss of education, loss of connections to peers and adults, and instability from the loss of security and safety. This has been compounded by the COVID-19 pandemic and a polio outbreak. Many adolescents have fled to neighboring countries, including Poland and Romania, and are removed from their culture and language. While it is too early to understand the outcomes for Ukrainian adolescents, there are studies from past wars that might predict the future for these youth.[6]

Technological advancements including smartphones, social media platforms, and laptops that continuously record and disseminate war-related violence footage may change the nature of war trauma. Research has suggested that media-based contact with terrorism affects children's emotions and results in substantial daily interference.[7]

Epidemiology

It is believed that more than 1 in 10 children worldwide are affected by armed conflict, and that makes it a public health issue. Approximately 250 million children live in areas affected by conflict.[8] The prevalence estimate of mental disorders in conflict settings for all ages has been estimated at 22.1 percent.[9]

According to the United Nations, conflict-related brutal violations against children in 2021 included 6310 children recruited and used as child soldiers, most notably in the Democratic Republic of the Congo and Syria. Over 8000 children were killed or maimed. Sexual violence was committed against 1326 children, and 872 attacks occurred against schools and hospitals. Other concerning trends included the detention of 2864 children and 299 incidents with schools and hospitals used by the military.[10]

Biopsychosocial Issues and War

Biological Issues and War

Sleep
Researchers from Pennsylvania and Norway studied nightmares, PTSD, and school functioning of adolescent residents of Gaza, which has been exposed to three wars in 2008–2009, 2012, and 2014, as well as an average of 10 limited escalations every year. Adolescents in this study had lived through the three wars, heard the intense noises of war, and viewed graphic television pictures of war scenes, some on social media. Many reported that family members or friends had been injured or died in the wars. Sixty-four students (63 percent female) ages 12 to 16 years (mean age 13.5 years)

were referred to the study because of sleep issues. Measures included self-reports of PTSD, nightmares, and school/social functioning. Teachers described the students' school/social functioning. The researchers learned that the students reported having nightmares an average of 4.7 nights per week. The nightmares were usually of violence with scenes of death or life threatening to them. Only female adolescents completed a PTSD survey, but 90 percent of them had scores in the PTSD range. The students demonstrated impairment in school functioning, and because they worried about nightmares, they had significant problems falling asleep and returning to sleep after being awakened by nightmares. There were behavioral and academic problems at school associated with nightmare frequency.[11]

Stress
Adolescents exposed to an acute stressor, such as war violence, may show physical symptoms such as palpitations, nausea, chest pain, or respiratory difficulties. They may also have short-term or long-term issues with sleep, anxiety, and irritability. Some adolescents minimize their concerns over the stressor but react with hypervigilance. Adolescent reactions to war are a dynamic process, and an adolescent's reaction is an interplay between the risk and protective factors. As a result, some will react immediately to the stress, and others will not manifest symptoms of distress until weeks or months later. When these emotional responses persist for more than a month and are accompanied by significant functional impairment, an adolescent may be diagnosed with PTSD.[12]

Psychological Issues and War

World events such as the war in Ukraine affect adolescents through their exposures to atrocities, organized violence, disintegration of social networks, injuries, death, and resettlement. Investigators in Ukraine, Finland, the United Kingdom, and Norway studied adolescents in the war-torn Donetsk region and in Kirovograd 2 years after the Russian invasion in 2014. The researchers evaluated a cross-section of adolescents for PTSD, depression, and anxiety. Those youth in the war-torn area had significantly increased risk for PTSD, severe anxiety, and moderately severe to severe depression. For those adolescents exposed to the 2022 war in Ukraine, one can expect increasing risks for these mental health issues. The long-term effect of war on these adolescents is not clear.[13]

To determine the prevalence of mental disorders among children exposed to war, researchers in Canada, Maryland, and Massachusetts conducted a systematic review. Using pooled data from 17 studies, including 7920 children, they determined that the prevalence of mental disorders was much higher in children who experienced war, with about 50 percent exhibiting PTSD as compared to less than 1 percent to 10 percent in the general youth population.[14]

Researchers from Georgia, Nepal, and the Netherlands examined the mental health status of 141 former Nepalese child soldiers and compared them to 141 children who had never served. The former soldiers were 53.2 percent female and had a mean age of 15.9 years; the control group was 51.8 percent female with a mean age of

15.0 years. A trained research assistant completed 60- to 90-minute interviews with study instruments to assess for symptoms of anxiety, depression, PTSD, and general psychological difficulties. The researchers learned that while the adolescents in both groups displayed a substantial burden of mental health and psychosocial problems, the prevalence was higher in the former child soldiers. While there was no difference between the groups in anxiety, on the other tested concerns, the former child soldiers had worse outcomes. These findings suggested that adolescents living through a war, regardless of their status as soldiers or civilians, have a generalized anxiety response.[15]

Anxiety and Depression

Researchers from the United Kingdom, Bosnia-Hercegovina, and Norway studied the levels of anxiety and depression in Bosnian municipalities around the city of Mostar. About 2 years after the 2-year war (1992–1994) ended, they sampled 2976 children with a mean age of 12.1 years; 51 percent were female. The questionnaire included demographic information and questions about the war trauma events the children may have witnessed, such as shellings, torture, and deceased victims, as well as scales to measure anxiety, grief, and depressive feelings. The researchers found that self-reports of anxiety and depression were not markedly raised, but they did see high levels of the symptoms of PTSD such as nightmares, anger, and irritability.[16]

These findings were corroborated by researchers in Lebanon and the United States who interviewed parents and their children and adolescents in southern Lebanon before a 15-day military operation, 3 weeks after the ceasefire, and 1 year later in May 1997. During the hostilities, the random sample of 143 students had a mean age of 11.5 years. About one in four of the students' homes was damaged. The results indicated that reports of anxiety and depression spiked shortly after the end of the war but 1 year later were similar to prewar values. The investigators felt that persistence of the disorders 1 year later was associated with prewar disorders and witnessing of war events.[17]

Eating Disorders

Because psychological trauma is a risk factor for eating disorders, exposure to war is thus included among those risk factors for adolescents. Researchers in Lebanon, France, and Brazil hypothesized that modifying eating behavior during wartime is linked to major stress and may increase the risk of developing an eating disorder. Seven months after the end of the Lebanese-Israeli war of July 2006, they performed a cross-sectional survey of university students in Lebanon. The sample of 303 students was 73.9 percent female, with a mean age of 19.0 years, and 13.9 percent had a body mass index of less than 18.5 (underweight). The survey included the "Sick Control One Fat Food" (SCOFF) questionnaire, which is a five-question screen targeting core features of anorexia nervosa and bulimia that is positive in almost 100 percent of individuals with an eating disorder and positive in 12.5 percent of the general population.[18] The researchers learned that SCOFF was positive in 31.4 percent of the students. Of those who were SCOFF positive, 70.5 percent indicated a need to change their eating behavior during the war—a figure that is in contrast to 48 percent who had a negative SCOFF ($p < .001$). The researchers concluded that a change in eating habits during the war was associated with an increased risk of developing an eating disorder in this population. Long-time stress from war appears to be a risk factor for an eating disorder in youth.[19]

Substance Use

In adolescents, exposure to war is related to the development of PTSD. Researchers from Israel and California examined the relationships between war and alcohol use in adolescents. They conducted the study 1 year after the second war with Lebanon (July 2006) among a representative sample of Israeli and Arab teens who lived in northern Israel. The cohort consisted of 4151 students of both genders and mixed Jewish and Arab ethnicities. During the war, this area received 4000 rocket attacks over 34 days. While in school, the students completed a questionnaire with measures that included exposure to war, PTSD, childhood adversity, substance abuse, and school violence. The researchers found that the students had very high rates of exposure to war events, such as hearing the shrieking of missiles. About 7 percent had symptoms consistent with PTSD. Forty percent reported consuming some alcohol; consumption was much higher in the Jewish students. A cumulative exposure to war events and posttraumatic symptoms from these events were significantly correlated with alcohol consumption ($p < .001$) for both groups. The results suggested that the effects of war events on adolescents included a broad scope of psychological distress and risk behaviors that lasted at least 1 year after the end of the war.[20]

Social Issues and War

Social Media

Social media or networks, which are now part of everyday life, may also be used to connect people during disasters, especially when people cannot come together in person. During traumatic events, classroom-based teachers have delivered intervention programs that have strengthened student resilience. Focusing on Israeli teachers and secondary school students who lived near the Israel-Gaza border during the 2014 war, researchers in Israel described using social network technology (SNT). During a 2-month period, the Israeli citizens were exposed to about 4500 rocket attacks. As the war was raging, the researchers collected data using an online open-ended survey completed by the adolescents and semistructured one-on-one interviews with the teachers. The most common student perception of the SNT intervention was that the teachers cared about them. They felt improvements in their anxiety, and the students were able to express and share their feelings. The teachers emphasized three themes—emotional support for the students, a mechanism to monitor students' distress, and an ability to maintain a civilized online discourse. The researchers observed that SNT enabled teachers to offer real-time proactive interventions to these adolescents during a stressful time. This finding supported their belief that in times of crisis, SNT may enhance the resilience of adolescents.[21]

However, social media may also contain false or misleading information that could unduly influence an adolescent's attitudes or thinking about war whether or not they reside in the war zone. TikTok is a social media platform that contains some videos concerning the war in Ukraine; a recent study determined that 20 percent of the search results on TikTok contained misinformation.[22]

Poverty

War or conflict violence in impoverished communities may have a special impact on adolescents. Researchers from Turkey investigated the psychological well-being of children living in three low-intensity conflict-affected cities in eastern Turkey. They collected data from 409 caregivers of children, primarily their mothers; there were 236 children, all female, between the ages of 5.5 and 18 years. Over 90 percent of the children came from intact families. All of the families had disadvantaged socioeconomic backgrounds; a notable 54 percent of the caregivers were illiterate, and 94.9 percent were unemployed. Twenty caregivers had paid work, and only 12 caregivers had a full-time job. Measures included children's background information, emotional and behavioral problems, income, family violence experiences, and armed conflict experiences. The researchers found that 88.5 percent of the children were directly exposed to conflict, 78.3 percent were frequently amid conflict, and 65 percent had at least one attack on their home. Almost half of the children had schools that were attacked or ruined, and 82 percent were deprived of basic needs, such as food, water, and shelter, because of the combat. In addition, 36 percent were exposed to family violence. So they witnessed violence within and outside their families and homes. The researchers learned that 14.3 percent of the children had either clinical or borderline clinical internalizing problems, 12.6 percent had either clinical or borderline externalizing problems, 15 percent were either clinical or borderline clinical for total problems, and 7.9 percent were clinical or borderline clinical for PTSD. When the researchers compared these scores to previous studies of children living in institutions or low-income families in central Turkey, they were significantly higher for internalizing, externalizing, and total problems. Living in a conflict zone exacerbated an already difficult physical and psychological life for these low-income children. The researchers advised the implementation of interventions in these areas to enhance the children's recovery and reduce the chances of them having long-term negative outcomes and becoming burdens to society.[23]

Researchers based in Massachusetts examined the impacts of war and displacement on executive function, or the higher order of cognitive skills necessary for abstract thinking in adolescents. Executive function is essential for focusing and completing daily tasks. The researchers were also interested in the contribution of poverty to working memory, which is important for reasoning, decision-making, and behavior. Their gender-balanced cohort consisted of 240 Syrian refugees and 210 Jordanian nonrefugees living in Jordan, ages 12 to 18 years. On average, the Syrian adolescents had been in Jordan for 2.97 years. Data were collected in four cities by Syrian and Jordanian research team members. Using tablets, researchers conducted assessments of inhibitory control and working memory, measures of executive function. As the researchers anticipated, the Syrian refugees experienced more adversity compared to nonrefugees, and they had less material wealth and more human insecurity and exposure to war-related trauma than their Jordanian peers. They had completed fewer years of education, and their mothers and fathers were more likely to have attained only a primary education. Females did worse than their male counterparts. The researchers observed that poverty worsened working memory. It appeared that the effects of poverty on young minds had a more negative impact than the exposure to war or conflict.[24]

Poverty appears to have an impact on maternal health in war areas. Researchers from Canada, the United States, and Brazil used data collected from 1990 to 2017 in 137 conflict and nonconflict low-income and middle-income countries to conduct a time-series multicountry ecological study. (Maternal death data were collected for the years 1990 to 2015.) The dataset included about 3.8 million surveyed mothers between the ages of 15 and 49 years and 1.1 million children and adolescents up to and including age 14 years. The researchers compared maternal and childhood health outcomes in conflict and nonconflict areas as well as the impact of poverty and a lack of financial resources. Annual mortality rates were obtained by adding the deaths across all countries in either conflict group and dividing by the total number of live births. Inequalities in intervention coverage were calculated for wealth, maternal education, and place of residence. The researchers learned that maternal and child mortality rates were higher in the countries with conflicts. The financially and socially disadvantaged mothers, children, and adolescents in the conflict countries suffered the most. They tended to have fewer health-related resources and less ability to travel to the resources that were available. While the researchers found that the adolescent mortality rates were "demonstrably higher" in many conflict countries, the figures may actually underestimate the correct numbers, such as children who were abducted, tortured, and forced to become child soldiers.[25]

Racism/Discrimination

Institutional racism during wartime can be traumatic for adolescents. Sarah Moskovitz, a psychologist who studied child survivors of the Holocaust, believed these individuals had three common attributes that helped them survive: adaptability, assertiveness, and appeal to adults.[26]

After the beginning of World War II, institutional racism occurred in the United States. Shortly after the United States declared war on Japan, President Franklin Roosevelt signed an executive order granting the secretary of war the authority to evacuate and incarcerate first-generation Japanese immigrants and their children. Between May 27, 1942, and March 20, 1946, over 120,000 people from the West Coast were placed in 1 of 10 internment camps.[27]

Though a citizen of the United States, Mary Matsuda Gruenewald was a child of immigrant Japanese parents. In 1942, when she was 17 years old, Mary, her parents, and her older brother were moved to Tule Lake Internment Camp in California. They lived in a 400-square-foot room with four cots and a potbelly stove, and were guarded by soldiers from the U.S. Army. By Mary's own admission, she suffered from bouts of depression and dreamed of violent blasts from machine guns. She wrote, "We had lost our right to be in the privacy of our own home, the right to come and go as we pleased, the right to voice our opinions openly without fear of retaliation.... The sudden loss of all these rights forced me to realize that this whole mass movement against the Japanese in America was the culmination of more than a half-century of anti-Asian prejudice." Despite her incarceration as an adolescent, Mary became a nurse, married, raised a family, and became a successful writer. An intact family, friends, and community enhanced her resilience during World War II.[28]

The Holocaust is an example of international wartime institutional racism. Researchers from Israel, the Netherlands, and Germany compared the anxiety and stress levels of 212 female children and adolescent Holocaust survivors to a comparable non-Jewish Polish survivor group who resided in Europe at the same time. The Jewish Holocaust survivors made up about one-third of the group and the remainder were Polish non-Jews. The research was conducted 60 years after the end of the war. Data were obtained from the members of both groups, who lived in Israel, with questionnaires and interviews. The groups were closely matched but differed by levels of education. Measures included anxiety, trauma-related stress, and posttraumatic stress indicators. From the results of their scores on the anxiety and traumatic stress measures, the researchers learned that the Holocaust still had an effect on the survivors six decades later. Current PTSD was two times higher in the Jewish group. Losing a parent in the war predicted a global decrease in well-being.[29]

Robert Knell, a child psychiatrist in Canada who was himself a child survivor of the Holocaust, described how some children were able to survive. To him, one key element was intellect. He wrote about Peter, an 11-year-old whose mother used an inverted rain barrel with water on top to protect him. From his hiding place in this barrel in Lodz, Poland, Peter witnessed his family and friends being taken away. Unfortunately, he was eventually discovered and marched with 200 other prisoners to a large ditch in the forest, where all of the prisoners were shot by machine guns. He fell into a ditch and later crawled out, even though he was wounded in the leg. Peter managed to escape further harm, and at the end of the war, he was the only member of his family to survive. Peter was fortunate to meet a man who guided him through his high school education that he completed in 2 years, and then he immigrated to Canada. Peter became a successful businessman, married, and had a family, all enhanced by his formidable intellect.[30]

Mortality

The loss of a parent is probably the most stressful trauma for an adolescent and is a strong predictor for psychopathology. The effects of such a loss may last well into adulthood, and it may impact a person's well-being. Researchers in Poland and Colorado examined how the loss of a parent during World War II altered the lives of adults. Between 2006 and 2007, the researchers interviewed 212 survivors; they had a mean age of 72.4 years and were between ages 5 and 17 at the end of the war, with a mean age of 10 years. About one-third of the group were Jewish Holocaust survivors, and the remainder were non-Jewish. The measures included PTSD symptoms, depression, social isolation, and one measure to determine exposure to trauma during the war, such as a parental death. The researchers determined that there was a direct link between all PTSD and social isolation measures and parental death. Those who lost a parent had poor well-being, and the degree of traumatic loss was greater for those in the Holocaust group. The researchers concluded that parental loss during childhood or adolescence may have altered the future well-being of World War II survivors, even 60 years after the war ended.[31]

Intervention and Prevention

It is imperative to protect the human rights of children and adolescents affected by war. This may be accomplished by mandating their unrestricted access to appropriate mental health services.[32] However, for adolescents in war areas, access to treatment services, programs, or aid may not be available. In recent decades treatment models have shifted to school- or community-based interventions. Newer programs have been identified that may be customized to different cultural groups, war areas, and languages.[33]

Trauma-focused cognitive behavioral therapy is one validated model of treatment. This protocol consists of eight components guided by a clinician and requires parental involvement in treatment in 90-minute weekly sessions. The program has been shown to reduce symptoms of PTSD, depression, and behavior problems after completion of the protocol.[34]

School- and community-based interventions have been shown to be effective, but their availability around the world varies considerably. These programs may include school-based group cognitive behavioral therapy or interventions to reduce PTSD, function impairment, somatic complaints, and anxiety.[35] One such program in Nepal demonstrated moderate short-term beneficial effects for improving social-behavioral and resilience indicators among subgroups of children exposed to armed conflict.[36]

Although adolescents may not have school or community resources in war zones, they may have access to the internet. This has the potential to help students, teachers, and schools. Bounce Back Now (BBN) is a free app designed to improve the emotional health of adults and their families affected by a disaster, including mass violence. It allows adolescents to choose an intervention for PTSD, depression, or substance use.[37] Through a randomized, controlled, population-based trial, researchers reached out to 2000 adolescents and parents from communities dealing with the aftereffects of tornadoes in Missouri and Alabama in 2011. During a 12-month follow-up, the researchers learned that the adolescents who had used the portal had fewer PTSD and depressive symptoms than the teens in the control group. The results supported the feasibility and efficacy of BBN as a technology-based, scalable mental health intervention for adolescents experiencing a disaster.[38]

Virtual reality games may also have a role as a treatment modality for adolescents experiencing mental health issues from war. In a military sample, virtual reality interventions were shown to reduce PTSD after as few as six sessions.[39] Additional research is needed to develop an effective virtual reality intervention for adolescents exposed to war and terrorism.

Interviews with adolescents during the Russia-Ukraine war showed that at the individual level, most of the adolescents demonstrated resilience that helped them cope with the disruption from the war. In addition, they reported receiving support from family, friends, and pets. Research has shown that the presence of a parent, especially the mother, during a traumatic experience is highly influential in the processing of war trauma.[40] The adolescents also described the importance of supporting relationships with peers. Moreover, one of the most helpful pillars of support was the ability to continue school during the war. And finally, they mentioned some social media platforms, including Telegram, which was a popular source of information even prior to the invasion. (Telegram is a cloud-based app that allows users to send and receive messages, calls, photos, videos, and audio and other files.) While social support did not totally relieve war-related trauma, it did help foster resilience within adolescents facing the horrors of war.[41]

Conclusion

"All wars, whether just or unjust, disastrous or victorious, are waged against the child," wrote Eglantyne Jebb, a British social reformer who founded Save the Children over 100 years ago. War impacts the biological, psychological, and social domains of adolescents, and these changes seem to often influence the remainder of the adolescent's life, whether they are victims, child soldiers, or indirectly affected by the conflict such as through social media accounts of the conflict. From World War II through Vietnam and the recent wars in Ukraine and Israel-Hamas, wars waged by older generations continue to violate the Convention of the Rights of the Child adopted by the United Nations. Ceasing armed conflicts will go far in preventing these harms to children, adolescents, and adults.

References

1   Bürgin D, Anagnostopoulos D, Board and Policy Division of ESCAP, et al. Impact of war and forced displacement on children's mental health-multilevel, needs-oriented, and trauma-informed approaches. *Eur Child Adolesc Psychiatry.* 2022;31:845–853.

2   Viner RM, Ozer EM, Denny S, et al. Adolescence and the social determinants of health. *Lancet.* 2012;379:1641–1652.

3   Maftei A, Dănilă O, Măirean C. The war next-door—a pilot study on Romanian adolescents' psychological reactions to potentially traumatic experiences generated by the Russian invasion of Ukraine. *Front Psychol.* 2022 Dec 5;13:1051152.

4   Lopatovska I, Arora K, Fernandes F. Experiences of the Ukrainian adolescents during the Russia-Ukraine 2022 war. *Inf Learn Sci.* 2022;123:666–704.

5   Etzel RA. Use of children as soldiers. *Pediatr Clin North Am.* 2021;68:437–447.

6   de Alencar Rodrigues JAR, Lima NNR, Neto MLR, Uchida RR. Ukraine: war, bullets, and bombs—millions of children and adolescents are in danger. *Child Abuse Negl.* 2022;128:105622.

7   Comer JS, Kendall PC. Terrorism: the psychological impact on youth. *Clin Psychol Sci Pract.* 2007;14:182–212.

8   Kadir A, Shenoda S, Goldhagen J, Pitterman S, Section on International Child Health. The effects of armed conflict on children. *Pediatrics.* 2018;142:e20182585.

9   Charlson F, van Ommeren M, Flaxman A, Cornett J, Whiteford H, Saxena S. New WHO prevalence estimates of mental disorders in conflict settings: a systematic review and meta-analysis. *Lancet.* 2019;394:240–248.

10 United Nations. *Children and Armed Conflict Annual Report of the Secretary-General.* United Nations; 2022.

11 Harb GC, Schutz JH. The nature of posttraumatic nightmares and school functioning in war-affected youth. *PLoS ONE.* 2020;15:e0242414.

12 Joshi PT, O'Donnell DA. Consequences of child exposure to war and terrorism. *Clin Child Fam Psychol Rev.* 2003;6:275–292.

13 Osokina O, Silwal S, Bohdanova T, Hodes M, Sourander A, Skokauskas N. Impact of the Russian invasion on mental health of adolescents in Ukraine. *J Am Acad Child Adolesc Psychiatry.* 2022;62:335–343.

14 Attanayake V, McKay R, Joffres M, Singh S, Burkle F, Mills E. Prevalence of mental disorders among children exposed to war: a systematic review of 7,920 children. *Med Confl Surviv.* 2009;25:4–19.

15 Kohrt BA, Jordans MJ, Tol WA, et al. Comparison of mental health between former child soldiers and children never conscripted by armed groups in Nepal. *JAMA.* 2008;300:691–702.

16 Smith P, Perris S, Yule W, Hacam B, Stuvland R. War exposure among children from Bosnia-Hercegovina psychological adjustment in a community sample. *J Trauma Stress.* 2002;2:147–156.

17 Karam EG, Fayyad J, Karam AN, et al. Outcome of depression and anxiety after war: a prospective epidemiologic study of children and adolescents. *J Trauma Stress.* 2014;27:192–199.

18 Morgan JF, Reid F, Lacey JH. The SCOFF questionnaire: a new screening tool for eating disorders. *West J Med.* 2000;172:164–165.

19 Aoun A, Garcia FD, Mounzer C, et al. War stress may be another risk factor for eating disorders in civilians: a study in Lebanese university students. *Gen Hosp Psychiatry.* 2013;35:393–397.

20 Schiff M, Pat-Horencyzk RR, Benbenishty R, Brom D, Baum N, Astor RA. High school students' posttraumatic symptoms, substance abuse and involvement in violence in the aftermath of war. *Soc Sci Med.* 2012;75:1321–1328.

21 Rosenberg H, Ophir Y, Asterhan C. A virtual safe zone: teachers supporting teenage student resilience through social media in times of war. *Teach Teach Educ.* 2018;73:35–42.

22 Brewster J, Arvanitis L, Pavilonis V, Wang M. Beware the "New Google": TikTok's Search Engine Pumps Toxic Misinformation To Its Young Users. NewsGuard; September 2022.

23 Kara B, Bilge S. Under poverty and conflict: well-being of children living in the east of Turkey. *Am J Orthopsychiatry.* 2020;90:246–258.

24 Chen A, Panter-Brick C, Hadfield K, Dajani R, Harmoudi A, Sheridan M. Minds under siege: cognitive signatures of poverty and trauma in refugee and non-refugee adolescents. *Child Dev.* 2019;90:1856–1865.

25 Akseer N, Wright J, Tasic H, et al. Women, children and adolescents in conflict countries: an assessment of inequalities in intervention coverage and survival. *BMJ Glob Health.* 2020;5:e002214.

26 Moskovitz S. Longitudinal follow-up of child survivors of the Holocaust. *J Am Acad Child Psychiatry.* 1985;24:401–407.

27 Yamashiro JP. More than half: multiracial families in the World War II Japanese American incarceration camps. *J Child Fam Studies.* 2022;31:721–734.

28 Gruenewal MM. *Looking Like the Enemy: My Story of Imprisonment in Japanese-American Internment Camps.* New Sage Press; 2005.

29 Lis-Turlejska M, Luszczynska A, Plichta A, Benight CC. Jewish and non-Jewish World War II child and adolescent survivors at 60 years after war: effects of parental loss and age at exposure on well-being. *Am J Orthopsychiatry.* 2008;78:369–377.

30 Krell R. Child survivors of the Holocaust—strategies of adaptation. *Can J Psychiatry.* 1993;38:384–389.

31 Lis-Turlejska M, Luszczynska A, Plichta A, Benight CC. Jewish and non-Jewish World War II child and adolescent survivors at 60 years after war: effects of parental loss and age at exposure on well-being. *Am J Orthopsychiatry.* 2008;78:369–377.

32 United Nations General Assembly. *Convention on the Rights of the Child. Treaty Series (1577).* United Nations; 1989.

33 Saltzman LY, Solomyak L, Pat-Horenczyk R. Addressing the needs of children and youth in the context of war and terrorism: the technological frontier. *Curr Psychiatry Rep.* 2017;19:30–38.

34 Cary CE, McMillen JC. The data behind the dissemination: a systematic review of trauma-focused cognitive behavioral therapy for use with children and youth. *Child Youth Serv Rev.* 2012;34:748–757.

35 Saltzman LY, Solomyak L, Pat-Horenczyk R. Addressing the needs of children and youth in the context of war and terrorism: the technological frontier. *Curr Psychiatry Rep.* 2017;19:30–38.

36 Jordans MJ, Komproe IH, Tol WA, et al. Evaluation of a classroom-based psychosocial intervention in conflict-affected Nepal: a cluster randomized controlled trial. *J Child Psychol Psychiatry.* 2010;51:818–826.

37 Amstadter AB, Broman-Fulks J, Zinzow H, Ruggiero KJ, Cercone J. Internet-based interventions for traumatic stress-related mental health problems: a review and suggestion for further research. *Clin Psych Rev.* 2009;29:410–420.

38 Ruggiero KJ, Price M, Adams Z, et al. Web intervention for adolescents affected by disaster: population-based randomized controlled trial. *J Am Acad Child Adolesc Psychiatry.* 2015;54:709–717.

39 Rothbaum BO, Price M, Jovanovic T, et al. A randomized, double-blind evaluation of D-cycloserine or alprazolam combined with virtual reality exposure therapy for posttraumatic stress disorder in Iraq and Afghanistan war veterans. *Am J Psychiatry.* 2014;171:640–648.

40 Masten AS, Narayan AJ. Child development in the context of disaster, war, and terrorism: pathways of risk and resilience. *Annu Rev Psychol.* 2012;63:227–257.

41 Lopatovska I, Arora K, Fernandes F. Experiences of the Ukrainian adolescents during the Russia-Ukraine 2022 war. *Inf Learn Sci.* 2022;123:666–704.

Glossary

Actigraphy: the monitoring of body movements with a small device to determine whether and how well a person is sleeping or resting

Adverse childhood experience: traumatic events that occur before a child reaches age 18, such as physical, sexual, or emotional abuse

Allostatic load: a measure of the cumulative burden of stress on the body

Amygdala: a portion of the brain involved in emotional learning, motivation, and processing of threats and emotions

Body mass index (BMI): a weight-to-height measure that can indicate if one has low, normal, or high body weight

Case-control study: a type of observational study used to look at factors associated with outcomes

Circadian rhythm: a 24-hour internal process that regulates the sleep-wake cycle

Cognitive behavioral therapy: a talk therapy that focuses on dealing with specific issues and is useful for such problems as anxiety, depression, eating disorders, and substance use

Congenital adrenal hyperplasia: a genetic disorder where the adrenal glands do not function properly

Continuous positive airway pressure (CPAP): a machine that uses mild air pressure to keep airways open during sleep

Cross-sectional study: an observational study looking at data at one point in time

Delayed sleep-wake phase disorder: a disorder in which a person's sleep is delayed by 2 or more hours beyond an acceptable or conventional bedtime

Epigenetics: a study of how behavior and environment control gene activity and expression without changing the sequence of DNA

Externalizing symptoms: behavioral symptoms including overactivity, poor impulse control, noncompliance, and aggression

Functional magnetic resonance imaging (fMRI): a noninvasive and safe way to measure brain activity by detecting changes associated with blood flow

Gonadotropin-releasing hormone: a hormone made in a section of the brain called the hypothalamus that causes the pituitary gland to make follicle-stimulating hormone and luteinizing hormone, which regulate estrogen in females and testosterone in males

Hippocampus: a portion of the brain that supports learning and memory

Hypothalamic-pituitary-adrenal axis: a complex system of neuroendocrine pathways and feedback loops that function to maintain physiological homeostasis

Incidence: the rate at which an event or disease occurs during a certain period

Internalizing symptoms: internally focused symptoms including anxiety, sadness, social withdrawal, and fearfulness

Likert scale: a rating scale that assesses opinions, attitudes, or behaviors quantitatively

Longitudinal study: a study that follows subjects over time with repeated measurements of the variables

Meta-analysis: a type of research that combines and analyzes the results of multiple studies

Minority stress: chronic stress from situations and experiences due to one's race, ethnicity, or sexual or gender identity

Neuroticism: a personality trait where there is a tendency for the individual toward anxiety, depression, self-doubt, or other negative feelings

Odds ratio: a statistic that measures the strength between one event and another

p value: a statistic that measures the probability that an observed difference might have occurred by random chance

Population-based study: a study of a group of individuals who share a common characteristic, such as a health condition

Prefrontal cortex: a portion of the brain that supports higher-order planning, reasoning, and decision-making

Prevalence: the speed or frequency with which an event or disease occurs per unit of time, population, or other standard

Prospective study: a study of a group of individuals over time who are alike in many ways but differ by a certain characteristic, such as adolescents who smoke and do not smoke tobacco

Randomized controlled trial: a prospective study that measures an intervention or treatment in subjects over time and has a control group of individuals who do not utilize the intervention or treatment

Rapid eye movement (REM) sleep: the phase of sleep where dreams occur, the eyes move rapidly, and there is an increase in brain activity, breathing, heart rate, and blood pressure

Scoping review: a type of research synthesis that scopes a body of literature, identifies knowledge gaps, and clarifies concepts

Social determinants of health: nonmedical factors that influence an individual's health outcomes including racism, discrimination, violence, poverty, climate change, housing, neighborhood, education, access to nutritious foods, and medical care

Sympathetic-adreno-medullary axis: a major component of the body's response to stress that leads to the release of epinephrine and norepinephrine

Systematic review: a type of research that uses reproducible methods to search studies and appraise and synthesize information on a specific issue

Trauma-focused cognitive behavioral therapy: a type of cognitive behavioral therapy that addresses children and adolescents suffering from the effects of early trauma

Index

For the benefit of digital users, indexed terms that span two pages (e.g., 52–53) may, on occasion, appear on only one of those pages.

Tables, figures, and boxes are indicated by an italic *t*, *f*, and *b* following the page/paragraph number